W9-BSA-752

THE PRICE OF GREATNESS

The Price of Greatness

Resolving the Creativity and Madness Controversy

Arnold M. Ludwig

THE GUILFORD PRESS
New York   London

A great presence may mold an age,
even as he is molded by it.

—THOMAS CARLYLE, *On Heroes, Hero
Worship, and the Heroic in History*

© 1995 Arnold M. Ludwig

Published by The Guilford Press
A Division of Guilford Publications, Inc.
72 Spring Street, New York, NY 10012

All rights reserved

No part of this book may be reproduced, stored in a retrieval system, or
transmitted, in any form or by any means, electronic, mechanical,
photocopying, microfilming, recording, or otherwise, without written
permission from the Publisher.

Printed in the United States of America

This book printed on acid-free paper.

Last digit is print number: 9 8 7 6 5 4 3 2 1

Library of Congress Cataloguing-in-Publication Data

Ludwig, Arnold M.
    The price of greatness: resolving the creativity and madness
controversy / by Arnold M. Ludwig
      p. cm.
    Includes bibliographical references and index.
    ISBN 0-89862-839-3
    1. Genius and mental illness. 2. Creative ability. I. Title.
BF423.L83 1995
153.3′5—dc20   94-44905
                                                   CIP

Preface

*I*n this book I present the findings of my 10-year investigation of the link between mental illness and exceptional creative achievement. During this investigation, I gathered extensive biographical information on over 1,000 extraordinary men and women who lived during the 20th century and achieved prominence in many areas, including the arts, the sciences, public office, the military, business, and social activism.

Besides having access to this enormous data bank, I also developed a scale that reliably measures creative achievement. This let me explore many uncharted areas, including the impact of broken homes, birth order, the death of parents, mental illness in the parents, precocity, nonconformity, career choice, sexual preference, religious beliefs, and social marginality on the emotional well-being and accomplishments of these people. As it turned out, it was possible to predict with great accuracy the lifetime creative achievements of persons on the basis of information about their personal characteristics and mental health. These findings offered a new perspective on the relationship between mental illness and creativity and dispelled much of the mystery that had previously existed.

In reporting my findings and observations, I wrestled with the dilemma of how technical to be, especially since I wanted this book to be accessible to anyone with an interest in this topic. Despite the extensive data, I tried to make the text comprehensible for readers without any knowledge of statistics. With this format, readers can either confine themselves exclusively to the narrative or, if they are scientifically or academically inclined, examine the extensive chapter notes, appendices, and statistical results presented at the end of the book.

Given the many issues involved, the scope of this book is broad. It is not possible to look into the connection between creativity and "madness" without delving into many of humanity's greatest achievements, the special attributes of the people responsible for these achievements, the unique circumstances of their lives, and the families that produced them. It is often difficult to separate these people from their personal struggles and their works.

Acknowledgments

Many people contributed directly and indirectly to this project and the preparation of this book. Over the years, Karen Cooke, Gregory Guenthner, Linda House, Janis Saylor, and Donald Jones served as research assistants. I am particularly grateful to Gregory Guenthner for his invaluable assistance and perceptive observations during this investigation. My secretary, Sandy Tipton, also played a key role.

I was most fortunate to have Richard Kryscio available for general statistical consultations and John V. Haley for consultation on a variety of matters. I also wish to express my thanks to several persons who critiqued an earlier version of my manuscript. These persons included Joshua Lederberg, Robert S. Root-Bernstein, Ruth Richards, Thomas Miller, Mark A. Runco, Jo Ann Reis, and my son, Daniel T. Ludwig. Kay R. Jamison warrants special thanks not only for her earlier encouragement of my project but, as an editorial referee, for pressing me to clarify certain notions. Although I have benefited immensely from all this input, I have not always followed suggestions. Therefore, I take full blame for any deficiencies in the book.

There are two people to whom I owe a special debt of gratitude. Kitty Moore, my editor, was a patient but hard taskmaster, who pushed me to undertake at least two more major drafts, even after I had vowed that the previous draft was the last. I am glad now that I made these revisions, for it is a much better book. I also want to thank my wife, Aline, for the countless ways she helped. Aside from her encouragement and support, I treasure our conversations about issues in this book during our many walks.

Contents

CHAPTER ONE

A Touch of Madness?

S alvador Dali said, "The only difference between me and a 'madman' is that I am not mad." This cryptic remark is as profound as it is paradoxical, a surrealistic insight into the relationship between creativity and madness.

The question of whether creativity and madness are related has been posed since antiquity. In the *Metaphysics*, Aristotle wrote that the creative act was a natural event, and, as such, conformed to natural law. In contrast, Plato claimed that a poet's inspiration arose during moments of "divine madness." But for the ancient Greeks, the notion of madness had a different meaning than it does today. Aside from the madness brought on by natural causes, such as delirium or melancholia, other forms were supposedly produced by the gods. Prophetic madness, induced by Apollo, enabled knowledge of the future. Ritual madness, precipitated by Dionysus, allowed emotional release and liberation from the self. Erotic madness, inspired by Aphrodite or Eros, stimulated rapture and love. And poetic madness, inspired by the Muse, gave rise to lyric expression. Almost any extraordinary performance or creative achievement—whether it be in writing, music, poetry, philosophy, dance, art, sculpture, or intellectual discovery—came from one or another of these divine forms of madness.[1]

The belief in the link between genius and madness persists. Advocates of this view point to the many famous people with mental aberrations. Virginia Woolf was sexually abused as a girl, suffered from severe mood swings as an adult, and later committed suicide. Sylvia Plath had episodes of psychotic depression and eventually ended her life. Ernest Hemingway drank excessively, suffered from extreme depression, and killed himself. Friedrich Nietzsche had fits of melancholia long before becoming deranged from syphilis of the brain. Eugene O'Neill was a severe alcoholic. Jean-Paul Sartre relied on stimulants, sedatives, and alcohol to regulate his mood swings and sleep patterns. Edvard Munch experienced attacks of severe anxiety. Hart Crane, who was manic–depressive and alcoholic, eventually killed himself by jumping off a ship. Wilhelm Reich, a renegade psychoanalyst, developed the paranoid delusion that deadly orgone energy would incapacitate him and, in order to elude it, he could not sleep more than two nights in a row in the same place. Paul Robeson had severe psychotic depressions and made several suicide attempts. Robert Lowell struggled with mania and depression throughout his adult life. Max Beerbohm, the caricaturist, had paralyzing anxieties and fears.

In the past, schizophrenia and melancholia, among the many forms of mental illness, were seen as the main sources for creativity. Recent research has emphasized the role of depression, and manic depression.[2] To a large extent, this shift was prompted by the results of a landmark study on 30 writers (27 of whom were men) attending the University of Iowa Writers Workshop. The results revealed that 80% of these writers, compared to 30% of those in a control group, reported suffering from some type of mood disorder. Although depression was the most common condition, over 40% of the writers had manic-depressive disorders, more than four times the rate in the control group.[3]

The results of my own past research on 59 women writers, recruited from participants in a Women Writers Conference at the University of Kentucky, support and extend these findings,[4] but they also allow for other interpretations. As in the Iowa study, I found that writers had much higher rates of depression and mania than the 59 matched controls who belonged either to the statewide homemakers association, the medical auxiliary, or the university women's club. But unlike the mostly male writers in the Iowa study, women writers showed certain differences as well. Compared to controls, they had higher rates of anxiety, panic attacks, drug abuse, eating disorders, and other nonspecific conditions. This suggested that, aside from depression and mania, almost any type of sustained emotional distress in women writers, provided it was not incapacitating, could be associated with creative activity. But what was more revealing was that the extent of creative activity in all 118 women, writers and controls alike, could be predicted on the basis of four factors: the extent of their mental problems, their reported exposure to sexual or physical abuse during childhood, mental difficulties in their mothers, and the degree of creativity in their parents. These results showed that any understanding of the relationship between mental illness and creative activity had to take familial, developmental, and environmental factors into account.

Anecdotal and research evidence of this sort suggests a definite relationship between creative achievement and madness. But any conclusion may be premature. Anecdotal accounts of emotional difficulties in famous people prove nothing. It is equally possible to find countless other examples of extraordinary artists, writers, poets, performers, composers, and scientists—people like Albert Einstein, Le Corbusier, John Dewey, Marie Curie, Edgar Degas, Henri Matisse, Arnold Schoenberg, Alexander Fleming, Orville Wright, Jules Henri Poincaré, Henry Moore, Edward Hopper, Carl Jung, Camille Pissarro, Neils Bohr, Fred Astaire, Margaret Mead, George Washington Carver, George Gershwin, or Duke Ellington—who seem to have led reasonably "sane," emotionally stable lives. As long as many people within the creative professions seem to be mentally healthy, we cannot claim that mental illness is necessary for creative achievement. As for the recent research studies, including my own on women writers, which show that a relationship exists between mental illness and creative activity, the findings are limited and inconclusive. What applies to writers or artists may not apply to people in the other creative arts professions or to creative persons in the social or natural sciences. Even more important, what applies to noneminent people, may not apply to those who are eminent.

Other issues having to do with the relationship between mental illness and creative achievement also remain unsettled. People engaged in the "creative arts" or drawn to the artistic lifestyle are not necessarily creative thinkers, nor are the works they produce necessarily inspired, extraordinary, or original. Even if those in the creative arts are found to be more "creative," we still do not know whether their mental disturbances are essential for creative activity or whether they affect each individual in various professions differently.

To talk of a relationship between mental illness and creativity also says nothing about what forms this relationship may take. Franz Kafka, for example, found writing therapeutic. "The existence of a writer," he commented, "is truly dependent on his desk. If he wants to escape madness, he really should never leave his desk. He must cling to it with his teeth." Truman Capote, in contrast, found his writing dangerous. "No one will ever know what *In Cold Blood* took out of me," he said. "It scraped me right down to the marrow of my bones. It nearly killed me. I think, in a way, it *did* kill me. Before I began it, I was a stable person, comparatively speaking. Afterward, something happened to me."

Just as creative activity may affect the mental health of persons for better or worse, mental illness may have a similar effect on creative activity. For Sylvia Plath, there was no question about the detrimental effects of mental illness on her work. "When you are insane," she said, "you are busy being insane—all the time. . . . When I was crazy, that was all I was." In contrast, Alberto Giacometti used his panicky spells of fear, shaking, and depersonalization as inspiration for his work. It was during these spells that he saw people "coming and going, a little like ants; everybody seemed to have a goal and be going in a direction, alone, that the others were ignorant of." His preoccupation with grays also seemed to come from these experiences. "When I see everything in gray . . . then why should I use any other color?. . . . Gray! Gray! Gray! My experience is that the color . . . means life itself to me." These different accounts suggest that any adequate explanation of the relationship between mental illness and creative activity needs to take both the positive and negative interactions between them into account.

Aside from the limitations of past scientific research, the main reason why the relationship between mental illness and creative activity remained murky was that the very question was misleading, prompting Procrustean answers of a "yes" or "no" nature, neither of which could be right. Attempts to find a correlation were doomed to failure because no one asked what kinds of people, what kinds of professions, what kinds of creative activity, and what kinds of mental illness this question referred to. However, as I show in this book, once we take these issues into account, much of the mystery about the relationship between mental illness and creative achievement disappears.

In what follows, I pose and then answer a series of interrelated questions, each of which bears on these issues. All of my answers are based on the findings of my studies. Together, my observations suggest that Seneca was right in claiming, "There is no great genius without some touch of madness," but only in a sense he did not foresee. I recognize that presenting my general conclusions first may detract from the suspense of the book. This is a risk I have decided to take, believing that readers who find my conclusions intriguing will want to know how I arrived at them and more about the people on whom they are based.

Are members of the creative arts more likely to suffer from mental disturbances than those in other professions?

My findings show consistently and clearly that members of the artistic professions or creative arts as a whole—architecture, design, art, composing, musical entertainment, theater, and all forms of writing—suffer from more types of mental difficulties and do so over longer periods of their lives than members of the other professions. However, no single pattern of mental illness characterizes all of the creative arts professions. Although alcoholism and depression are widespread within the creative arts, each profession in its own way shows a distinctive pattern of psychopathology. Illicit drug use is more common among musical performers and actors. Musical composers, artists, and nonfiction writers suffer mostly from alcoholism and depression throughout their lives. Musical entertainers, architects, and actors are relatively free from depression. Poets show a high prevalence of both mania and psychoses. Poets, actors, fiction writers, and musical entertainers are more likely to attempt suicide. Among all those in the creative arts, only architects and designers, and to some extent nonfiction writers, show few signs of mental instability. Overall, the findings suggest that members of those creative arts professions that rely more on precision, reason, and logic (e.g., architects, designers, journalists, essayists, literary critics) are less prone to mental disturbances, and those that rely more on emotive expression, personal experiences, and vivid imagery as sources of inspiration (e.g., poets, novelists, actors, and musical entertainers) are more prone.

Why do those in the artistic professions experience so much emotional distress? At this point, we can put to rest the notion that emotional suffering represents a Promethean punishment for expression of the gift of creativity. The findings show that for substantial numbers of these individuals, their predisposition for mental disorders is established long before they launch their careers. Not only do they display a greater family tendency for mental illness, which also appears to influence what forms their own emotional difficulties take, but they also already show more emotional problems during childhood and especially adolescence than members in the nonartistic professions. If emotional suffering is a prerequisite for creative achievement, then many of these individuals get off to a running start.

Why, then, should so many emotionally disturbed persons be drawn to the creative arts? The reasons are complex. Unlike other professions, the artistic occupations (with notable exceptions) simply lack the capacity to keep "unstable" persons out. It is not that these professions welcome people who are emotionally unstable, but without as many formal training requirements or licensing boards as most nonartistic professions, they are less able to police their professional borders. Nor are they inclined to do so. The creative arts professions also seem to place a higher premium on the creative products of persons than on their personal behaviors. This opens a window of opportunity to many people who rebel against the constraints of traditional training or, because of their psychological makeup, find it hard to comply with formal rules. Small wonder then that those who are more nonconformist, eccentric, rebellious, socially alienated, or emotionally troubled (as well as those who are socially stigmatized) should find the creative arts so attractive. These professions, for the most part, represent an occupational haven for those who wrestle with their personal demons or, at the least, try to contain them through their creative activities.

Besides the emotional conflicts that individuals bring to their particular professions, the professions themselves exert powerful shaping influences on them, encouraging certain behaviors and discouraging others. For example, for poets to be taken seriously, they may need to reveal pain, anguish, and desperation in their writings. Many artists may feel compelled to portray the image of the mad genius or at least to cultivate their eccentricities to increase their public appeal. Margaret Atwood, in *Cat's Eye*,[5] aptly has an artist say, "If I cut off my ear, would the market value (of my paintings) go up? Better still, stick my head in the oven, blow out my brains. What rich art collectors like to buy, among other things, is a little vicarious craziness." Musical entertainers may find that drinking heavily and using drugs seems to help them give the uninhibited performances expected by their audiences. Journalists, biographers, and literary critics may experience a greater need than fiction writers or poets to appear rational, erudite, and objective in both their writings and personal lives to maintain their credibility. Actors may need a degree of psychological instability that enables them to fall in and out of love and to experience the gamut of emotions so that they can draw from these experiences when they play various parts. Architects may need to be more emotionally stable and businesslike than others in the creative arts because of their dealings with engineers, builders, business people, public officials, and prospective clients.

These professional influences and constraints apply to the nonartistic professions as well. Military officers need to be reliable, conforming, respectful toward authority, courageous, and emotionally stable to be effective leaders. Politicians need to be sociable, conventional, and religious—or at least to give the appearance of being so—in order to gain the support of voters. The intensely solitary nature of investigative pursuits suggests that scientists must be solitary, nonaffiliative, emotionally stable, and unlikely to be swept away by romantic passions.

Given the powerful shaping influence of these expectations on behavior, the personal identities and professional roles of people often merge. For many, being an artist cannot be separated from the artistic life-style.[6] Romantic images that associate drinking, for example, with the creative life hold powerful appeal for many: famous writers, poets, and artists gathered at cafes on Paris' Left Bank, at the exclusive Algonquin Club, or at a bar on the Florida Keys, sipping on their drinks, smoking, and engaging in deep conversation; writers sitting alone at their typewriters and staring at a blank sheet of paper with a glass of gin or scotch nearby, trying to overcome a writing block.

These professional expectations not only draw certain types of individuals but also determine whether individuals reveal their emotional difficulties and seek help for them. People in the creative arts, for example, may flaunt these difficulties as badges of honor. In other professions, such as the military, science, or politics, individuals often disguise their emotional difficulties because any signs of mental instability or social deviancy are taboo. Professions that operate in the public domain are more likely to be selective for people who are reasonably stable or who have the capacity to hide their particular psychopathologies, perhaps even from themselves. When the public expects people in certain professions to conform to certain images, people usually try to comply.

These observations, however, require qualification. Some may argue that because members of the creative arts are inclined to exaggerate emotional difficulties and members of the enterprising or investigative professions are inclined to cover them up, the differences in the rates of emotional disorders for these groups may be overblown. Although this argument is legitimate, it is also flawed. Not only does it ignore the clear pattern of differences in psychopathology between members of the artistic and other professions; it also ignores the convincing differences in their family and childhood backgrounds as well. If differences in their rates of mental disturbance are overblown, then so too are their rates for everything else. This clearly cannot be the case with such objective differences between members of the various professions as their longevity, suicide rate, divorce rates, sexual orientation, family size, and many other characteristics as well.

There is another matter that, although obvious, needs emphasis. Simply because greater percentages of those in the creative arts suffer from mental illness than those in other professions does not mean that all creative artists do. Members of certain of the creative arts professions, such as architecture, design, composing, and nonfiction writing have lower rates of certain mental illnesses than those of other creative arts professions. And all creative arts professions, with the possible exception of poetry, have substantial percentages of persons who are emotionally stable throughout their lives, showing that mental illness is not essential for artistic success.

What is the relationship, if any, between mental disturbances and the creative accomplishments of eminent people?

To answer this question, we need to make a distinction between creative activity and creative achievement. Creative activity refers to the mental and physical effort involved in producing new works, products or perform-ances. As such, it occurs not only in the arts and sciences but also in any fields in which originality and innovation are important. Creative achieve-ment represents the works, products, or performances resulting from the creative activity. Creative activity, when unsuccessful, need not result in creative achievement, but creative achievement is always predicated on creative activity. Because of this distinction, it is possible that the presence of psychopathology may be important for one and not for the other.

What we find is that a complex relationship exists between creative activity and the presence of emotional difficulties. To understand the nature of this relationship, we need to recognize that emotional difficulties can occur during different phases of the creative activity. Mental problems may arise long before the activity and be resolved long before it begins. They may precede and continue during the activity. They may arise during the activity and cease when the activity ends. They may become an integral part of the activity when the professional and personal lives of people merge. Or they may arise long after the creative activity is over. The potential impact of mental disturbances and creative activity on one another differs for each of these situations.

The mental difficulties of people do not always affect creative expres-sion in the same way. For long stretches of time, as in the early stages of alcoholism or drug use, these mental difficulties may have little effect on creative output. In certain documented instances, they may actually in-crease productivity and improve the quality of the creative work. This is especially so for milder or subclinical forms of psychopathology. As noted by others, an "inverted-U" shaped relationship likely exists between mania and creativity, with hypomania leading to a moderate increase in creativity and severe mania leading to a decrease.[7] A similar relationship probably holds for most forms of psychopathology. A mild degree of depression, a few drinks, a mild level of anxiety, or a moderate amount of drugs may allow certain people to be more creative at times than if they were perfectly relaxed or more severely depressed, anxious, or intoxicated. For the most part, however, when mental difficulties persist or are severe enough, and are not tempered by other factors, they tend to be destructive, adversely affecting the quantity or quality of the creative output.

Just as mental disturbances can influence creative activity, creative activity can influence mental disturbances. Usually when this relationship exists, work or creative activity has a beneficial effect on psychological conflicts, often serving as a form of self therapy. For many, creative activity is self-reinforcing. Like a drug, individuals may become "addicted" to it because of its capacity to relieve emotional distress or to produce highly pleasurable states. Some even view creative activity as vital for their emotional survival. "Sometimes I wonder," Graham Greene wrote, "how all those who do not write, compose or paint can manage to escape the madness, the melancholia, the panic fear, which is inherent in the human situation."[8] But creative activity also may unleash buried emotional conflicts that linger on after the artistic endeavor is over. Something of this nature may happen with poets who, when overwrought, dredge up emotions that overwhelm them. Reawakening painful memories or examining a difficult past is like playing with fire. It allows many poets and fiction writers to perceive the world with an intensity, coloration, and passion unavailable to those who avoid tampering with their emotions. But they sometimes do so at the risk of being unable to put their "psychological lids" back on once their creative activities are over.

We also need to recognize that different types of mental disturbances can affect creative expression in different ways. Mania, for instance, may affect the rate and flow of speech, give rise to prolixity and word play, produce discursive and tangential thought, foster expansiveness and grandiosity, and contribute to enormous output or productivity. Depression may decrease verbal associations, constrict coloration, foster nihilism and sadness, shift the focus to dying rather than living, and reduce work output. Schizophrenia may lead to disorganization and relative incoherence in writing, musical composition, or painting or provide the adamancy of delusional convictions. Temperate amounts of alcohol and drugs may overcome creative blocks, decrease inhibitions and performance anxiety, raise confidence, or offer new visions of reality, but when used in excess, they may lead to a garbled and stumbling presentation of ideas and a deterioration in productivity and execution.

Mental disturbances also may provide the motivational juice for creative activity. Anecdotal accounts are common about geniuses who claimed to be obsessed with their work, unable to attend to little else, or who came to believe their work controlled them. William Faulkner wondered whether it was he who created all the characters who peopled Yoknapatawpha County or they who created him. For many others, their very existence may become defined by their art. The wife of Eugene O'Neill, for instance, claimed that her real husband died when his hand tremor kept him from writing, though he continued to live on for many years.

Mental disturbances also may serve as a source of inspiration for people and provide them with the raw material for what they later choose to express. For poets, novelists, composers, and actors, these disturbances may be as essential for their work as is the paint on the palette for an artist. This raises the question of whether we should regard all mental disturbances as "pathological." Many writers have described their personal struggles with alcoholism, drugs, or emotional difficulties through their characters or have gained insights about the human condition through their own experiences with mental illness. Composers have transformed past encounters with depression or mania into powerful symphonic music. Great actors have drawn upon their own struggles with alcoholism or depression to portray what their characters feel. Artists often attempt to translate their intense passions or conflicts onto canvas. Perhaps this is what George Bernard Shaw meant when he wrote that if you could not get rid of the family skeleton, you might as well make it dance.

Despite the intricacies of the relationship between emotional difficulties and creative activity, the results are clear on one important point. While the presence or absence of emotional difficulties may affect the daily creative activities of eminent people in different ways, these difficulties, experienced over their entire lives, have little direct bearing on the extent of their lifetime creative achievements. Even when I examined this relationship for the artistic, investigative, social, and enterprising professions separately, the few significant predictors of creative achievement that emerge only account for a negligible portion of the variation. This lack of a meaningful, simple relationship between the presence or absence of mental disturbances and lifetime creative achievement should not be surprising. When eminent people who are emotionally stable are as capable of making major creative achievements over the course of their lives as those who are unstable, and when mental disturbances can hinder or help daily creative activity, we should not expect the various forms of mental illness to be predictive of creative achievement to any substantial degree. But, as I show, a different situation applies to the extraordinary creative individuals.

Do differences exist between people in the upper and lower rungs of eminence, and if so, what implications do these differences have for understanding the nature of the relationship between mental illness and greatness?

While we cannot compare eminent to noneminent people, mainly because appropriate biographical material is not available on those who are unknown, we *can* compare people of lesser eminence to those of greater eminence. In a comparison of this sort, we find that these two groups differ markedly in their family backgrounds, certain childhood features, and many adult attributes as well. Using a statistical regression model, we can predict with remarkable accuracy whether individuals belong to the upper or lower quartiles of creative achievement based on information about their personal lives and backgrounds. These findings, along with other observations of the very eminent, suggest that a template for greatness exists that predisposes individuals to exceptional creative achievement. The key elements of this template include an innate ability or precociousness tempered by suitable education and training, the "right kind" of parents and family resources, a certain irreverence toward authority, self-sufficiency and independence, a sense of physical vulnerability, the existence of psychological "unease," works that bear a "personal seal," and a striving for dominance or power. While possession of this template appears to increase the potential for lasting posthumous fame among the eminent, complex social and historical forces, many of which remain unknown, likely decide whether it will be realized.[9]

What about the role of psychopathology in this process? While those who are considered more eminent are more likely to suffer from certain emotional difficulties over the course of their lives than those at the lower rung, we cannot assume that these emotional difficulties alone are vital to their accomplishments, even though they are important predictors. For example, when we rely only on the presence of emotional difficulties, we can correctly classify over 60% of those in the upper or lower quartiles of creative achievement. But when we include other elements of this template in the predictive equation, our predictive power rises to over 90%. What this suggests, as I explain below, is that certain emotional difficulties only become important for creative achievement when they are embedded in a matrix of other attributes or circumstances as well, and that they can prove either helpful or harmful, depending upon the context in which they occur and the uses to which they are put.

These, then, represent my main conclusions about the relationship between mental illness and creative achievement, the distillate of more than 10 years of research and thought on the topic. In the chapters that follow, I explain how I arrived at these conclusions, fill in gaps, and address other important issues. First, however, I need to delineate what greatness means, since it was a requirement for the 1,004 extraordinary men and women who were in my study.

CHAPTER TWO

Determining Greatness

P eople often use the notions of "greatness," "eminence," and "genius" interchangeably, as do I. Webster's Dictionary offers justification for these substitutions, defining greatness as eminence, eminence as a position of prominence or superiority, and genius as extraordinary intellectual power, especially in the creative arts. Despite their slightly different connotations, these notions have common denominators. All are predicated on the exceptional personal, professional, or creative achievements of individuals. And all require cultures to recognize the achievements of individuals as great.[1]

Understanding the potential relationship between mental illness and greatness requires knowledge about how people get to be great. Paths taken to greatness reveal a lot about the kinds of opportunities society provides, the type of people who respond to them, and the kinds of activities and achievements that are rewarded. As with so many other areas, Shakespeare penetrated to the heart of the issue when he observed, "Some are born to greatness, some achieve greatness, and some have greatness thrust upon them." This observation has important implications, but as I show below, it also can be misleading.

DIFFERENT PATHS TO GREATNESS

Among the notable people in my sample, there undoubtedly are those who seem born to greatness, entering the world with the proverbial caul about their heads. These are the persons who have everything going for them. Their parents are highly literate, professionally accomplished, personally gifted and creative, and belong to the cultural elite. Socially and financially advantaged, they have the resources to pursue their goals. With outstanding natural endowments, they are precocious and gifted children. Achievements come easily and early in their careers. Their bearing and manner often reflect their self-assurance. By virtue of their towering intellects or superior abilities, they gravitate toward positions of leadership and power. Their success appears inevitable, with obstacles disappearing before them, like the waters parting before Moses.

Charles de Gaulle, for example, seemed fated to lead France. Even his surname presaged this. His father, a gifted teacher at the College of the Immaculate Conception, schooled him in France's history, and his mother imparted to him an intense love of France. As a child, de Gaulle was stubborn and always wanted to be in charge. When he played war games with his brothers, he insisted on representing France. As an adult, with his incredible memory, self-confidence and intransigence, he let little get in his way. When World War II broke out it seemed inevitable that he be called upon to save France—as, with his almost prescient sense of destiny, he always believed he would be.

Even as a youth, Jean-Paul Sartre had greatness written all over him. He came from a distinguished, upper-class family. His maternal grandfather was a minister, musician, and educator, his paternal grandfather a physician. His father was a brilliant naval officer, while his mother was brought up to be a proper young lady, trained in piano and voice. As a child, Sartre was precocious, learning to read at age 3 and already writing novels at age 7. Not surprisingly, he soon came to regard himself as a genius and, over the years, increasingly dominated conversations, regaling his many admirers with his daring ideas and unorthodox views. His talent and versatility were extrordinary. At different points in his life, he was an actor, singer, pianist, critic, composer, poet, novelist, editor, and philosopher, showing brilliance in much of what he did. His nomination for the Nobel Prize seemed an inevitable consequence of his life's work, while his refusal to accept it seemed an inevitable consequence of his personality.

Despite his being black in a white society, Paul Robeson seemed to embody greatness. His father, William Drew Robeson, was born a slave, and after escaping to Pennsylvania at the age of 15, went on to receive a bachelor's degree in sacred theology from Lincoln University. He then became the pastor of a black Presbyterian church in Princeton, New Jersey. As a youth, Paul excelled in sports, in singing, in academic studies, and in debating. At Rutgers, he was an All-American in football (the second black player to achieve that honor), won 15 varsity letters in four different sports, won the oratorical prize 4 years in succession, was admitted to Phi Beta Kappa, and was valedictorian of his class. After his graduation, he starred in various stage productions and films and then launched a highly successful singing career, performing in concerts throughout the world. Because of his phenomenal accomplishments and his commitment to civil rights and social causes, *Ebony* magazine named him as one of the "10 greats in black history."

David Ben-Gurion, another person who seemed to be born to greatness, always had a sense of destiny. His father was an ardent Zionist who inculcated in his son the desire for a Jewish state. By the age of five, David could read and speak Hebrew and had an incredible memory. At age 10, he founded a young people's Zionist Society but his parents forced him to dissolve it, regarding him as too young for such an undertaking. Though taciturn and introspective, in his teenage years he showed the ability to rouse people. At the age of 14 he founded the Ezra Society, to teach Hebrew to children and have them hear Zionist poems. By the age of 19 he was a well-known figure in local labor activities and the Zionist movement. With his inexhaustible energies and single-minded vision, he chipped away at centuries of inertia and mobilized fellow Jews in their fight for a Jewish state. By 1933 he was the world's most famous Zionist. From 1948 to 1953, as seemed almost inevitable, he was the first Prime Minister and beloved leader of Israel.

Unlike these individuals, others achieve greatness by dint of their phenomenal accomplishments, discoveries, or original contributions. Without obvious natural gifts or cultural advantages, these individuals show little in their early lives to suggest the magnitude of their later achievements. Although they tend to pursue their goals with a single-mindedness of purpose, they would most probably never have become known if their efforts had proved unsuccessful or if their distinctive life-styles or manner of death had failed to capture the public imagination. Although success may not come easily and automatically to them, these individuals tend to display remarkable opportunism, capitalizing on whatever their circumstances have to offer. They may not be born to success, but they are not daunted by failure.

On the surface, there was little about Alexander Fleming, the discoverer of penicillin, to suggest that he was an exceptional scientist, and especially no inkling that he one day would be credited with what is arguably the greatest medical discovery of all time. Even-tempered, gregarious, and sociable, he was seemingly without ambition. He made no effort to be promoted from the rank of private in the London Scottish army, where he served for over 14 years. He enjoyed his 9 to 5 workdays and his evenings at the club. And he loved all forms of games, including billiards, snookers, chess, golf, and shooting. Despite his earlier discovery of lysozyme, a natural antibacterial agent in bodily tissues, only his fortunate observation in 1928 that bacteria failed to grow around a contaminating Penicillium mold kept him from obscurity.

Born to aristocratic parents and coming into great wealth as a young man, Leo Tolstoy showed few signs that he would either become one of Russia's greatest writers or eventually found a new religion. As an adolescent, Tolstoy was aimless and lazy. Until he began to write, his general conformity to the aristocratic tradition suggested neither his later unconventional and revolutionary behavior nor his heretical views, which eventually led the Church to excommunicate him.

Other people, in contrast, have greatness thrust upon them. These individuals achieve a measure of fame because they are at the right place at the right time and take advantage of the situation. Their achievements in and of themselves may not be great, but they become critically important within the context in which they occur. These persons are often the trailblazers and precedent setters, serving as inspirational symbols. Often, they would not have been considered great if an accident or incident not of their making had not brought them to prominence. They assume greatness because of their leadership during a crisis or their appearance at a critical time in a social development or cause. Their lives more than their actual achievements may achieve monumental status. They represent heroes of a sort, cultural icons, sometimes immortalized by their tragic lives, their struggles with personal adversity, or their martyred deaths.

George Washington Carver, for example, is revered today more for what he represents—as an inspirational symbol of the ability to overcome great disadvantage and adversity—than for any lasting scientific breakthroughs he may have made. Raised as a slave on the Moses Carver farm, he taught himself to read and, despite the difficulty of pursuing his education because of his race, he eventually earned his bachelor's degree in 1894 and master's degree 2 years later. From these humble beginnings, he went on to make significant contributions through his research in agriculture, developing more than 300 by-products from the peanut and sweet potato, and helping to revitalize the economy of the South.

When Harry Truman was president, few could have predicted he would ascend posthumously to the ranks of the eminent. An uninspiring vice-president and unsuccessful haberdasher from Missouri, Truman succeeded the immensely popular Franklin Delano Roosevelt, who died in office. He left his historical mark by ordering atomic bombs dropped on

Hiroshima and Nagasaki, formulating the Truman Doctrine, which marked the beginning of the U.S. effort to contain communist expansion in Korea and Europe, firing General Douglas MacArthur, advancing the cause of civil rights, and overseeing the evolution of the New Deal into the Fair Deal.

Marcel Duchamp would have found his posthumous fame the height of irony, since he spent much of his life parodying the very art establishment that eventually would revere him. With the exception of his "Nude Descending a Staircase, No. 2" in 1913, the public ignored his works throughout most of his life, regarding him as an eccentric and a failure. Perhaps this was because Duchamp did not seem to take his work seriously, submitting his urinal, called "Fountain," as a work of art for an exhibit, introducing "ready mades" or three-dimensional puns, and painting a sacrilegious mustache and beard on a picture of Mona Lisa. He tried to develop an "antimasterpiece," a painting without a canvas, brushes, an external model, or identifiable colors. He defined himself as an antiartist and produced relatively few works. Nevertheless, because of the time and context in which he worked, he came to receive a measure of greatness as an initiator of what has been called "Pop art" or "Op art."

Margaret Sanger is remembered as much for her independent, free-spirited life, which flew in the face of Victorian mores, as she is for the importance of her causes. Little in her background or personality presaged her later achievements and renown. Her mother was a devout Catholic who was firmly against birth control, and her father spent much time in the local pub, drinking and talking about socialism and free thought. Some thought her to be a timid, nervous speaker, without any natural ability to inspire others. Yet this determined woman, who was forced to drop out of nurse's training in order to marry, became the founder of the birth-control movement in the United States and an international leader in the field. It was not that her ideas were novel or original, for others had maintained many of them before, but she was one of the first to fight courageously for these ideas and openly to live her life in accord with them at a time when their upholders faced great opposition.

This overview of different paths to greatness is obviously oversimplified: for most persons there is considerable overlap among these paths, and all tend to be represented in varying degrees. Nevertheless, the notion of different routes to eminence is important because it shows that different clusters of personal attributes seem essential for different forms of greatness, and that no single set of external circumstances accounts for all of those deemed great by their culture.

THE PREVALENCE OF EMINENCE

Having noted the existence of different paths to greatness, we have yet to identify a suitable sample of people who become great. Ideally, the sample should include sufficient numbers of people to permit comparisons among those in the arts, the sciences, and other fields. But identifying a potential "pool" of eminent people within the general population is difficult. Because of the transiency of fame, many of those who qualify as eminent at one time may not at another. Other potential geniuses languish in relative obscurity, their reputations lost to posterity because of insufficient media coverage, indifferent public reception of their contributions, newer technological developments supplanting their own, or changing economic or social conditions that reduce the value of their achievements.

In a sense, the problem of identifying unrecognized genius is not so unlike the mystery of what happened to the .400 hitters in baseball. In an essay on this topic,[2] Stephen Jay Gould argues that the reason for the drop in the top batting averages in modern times has more to do with refinements and adjustments in the game—such as increased knowledge of how to pitch to or position oneself more effectively against the batter—than to a deterioration in the quality of hitting. This may be so, but his argument begs the question about whether .400 hitters exist in baseball today who potentially can bat .400 but never will. The answer to this absurd question is, of course, no.

Just as being a .400 hitter means hitting .400, being eminent means being judged as eminent. Since eminence represents a judgment conferred upon people by their followers, professions, or societies, it cannot exist unless it is recognized as such. This does not mean that others with comparable intelligence, talent, cleverness, or creativity whose fame is limited are less deserving of eminence than those who gain it. It only means that they have not received comparable recognition for their achievements. But this is no small difference.

Any serious discussion of greatness must start with the hallmark writings on this topic by Francis Galton. In his book, *Hereditary Genius*, Galton claimed that a measure of a man's genius derived from his degree of eminence, which, in turn, rested on his reputation. By reputation he meant "the opinion of contemporaries, revised by posterity . . . based upon a favorable appraisal of a man's character and natural abilities." Natural ability represented those qualities of intellect and disposition "which urge and qualify a man to perform acts that lead to reputation." An individual with this natural ability pursued his goals zealously and persevered until all obstacles were overcome. A genius, therefore, could not be thwarted.[3]

While other prominent views acknowledge the importance of reputation for greatness, they emphasize different qualities as well, such as leadership, creativity, or productivity. Despite the diversity of views, all seem to agree that social recognition is a key element of eminence or greatness. Other potential geniuses may have equal intelligence, talent, cleverness, or creativity and be as deserving of fame, but they cannot qualify as eminent unless their societies judge them to be. There can be no undiscovered geniuses.[4]

Since my study deals with the mental health and achievements of eminent people, it is important to ascertain how rare or common eminence is. Understandably, reliable figures of this sort are difficult to obtain, but perhaps the best estimates are available on scientists. Harriet Zuckerman, in her classic study on the prevalence of scientific eminence,[5] noted that for every Nobel laureate in the United States, the "ultraelite" of science, there were 13 members of the prestigious National Academy of Sciences, 2,600 scientists of sufficient stature to be included in *American Men and Women of Science*, 4,300 professionally successful scientists identified in the *National Register*, and 6,800 self-defined scientists. If we extend these analyses and, for the sake of simplicity, set the number of members of the National Academy of Sciences and Nobel laureates in science at 1,000 and round off the U.S. population for 1970 at 200,000,000, we arrive at a rate of one prominent scientist per 200,000 individuals of the general population or about five per million, a rate approximating that proposed by Francis Galton many years before in his study *English Men of Science*.[6]

While reliable statistics are not available for eminent persons who are not scientists, we may assume that they are equally as uncommon. Although they are seriously flawed, older studies offer ballpark estimates. One study calculated that about 250 people per million were eminent, 15 per million "more illustrious," and about one per million "true geniuses"— those "whom the whole intelligent part of a nation mourns when they die; who have or deserve to have, a public funeral; and who rank in future ages as historical characters."[7] Another study, relying on different sources of information, arrived at remarkably similar results, with an estimated rate of eminence of 12 people per million.[8]

Whatever the true rate may be, all available evidence suggests that it is low. There simply are not that many people who exert profound influences on their disciplines, their societies, and their times.

The Star System

There are, however, reasons other than the difficulty of accomplishment that explain the rarity of genius. It is rare for social and organizational reasons as well, because the elites seem to fulfill certain distinctive functions in society. As leaders, trend setters, role models, spokesmen, and pioneers, they occupy the top positions of fame, power, and wealth in society, and exercise authority and influence in their fields. They formulate policies, set standards, and establish future directions in government, science, art, education, and culture.

The notion of elites, though it extends as far back as Plato, appeared in social science in the early 20th century through the writings of two Italian scholars, Vilfredo Pareto and Gaetano Mosca. Pareto's law of universal inequality held that in any area of human activity, whether in the arts, sciences, politics, business, or other endeavor, the highest achievers formed the elites who possessed special psychological qualities. The remainder comprised the masses. While agreeing that the elite possessed special personal qualities, Mosca stressed the importance of organizational and social factors as the basis for a ruling class. Elite rule represented an inevitable feature of social life. Beneath a highly organized group of elites was a much larger group of subelites, composed of technocrats, intellectuals, civil servants, managers, and the like, whose task it was to carry out, translate, and explain the wishes of the elites to the masses. The very stratification of Western society implied a hierarchy of power, with those at the very top in their fields wielding the greatest influence and those at the bottom the least.[9]

It is not my intention here to delve into the sociology of power and authority. I simply want to point out that there may be reasons for eminence and elitism other than those of personal achievement. Social institutions in general and the arts and sciences in particular seem to need only limited numbers of leaders entrusted with moral, aesthetic, intellectual, legal, or political authority to establish standards and set directions within different fields. A "star system" of this sort provides general stability and order for the field as a whole.[10] The stars in a particular field not only decide which ideas are acceptable and which are not but also exert control over the allocation of scarce financial resources and access to the media. In the case of science, if other scientists did not grant intellectual authority to these stars, science would probably go off in many different directions and lose its cumulative character. This holds for other fields as well.

For those of us who do not fulfill the criteria for eminence, it would be comforting to believe that our contributions to science, art, or society are important, no matter how minor, trivial, or mediocre they may be. This belief has been called the "Ortega hypothesis" because of the claim made by Jose Ortega y Gasset, the famous Spanish writer, philosopher, and diplomat, that "experimental science has progressed thanks in part to the work of men astoundingly mediocre, and even less than mediocre. That is to say, modern science, the root and symbol of our actual civilization, finds a place for the intellectually commonplace man and allows him to work therein with success." Without the minor contributions and minor discoveries by a mass of average scientists working on unambitious or unimaginative projects, the breakthroughs of the truly inspired scientists would not be possible.[11] This is a comforting, egalitarian claim. Unfortunately, it does not seem to be borne out by the evidence.

Evidence against the Ortega hypothesis is convincing. The most highly cited and influential papers in physics, for example, come almost exclusively from the most distinguished physics departments or research laboratories; the best papers tend to quote only other significant papers; and even relatively minor discoveries or breakthroughs are made by the more distinguished scientists. These and other findings argue more for an elitism than for an equality in science.[12]

What applies to science also seems to apply to the arts. Take the case of classical music. According to one survey, only about 250 of the thousands of classical composers are responsible for all the compositions that are performed regularly in the concert and recital halls.[13] Of the total of 250 composers, the first 40 account for three-fourths of the works played; the first 16 account for one-half; and the first 10 account for about 40%. Amazingly, the first five composers—Mozart, Beethoven, Bach, Wagner, and Brahms—account for over one-quarter of all the works performed. Although comparable figures are not readily available for the public's appreciation of art, sculpture, poetry, or architecture, I suspect that they would be similar.

The finding that only small numbers of people have a disproportionately large influence on their fields or societies may show not only the relative scarcity of exceptional persons but also the rarity of suitable slots of influence, prestige, or power for them to fill. They probably could not exercise their authority well if there were too many of them. Too many elites detract from the specialness of their privileged status. This represents the "phenomenon of the 41st chair," named after the practice of The French Academy of Science to elect only 40 distinguished members to its ranks of "immortals." By default, even though they may have made important contributions in their fields, those persons failing to be elected are metaphorically relegated to the 41st chair.[14] A similar situation seems to hold for runners-up for the Nobel Prize, losers of major elections, second-place finishers in important events, and those not appointed to prestigious posts. Ordinarily, we should expect many of these deserving and capable runners-up, uncrowned laureates, nominees, or silver medalists to exert an influence in their respective fields proportionate to their achievements and to receive their proportionate share of awards. They are, after all, exceptional and worthy people. Apparently it makes little difference. Even with the recent proliferation of available prizes to offset the scarcity of the most prestigious awards[15] and the establishment of new organizations to honor lesser luminaries, runners-up do much worse proportionately in terms of endorsements, reputations, influence, and awards than those chosen for the most select roles.

The cumulative advantage of the "immortals" over the occupants of the 41st chair can be seen in many areas. Marked disparities in reputation exist between those more and those less eminent, disparities far greater than the differences in their talents or even accomplishments seem to warrant.

Why is it, for example, that Sigmund Freud is far better known today than Havelock Ellis, when both had so much in common? Ellis, an English physician, wrote a seven-volume magnum opus, *Studies in the Psychology of Sex*, which was as startling and enlightened at the time as were Freud's writings on human sexuality. He was equally productive, writing over 200 articles and many books, and equally versatile, with interests in poetry and anthropology. In many ways, with his imposing looks and eccentric dress, he was far more colorful, proclaiming the naturalness of nudity and masturbation and even admitting to possessing the perversion, "urolagnia," a morbid fascination with the urinary activities of others.

As another example, we find that Judy Holliday is all but forgotten while Marilyn Monroe lives on as a cult figure, with many biographies written about her over the years. Judy Holliday was an attractive, talented actress and comedienne, winning an Academy Award in 1946 for *Born Yesterday* and a Tony Award in 1950 for *Bells Are Ringing*. Although she may not have exuded that same aura of innocence and sexuality or died in as mysterious a way as Monroe, Judy Holliday possessed a magnetism of her own, and her early death from cancer was just as tragic.

Again, why is it that Leon Blum, the first Socialist premier of France and the first Jewish person to hold that position, should become a footnote in history while his contemporary Winston Churchill, the former head of the Conservative Party and later prime minister of Britain during World War II, remains widely known? No doubt, Churchill is deserving of his fame for his inspiring leadership during a time of worldwide crises, but Blum does not seem to warrant his growing obscurity. Elected to office three times, Blum made important reforms for labor, including laws on collective bargaining, the 40-hour work week, and paid vacation. As an essayist, poet, literary critic, and editor of Le Populaire, he was as prolific and gifted a writer as Churchill, and his wartime essay, For All Mankind, written in 1946, was arguably as magnificent as Churchill's chronicles of World War II. In his own way, Blum was a war hero, too. Arrested in 1940 after the German defeat of France and tried in 1942 by the Vichy government, he staged a courageous defense that caused his trial to collapse. Afterward, he was transferred to a German concentration camp and remained there as a symbol of occupied France until U.S. troops liberated him in 1945.

The obvious explanation for these widening discrepancies in fame is that they reflect true differences in the accomplishments of these people. There are differences in accomplishments, to be sure, but this explanation still does not account for why reputations of those who are better known often grow to mythic proportions while reputations of those who are lesser known fade into oblivion. What the discrepancy in fame really reflects is a tendency for the most eminent within each field to gain a cumulative advantage over those accorded lesser stature. Over time, they become the standard bearers within their professions or societies. They have favored access to the media, attract more followers, and command greater resources, all of which leads to even greater fame and renown.

What this confirms is that the designation of greatness is not solely determined by an individual's accomplishments. From available estimates, it appears that greatness is an uncommon phenomenon, limited only to a select few in each field. But it also represents a dynamic process, like a grain of sand that seeds a pearl, because of its cumulative nature. The better known people are, the better known they are likely to become. In many instances, they may become so prominent and revered that their reputations live on well after their deaths.

As part of this dynamic process, certain other forces are at work, which go beyond the actual accomplishments of the individuals themselves. These forces decide, to a large extent, the number of slots available for eminence in the various fields and in society at large. This seems to serve an important stabilizing function that contributes to the cumulative nature of science and to the progression and development of other fields. Just as too many cooks can spoil the broth, too many authorities can cause confusion. What this quota on eminence suggests is that the eminent not only are select people but they also have been selected for their roles. Eminence, then, represents a complex interaction between the person, his or her works, his or her field, and his or her audience.

THE SELECTION PROCESS

With this clarification as background, we now can turn to the issue of how best to identify a large sample of eminent people and how best to gather information about them. Several concerns governed my approach to this issue. The people selected for study had to be eminent; the information base had to cover their entire life span; and the sources of information had to deal with how the eminent people viewed themselves and how they were viewed by others.

The Biographical Approach

At best, any approach to information gathering about the private lives of people is imperfect, and certain trade-offs need to be made, depending on who or what is under investigation. For example, while direct interviews with people allow systematic probes into their feelings and attitudes, the information obtained is colored by what people choose to reveal, how they interpret their experiences, the selective focus of the interviews or questionnaires, the retrospective nature of their responses, and the biases of their interviewers. In addition, the information does not cover an entire lifetime, from birth to death, and offers no gauge of posthumous fame.

After evaluating all the potential approaches to information gathering I could think of, I decided that the biographical method was best suited for answering the questions I posed. I was well aware of the limitations of relying on biographical materials, which included potential biographer bias in the selection and interpretation of facts, the inability to pry into certain personal areas and question individuals directly, and the retrospective nature of the information. However, for my purposes, whatever disadvantages were inherent in the use of biographical materials seemed to be more than offset by the richness of the information (e.g., memoirs, autobiographies, interviews with the person and knowledgeable informants, observations by others, intimate accounts, and judgments by authorities), as well as by the placement of lives within a cultural and historical context.[16] Also, even the most detailed personal interviews and comprehensive inventories could not match the time and effort expended by responsible biographers in the study of their subjects. For instance, in personal communications with me, Leon Edel revealed that he spent over 20 years on Henry James, William Manchester over 13 years on Winston Churchill, David McCullough over 10 years on Harry Truman, Donald Spoto over 6 years on Alfred Hitchcock, Diane Middlebrook over 8 years on Anne Sexton, and Christopher Benfey over 5 years on Stephen Crane. From my interviews with more than 20 distinguished biographers, I estimate that they devoted on average about 3 to 4 years for each of their subjects. In many instances, I suspect, these biographers got to know their subjects in certain ways better than the subjects knew themselves.

No form of information gathering, however, is suitable unless safeguards exist to insure its reliability and validity. Whatever the information extracted from biographical sources, it should be consistent, reproducible, and hold similar meaning for trained raters or informed observers.[17] We also cannot assume that because someone reports something it is necessarily "true." John Cheever, for instance, boasted that he never told the truth to psychiatrists. Marilyn Monroe supposedly made a similar claim. From a scientific standpoint, the most "valid" types of information are "objective" data—that is, documented behaviors, such as publications, performances, medical or psychiatric illnesses, handicaps, years of schooling, or demographic variables, such as age, gender, race, place of birth, birth order, occupation, and marital status—because they are capable of independent corroboration or proof. The more abstract, interpretive, general, experiential, subjective, or inferential the information, the more difficult it is to establish its reliability and its actual correspondence to something objective in the real world. This is the kind of information of which we need to be wary.

Representativeness of Sample

Having decided on the use of biographies, I had other decisions to make. What source should I use to gather suitable names? What selection criteria should I use? And how could I establish the representativeness of my sample?

As my source for suitable names, I settled on the *New York Times Book Review*, since I believed it offered the best coverage of biographies. All individuals qualified for my sample who met my selection criteria and whose biographies were reviewed between 1960 and 1990 (an interval when more intimate and personal material about people was more likely to be included in biographies than previously). Concerned that changing cultural and historical factors would confound the nature of creative achievement and judgments about professional success, I included only those people who belonged to Western culture and had lived during the 20th century. This allowed a much higher representation of women in the sample, since their opportunities for prominence before the turn of the century and in most non-Western societies were almost nil. I also chose individuals who had died, so as to insure complete information about their entire lives and their posthumous reputations. They also must have had at least one well-documented, comprehensive biography published about them (not necessarily the one reviewed by the *New York Times Book Review*). Those who gained fame or notoriety because of criminal activities, catastrophes, wars, or other sensational events (such as overcoming handicaps, illness, drug addiction, or other adversities), were excluded from the study.

With these criteria, I was able to select a sample of 1,004 eminent people, about three-fourths of whom were men and one-fourth of whom were women. These people gained eminence in a wide variety of professions: not only the arts and sciences but also business, sports, exploration, public office, philanthropy, and the military. Appendix A lists their names and professions. Although there were over 25 countries represented, the large majority of these people came from English-speaking nations.[18] Depending upon the adequacy of the primary source, from one to four complete biographies were read on every subject, supplemented by entries from encyclopedias or biographical dictionaries. Nearly 2,200 biographical sources were used.[19]

Once I had selected this sample, my next step was to test its representativeness—namely, how comparable my sample was to those that could be gathered through other sources or means. The more representative my sample, the more my findings should apply to eminent people in general, or at least to those who became famous enough to have biographies written about them. Since my sample of eminent people was drawn only from biographies reviewed in the *New York Times Book Review* between 1960 and 1990, I did not expect it to include eminent people whose biographies were reviewed before those years. I estimated that if my sample contained at least 50% of the names of those in other samples of eminent persons of the 20th century, then its representativeness would be adequate. As measures for comparison, I chose (1) the lists of suitable names in the *Book Review Digest*, which contains citations for all current biographies written in English, published in the United States, England, or Canada, and reviewed by at least two of its periodicals or journals; (2) the names of eminent people in the 1962 and 1978 Goetzel studies; (3) S. M. Stievater's *Biographies of Creative Artists: An Annotated Bibliography*; and (4) P. E. Shellinger's *St. James Guide to Biography*.[20] The percentages of people from these different sources included in my own sample ranged from 67% to 85%. Also, of those who met my selection criteria in the 1990 listing by *Life* magazine of the "100 Most Influential People of the 20th Century," 68% were in my sample. These assorted results established that my sample of eminent people was representative of all eminent people who came from Western countries, lived some portion of their lives in the 20th century, and had biographies written about them.

Classifying Professions

It is not sufficient to have a representative sample of eminent persons without also having an ample number of professions represented. Without being able to compare people in different professional groups, we could not tell whether various findings are characteristic of eminence *per se* or are mainly associated with certain kinds of vocational activities. This means that we not only must understand the nature of professions but also use suitable methods to classify them.

Professions serve many functions. They allow people to earn a living. They offer opportunities for communication with colleagues and fellow employees. They provide outlets for physical and emotional energies. They help consolidate a sense of personal identity and self-worth. They allow people to gain social recognition. They also offer people a vehicle to express their creativity and aspirations and possibly to reshape their societies and world.

A complex interaction exists between people and their professions. While people often view their professions as personal extensions of themselves, they sometimes become servants to their professions. In obvious and not-so-obvious ways, their professions decide what types of occupational activities are permissible and the relative values placed on them. The more professions are accountable to the public, the more they regulate the behavior of their members.[21] Professions such as medicine, law, architecture, dentistry, teaching, science, and the military have licensing boards, credentialing bodies, or certification procedures to establish educational requirements, training experiences, knowledge base and performance standards, and codes of ethical and appropriate behavior (i.e., the Hippocratic oath, confidentiality requirements, etc.). If members do not comply with these expectations or violate certain laws, rules, or regula-tions, they face disciplinary action, special sanctions, loss of licensure, limitations in practice, disbarment, suspension, and/or professional cen-sure. Professions such as visual art, musical entertainment, acting, or composing, which have little impact on public safety or welfare, have more lax standards for the personal and occupational conduct of their members. Although they may offend public taste, members need not fear official, professional censure.

In general, professions arise to meet certain social needs. In a changing society, occupations evolve and change over time, some thriving and others disappearing under different political, economic, and technological conditions. Sometimes a particular field evolves and differentiates slowly from within through the incorporation of new technology and informa-tion. Sometimes new fields emerge suddenly after major discoveries or breakthroughs, the introduction of new media of expression, the develop-ment of new technologies, or in response to new social needs.

As it happens, there are many ways to categorize professions.[22] To an extent, any classification of professions is arbitrary and based on certain practical and theoretical considerations. It becomes risky, then, to rely entirely on one classification system that does not allow for more specific conclusions about certain professions or more general observations about several related professions.

Given the potential importance of professional affiliation on creative achievement and general behavior, I decided to use three different profes-sional classifications in the interpretation of results, each classification corresponding to a different level of "magnification." The highest level of magnification involves empirically grouping the people in my sample into 18 general professions, each combining certain related professions (e.g., art includes painting, sculpting, and photography; public office includes politics, appointed office, and law).[23] This classification yields eight crea-tive arts professions (e.g., architecture, art, composing, musical perform-ance, theater, fiction, nonfiction, and poetry) and ten other professions or primary activities (e.g., business, exploration, public office, the natural sciences, the social sciences, companionship, the military, social figure, sports, and social activism) (see Table 2.1).[24]

The next level of magnification—which I call moderate—involves the use of the Holland classification.[25] Not only does it offer a simple way to categorize professions and to describe the kinds of people who are drawn to them, but it also has ample research support.[26] Although this classifica-tion of professions lists six general types—artistic, enterprising, investiga-

Table 2.1. Primary Professions of Sample

Profession	Number	Percentage
Architecture/Design	23	2.3
Art	70	7.0
Business	70	7.0
Companion	19	1.9
Exploration	11	1.1
Fiction	180	17.9
Military	20	2.0
Musical composition	48	4.8
Musical performance	47	4.7
Natural sciences	39	3.9
Nonfiction	64	6.4
Poetry	53	5.3
Public office	108	10.7
Social activism	61	6.1
Social figure	30	3.0
Social sciences	73	7.3
Sports	19	1.9
Theater	70	7.0
Total	1,004	100

tive, social, conventional, and realistic—only the first four apply to our subjects. This is because the *conventional*-type occupations largely have to do with operating business machines, record keeping, secretarial, or clerical work, and the *realistic*-type largely have to do with factory work, raising animals, construction, farming, or the operation of heavy machinery. No eminent people have gained professional fame in these ways.

The theory underlying this classification system holds that different types of occupations attract corresponding types of people. *Investigative types* seek activities that allow them to understand, investigate and control physical, biological, and cultural phenomena, and avoid those that require persuasive and social skills. They portray themselves as reserved, rational, unpopular, unassuming, scholarly, intellectual, mathematical, and scientific, and as lacking in leadership abilities. *Artistic types* prefer ambiguous, free, unsystematized activities that involve the manipulation of physical, verbal, or human materials to create artistic products, and dislike explicit,

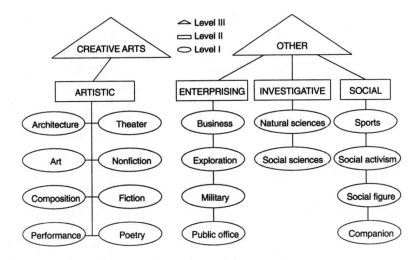

Figure 2.1. Classification of professions by levels.

systematic and ordered activities that require organization, documentation and precision. They perceive themselves as expressive, original, intuitive, nonconformist, introspective, independent, disorderly, emotional, and creative. *Social types* enjoy activities that involve training, helping, or enlightening others, and avoid explicit, ordered, systematic activities that involve the use of materials, tools, or machines. They see themselves as helpful, understanding, friendly, sociable, and persuasive, and as lacking in mechanical and scientific abilities. *Enterprising types* prefer activities that involve the manipulation of others to attain organizational goals or economic gain, and dislike activities that rely on observational, introspective, or symbolic processes. They see themselves as aggressive, popular, self-confident, sociable, adventuresome, extroverted, having leadership and speaking abilities, and lacking in scientific talent. They also value political and economic achievement.

Based on this schema, the highest vocational aspirations and achievements should be associated with the enterprising and social occupations, the highest educational and interpersonal achievements with the investigative and social professions, the highest competence in interpersonal relations with the social and enterprising professions, and the highest creative performance with the artistic and investigative professions. Fortunately, we are able to test these assumptions.

Finally, at the lowest level of magnification, when gross generalizations are feasible, we can collect all the groups into two separate categories and use the conventional distinction between the creative arts and non-creative arts professions. With this classification, people are grouped according to whether they use subjective media of expression and create personal products or whether they do not. The relationship among these three different levels of classification can be seen in Figure 2.1.

So far we have noted that vocational activities are a vital part of people's existence. They represent not only a way for people to earn a living but, for many, a way to satisfy many of their needs for personal and creative expression. Most ordinary people usually operate within the general constraints and boundaries of their fields. If there is any distinctive feature of eminent people, especially the truly great, it is their ability not only to set the standards within their fields but also to alter radically the boundaries of their fields, and sometimes even to create entire new disciplines and specialties. The goal now is to learn what kinds of people are able to do this and what factors govern their choice of career.

CHAPTER THREE

The Early Years

W ith the benefit of hindsight, the career choices of eminent persons
seem inevitable. They appear to have found their perfect niche, a proper
fit between their personalities and talents and the demands of their
professions. But what is so obvious with hindsight may not be evident
before it occurs, during their youths, when their entire lives lie ahead of
them. Who, for example, could have predicted the ultimate careers into
which the remarkable James brothers would settle? Henry, who was to
become one of the most influential figures in American literature, was first
drawn to art and then to law. William, his brother, first studied art in Paris,
then chemistry and comparative anatomy for 3 years before enrolling in
Harvard Medical School. He interrupted his medical studies twice to
pursue certain research opportunities, and then, after earning his M.D.,
began teaching as an instructor in anatomy and physiology at Harvard. He
was 32 years old before he set up the first psychological laboratory and
taught psychology, the field in which he eventually would gain a measure
of immortality.

Nevertheless, if individuals are to a large extent the products of their
pasts, the critical information about their later selection of a career should
be identifiable during their youths, provided we know where to look. It
should not make much difference whether youths zero in on their eventual
professional destinations at an early age or get there after pursuing a zigzag
career course.

Sometimes how adults were influenced as children is obvious, but
more often it is obscure. In children with prodigious talent, these early
influences usually are clear. Pablo Casals, for instance, began taking piano
lessons at the age of 4 from his father, an organist, composer, and choir
master at the church. At age 7 his father arranged for him to take violin
lessons. By the age of 13, thanks to the continuous involvement of his

father, his career was well established. He played the cello professionally as part of a trio, began composing a few years later, and gave his first solo performance as a cellist at the age of 21.

In the case of someone like Che Guevera, early family influences are uncertain. Although we probably will never know all the early factors that contributed to him becoming a physician, revolutionary, and politician and eventually being killed in the remote hills of Bolivia while waging guerilla warfare, we could not be too far wrong to identify at least one influence from his childhood. His radical, free-thinking parents, both of whom were fervent anti-Peronists, very likely contributed to his rebelliousness, social consciousness, and commitment to revolutionary causes.

It is hard to isolate particular factors that lead individuals to particular achievements. Indeed, entire biographies are written to explain how early childhood influences later life choices. Fortunately, when we try to identify the important early influences on children who later become eminent, we have recourse to an important developmental theory of eminence, which offers a useful framework for organizing information about the early lives of extraordinary people.[1] This theory holds that the special talents and gifts of children serve as "organizers" of behavior, which shape their personal development and their immediate social environments. In other words, these children "serve" their talent, just as their talent comes to serve them. They want to do well and be special in the eyes of their parents, teachers, and peers. Since their unique abilities gain them special attention and praise, they tend to seek out opportunities to exhibit them. They begin to surround themselves with people who have similar talents and interests. Over time, their life revolves around their gifts and they spend more and more of their time exercising them.

If their parents recognize that their children are gifted and special, and are able to do so, they provide the necessary financial resources and make sacrifices to insure that these gifts develop and thrive. Gifted youths attract mentors who offer guidance and direct them to masters or the best institutions. The institutions themselves encourage these youths to display their abilities and be rewarded for them.

In a sense, the exceptional talents of children serve as powerful organizers for their own behaviors and the behaviors of those around them. The talents progressively shape the immediate environment of children into one in which their gifts are central. Their world becomes one in which the youths themselves, as well as their parents, teachers, mentors, other important people in their lives, and the institutions in which they train reinforce these talents and enable them to grow. When a "fit" exists among all these elements, gifted youths have optimal chances for career success.

What this developmental theory of eminence reveals is that the most important influences operating on these children are those that potentially aid or hinder the expressions of their talents. Such potential early influences should include family backgrounds, certain characteristics of the parents, early traumatic experiences, physical health, natural talents and endowments, and educational experiences. The more we know about the responses of children to these influences, the better able we should be to determine whether certain kinds of youths are likely to choose certain kinds of career paths to express their particular talents.[2] Of these many potential influences, the first experiences come, of course, from their families.

FAMILY BACKGROUND

Characteristics of Parents

Past studies of eminent persons have found that most come from families in which their fathers are professionals and businessmen. My own findings, based on several related measures, support this conclusion.[3,S1] The vast majority of eminent persons in my sample seem to have a decided edge over less advantaged people because of the financial and cultural resources available to them and the success-oriented value systems to which they were exposed. About two-thirds of all wage-earning parents were professionals (e.g., doctor, lawyer, teacher, minister, artist, entertainer, businessperson, writer, soldier) and the remainder were either aristocrats, tycoons, or members of royalty (11%), or unskilled laborers (22%). About two-thirds of their fathers completed college or obtained graduate degrees, compared to about one-fourth of their mothers.

The parents' social status clearly bears upon the career choice made by their offspring. Social figures, famous companions, or public officials, for instance, mostly come from sophisticated, cultured families, which afford them the necessary resources and experiences for fulfilling these roles. Those individuals who enter professions that require extensive formal training, such as scientists and academicians, come from upper middle-class, professional families. Athletes and musical entertainers, who rely more on natural talent and physical skills than formal education, are more likely to come from less well-to-do families and have unskilled or unsuccessful fathers.[S2–S5]

Parents' social attitudes also affect their children's vocational interests. Freethinking parents, especially fathers, are more likely to raise nonconforming children who enter nonconforming professions, such as the arts, theater, or writing. Angelica de Kostrowsitsky, mother of Apollinaire, for example, worked in a gambling house in Monaco and had two illegitimate children, despite her upper-class background. Lenny Bruce's mother worked in bars as a master of ceremonies and a comic and led a very unconventional life. Charlie Chaplin's mother, Hannah Hill, was a great pantomime who sang and performed in music halls. Jack London's father, William H. Chaney, was a footloose astrologer and freelance philosopher who claimed to have had six "wives," several of whom he never married. Condé Nast's father rebelled against his own father's rigid puritanism and "vanished" for 13 years, ending up in Europe where he sought his fortune. Waldo Barnes Buddington, the father of Djuna Barnes, raised his family, educated his children, and attempted to achieve self-sufficiency on a 105-acre farm as the expression of a messianic impulse to create a more natural society. Count Alphonse de Toulouse-Lautrec, the father of Henri, lived in a world of his own creation, jumping horses all day, going dancing, coming to dinner in a tutu, or giving his hawks holy water to drink—in order, he said, not to deprive them of religion.

In contrast, socially conformist parents are less likely to raise offspring who enter the creative arts[S6] and their children are more likely to follow professionally in their father's footsteps.[S7] The eventual career choice of Lyndon Baines Johnson, for instance, seems to reflect this type of parental influence. His father served in the Texas State Legislature, and his mother was the daughter of the person his father defeated for office. By the time he was in the ninth grade, Lyndon was devouring newspapers and constantly reading the *Congressional Record*. Although he was skilled at debate and his high-school classmates predicted that he someday would be governor of Texas, Johnson took several career detours before fulfilling familial expectations. After his graduation he was fired from a clerical job, taught school after obtaining a 2-year certificate, entered law school, and worked later as a private secretary for a U.S. Representative—before ever running for election.

Not surprisingly, along with the extent of their conformity, the creative and aesthetic interests of the parents also exert an influence on their children's career choices. Parents actively involved in music, art, handicrafts, writing, or the theater are more likely to pass on an aesthetic appreciation to their offspring and orient them toward the creative arts. The artistic types, such as musical entertainers, poets, composers, artists, actors, and architects (roughly 40 to 70%), are far more likely than the enterprising types, such as soldiers, social activists, businesspeople and sports figures (roughly up to 20%), to have mothers and fathers with strong aesthetic interests. Artistic types are also more likely to have at least one sibling with creative interests.[58] Clearly, creative activity and aesthetic interests tend to run in families.

Death of Parents

Various developmental theories of eminence point to certain traumatic events during childhood, such as the loss of a parent, as the basis for later achievement and mental illness. Presumably, an event of this sort, happening at a time when individuals are most vulnerable, helpless, and impressionable, should have a devastating impact on them, psychologically scarring them for life and, for certain of them, spurring them on to compensate for this loss through constant creative activity. This makes conceptual sense. Unfortunately, authoritative claims to the contrary, no solid scientific evidence exists that proves this to be so.

In her study of 24 consecutive British Prime Ministers, beginning with Spencer Perceval in 1809 and ending with Neville Chamberlain in 1937, Lucille Iremonger[4] noted that 15 had lost one or the other parent before the age of 15, about a 63% rate, compared to an estimated 17% rate of orphanhood before age 14 for the general population, according to the 1921 Census for England and Wales. On further study of this phenomenally high rate of orphaned Prime Ministers, Iremonger observed what she thought to be a characteristic set of attributes among them, which she called the *Phaëthon complex*. These attributes consisted of an insatiable need for love and attention, a recklessness in seeking this love and attention, an isolation and reserve, an abnormal degree of sensitivity, depression, superstitiousness, austerity, and aggressiveness, an overreaction to bereavement, and an intense devotion to one's own children.

The Phaëthon complex is named after a Greek mythological figure. Phaëthon, loved by Venus, was a handsome, vain, and arrogant young man who was disturbed by insinuations about his birth. With the approval of his mother, he sought out Phoebus in his Palace of the Sun and insisted on proof that he was his father and loved him. As a sign of his fatherly devotion, Phoebus swore an oath by the Styx that he would grant Phaëthon whatever he asked. Phaëthon immediately demanded to drive his father's fiery chariot, the sun itself. Worried about the danger of this request Phoebus tried to talk Phaëthon out of it, but Phaëthon insisted. No sooner did he grab the reins of the chariot than the flying horses plunged from the track. At that point Jupiter struck him with a thunderbolt to keep the world from being set afire.

One message of this myth is clear. Because of the past absence of a father, Phaëthon wanted to be acknowledged and legitimatized in a way that the entire world would notice, even if it meant risking his life.

Other authors also claim that being orphaned or abandoned by a parent represents an important determinant of eminence. In his study of 573 eminent subjects who lived between 500 B.C. and on through the 20th century—subjects whose names he secured from the *Encyclopaedia Britannica* and the *Encyclopedia Americana*—J. Marvin Eisenstadt found that by age 10, 25% of the subjects had one parent dead, by age 15, about 35% had at least one parent dead, and by age 20, 45% had at least one parent dead. By age 10, 3% of the subjects had lost both parents, and by age 15, 6% had lost both. This contrasted with the rates given in the 1921 Census for England and Wales, showing that about 12% of the people experienced the death of one parent during their first 9 years, and 17% during the first 14 years—rates that were about one-half those obtained for his sample of eminent people. But as Eisenstadt acknowledged, although perhaps not forcefully enough, the comparison of the death rates of a sample of eminent people whose lives spanned 2,500 years of recorded history to the 1921 Census data for England and Wales might not be appropriate.[5]

The reports of high rates of early parental loss among the eminent are plentiful. One researcher reported that about 30% of the poets studied lost their fathers before age 15. Another researcher discovered that 15% of her sample of eminent scientists lost a parent before the age of 10. Yet another researcher reported a threefold increase in early parental loss in eminent or historical geniuses compared to that of a gifted college population.[6] Unfortunately, none of these authors, including Eisenstadt, compared these percentages with those of time-matched controls, in whom the longevity and mortality rates could be expected to be similar. This keeps us from drawing any meaningful conclusions from them.

The current study records the rates of early parental loss in members of the different professions during their first 6 years of age, ages 7 to 13, ages 14 to 20, and after age 21. For the 618 mothers and 645 fathers on whom reliable information was available, the most important finding was that no significant differences existed among members of the different professions for the death rates of either parent at different ages in their lives. The death rates for mothers and fathers also appeared roughly the same. Six percent of the mothers, 8% of the fathers, and 11% of *either* the mothers or fathers died when their children were under age 7; 9% of the mothers, 8% of the fathers, and 13% of *either* the mothers or fathers died when their children were 7 to 14 years of age; 8% of mothers and 12% of fathers and 9% of *either* mothers or fathers died when their children were between the ages of 14 and 21; and the remainder of the mothers and fathers died after that.[S9]

Whether these rates of early parental loss are exceptionally high for eminent persons is unknown. Although it is difficult to obtain appropriate population statistics for comparison, largely because of the many countries represented in the sample and the time span involved, the 1921 Census data for England and Wales (taken at a time when the average for members of my sample was about 40 years) showed that about 17% of the population experienced the death of one parent during their first 14 years, a lower rate than the cumulative 24% for my own sample. However, available U.S. statistics on orphans under the age of 18 reveal a steady decline from 16% in 1920 to 12% in 1930, 10% in 1949, and 5% in 1959. Extrapolating from these figures, I find it reasonable to expect that the rate of orphanhood among children would have been well over 20% in 1900, a figure approximating that for my sample as a whole.[7]

Still to be discovered was the impact of early parental loss on later mental illness and creative achievement. Surprisingly, the results of statistical analyses did not support the common belief that the lifetime mental difficulties of eminent persons were due to the loss of a parent during childhood. There was no relationship between the age periods at which people lost their mothers or fathers and their later difficulties with alcohol, drugs, depression, mania, psychoses, severe anxiety, adjustment disorders, or the length of time they experienced them.[S10] The reasons for this lack of relationship become obvious when we examine the early lives of those who should have been the most emotionally crippled: those who lost both of their parents by the age of 13. As we see below from this selection of people, the reasons mostly have to do with the different ways that these children reacted to the loss of their parents and other circumstances in their lives. Contrary to conventional expectations, not all people are permanently devastated or damaged by such a loss.

For the entire sample of subjects, only two lost both parents before they were 6 years of age—Bill Robinson and Bertrand Russell—and another 14 before the age of 14. Among the latter were six fiction writers (Maxim Gorky, J. R. R. Tolkien, Leo Tolstoy, Joseph Conrad, Frederick Faust, and Somerset Maugham), one poet (Conrad Aiken), two public figures (Key Pittman, Herbert Hoover), two businesspeople or promoters

(Alfred I. Du Pont, Sergei Diaghilev), one social activist (Roger Case-ment), one musical entertainer (Bessie Smith), and one famous spouse (Eleanor Roosevelt). Although there were certain common features, the deaths of their parents affected each of these people differently.

Some children experienced worsening in both their material and emotional lives after both of their parents died; resources were scarce and no close relatives took a personal interest in their welfare. Bill Robinson, sometimes known as "Mr. Bojangles," is a case in point. Reluctantly raised from infancy by his grandmother, a former slave, he began dancing on street corners as a child, dropped out of school at 7, ran away to Washington, D.C., and eventually appeared in his first show, The South Before the War, at 14. Although he gambled, drank heavily on occasion, and was once arrested for armed robbery, he eventually managed to rise to the top of his profession without ever being seriously incapacitated by any psychiatric illness.

Frederick Faust, best known for his novels about the West, is another example. Orphaned by the age of 13, he led a hard life, passed between distant relatives and forced to support himself by working on a succession of farms and ranches. During this time, he attended 19 different public schools, each time with a "series of fist fights until I had found my place." "I grew up," he recalled, "learning to withdraw from children my age, thrown utterly into a world of books and daydreaming." Eventually, he went on to graduate from high school and enter Berkeley, but he had to leave his senior year for disciplinary reasons. Although Faust suffered from alcoholism and periodic depressions throughout his life, he continued to be remarkably productive.

Some had been born into wealth, and didn't lose material advantages and educational opportunities after their parents' death. They also had relatives who took their guardianship seriously. Still, despite this strong support system, their lives were blighted by serious depressions.

Bertrand Russell, the British philosopher, mathematician, and social activist, lost both of his parents by the age of 3. His grandmother, a puritanical and strict woman, took over his care and instilled in him a strong sense of personal duty. Opposed to philosophical debate, she sup-posedly responded to the question, "What is mind?" with "Never matter," and then "What is matter?" with "Never mind." She raised her grandson in isolation from other children and provided tutors for him until he later went off to school. There was little indication at the time that this shy, conforming youth with a passion for reading would go on to win the Nobel Prize in literature and take many shocking social stands.

Leo Tolstoy, brought up in a wealthy, aristocratic family, lost not only both parents but also two other family members while he was young. His mother died when he was 2; his father, a prince and ex-army officer, died when he was 8; his grandmother, whom he went to live with, died when he was 9; and his aunt Alexandra, who next raised him, died when he was 13. He then went to live with another aunt, a countess, who became his guardian. Carefree and irresponsible as a youth, he eventually found his calling once he started to write.

Those children whose parents' death occurred under inauspicious circumstances remained haunted by their loss, despite adequate family support and sufficient finances. When Conrad Aiken was 11, his father, a prominent ophthalmologist and frustrated writer and artist, murdered Conrad's mother and then killed himself. Conrad's grandmother and grandfather, a Unitarian minister who was known for his "saintliness," sent him to private school and eventually to Harvard. Despite the care and concern of his guardians, Conrad remained solitary and rebellious, convinced that his parents' murder–suicide was a "black mark" against him, which he had to conceal. Later in life he became alcoholic and suffered from periodic depressions, problems that could be attributed to this early trauma, but that also may have been due to his inheriting his father's manic–depressive illness.

Some children had strong family support systems and somehow managed to survive the early deaths of their parents without any apparent, lasting detrimental effects on their mental health, creative achievements, or productivity. When Eleanor Roosevelt was 8, her mother, a glamorous society woman, died of diphtheria. Her alcoholic father, who had been separated from his wife, died of a fall 2 years later. Her grandmother, who became her guardian, arranged for her to be tutored and later to go to finishing school in Europe. Eleanor was a gentle and painfully shy child who was not allowed to visit friends. She eventually turned out to be a strong-willed and stubborn person who buried herself in other people's problems.

Herbert Hoover, the 31st President of the United States, came from a lower middle-class, Quaker background. His father, a village blacksmith, died of complications from typhoid fever when Hoover was 6, and his mother died of pneumonia 3 years later. After their deaths, he went to live with his uncle, a country doctor who was interested in education. Hoover attended a Quaker academy that his uncle helped direct, and then went on to receive an engineering degree from Stanford. From all accounts, he never suffered from serious emotional difficulties.

J. R. R. Tolkien, most famous for his trilogy, *Lord of the Rings*, came from a middle-class, literate background. His father, a banker, died of typhoid when Tolkien was 4, and his mother, who was talented in languages and drawing, died of diabetes when he was 12. His legal guardian, a Catholic priest, generally oversaw his care. Tolkien remained outwardly cheerful, even-tempered, and sociable and appeared to show no obvious mental repercussions from the death of his parents.

These selected vignettes illustrate how the early deaths of parents affect children in different ways and show that the common assumption that the loss of a parent at an early age has lasting adverse effects on most youths is fallacious, especially when the context within which the loss occurs is not considered.[8] Such factors as the age at which the loss occurs, the past relationship the child had with its parents, special circumstances surrounding the death, inherited tendencies for depression or alcoholism, the emotional disposition of the child, the availability of caring relatives or guardians and the influences they exert, the adequacy of the financial resources, the available educational and professional opportunities, and hosts of other variables seem to influence how the child will adapt to the loss. This shows that the long-term significance of the loss of a parent, while traumatic at the time, largely has to do with the significance the child attributes to the loss and its subsequent impact on the child's life.

I found no evidence either for the impact of early parental loss on lifetime creative achievement—a relationship that might be expected based on the Phaëthon complex. Correlation values between the period of their mother's or father's death and the extent of their lifetime achievements were essentially zero. Since the same considerations should hold for the effects of early parental loss on later creative achievement as on later mental health, this lack of any significant relationship also makes retrospective sense. Thus, in addition to his borrowed chariot, the complex named after Phaëthon likewise seems destined to go down in flames.

Broken Homes

Another potentially disruptive effect on the lives of youths before the age of 21 has to do with whether their parents separate or get divorced. Among our eminent persons, 88% of their parents stayed married, 4% got divorced, 6% separated, and 2% had other arrangements.[9]

The percentages of those who came from intact homes varied considerably among the different professions. Politicians, artists, natural scientists, social activists, and social scientists (92 to 97%) were most likely to come from intact homes, and musical entertainers, actors, sports figures and poets (71 to 77%) were less likely.[S11] Whether their parents remained married had no bearing on their eventual professional achievements.[S12]

The results, however, revealed that coming from a broken home seemed to have negative effects on the later mental health of the eminent. Those whose parents got divorced or separated had higher rates of alcoholism, drug use, psychoses, and suicide attempts later in life.[S13] Interpretation of these effects is complicated, however, by the finding that both the mothers and the fathers who separated or got divorced also happened to be significantly more emotionally disturbed than those whose marriages remained intact.[S14] This means that the increased rates of certain emotional disorders in eminent persons may have had less to do with their being raised in broken homes than with their being raised by mentally ill parents. Because of the implications of this finding, I examine it in detail later in the book.

Family Size and Birth Order

The eminent men and women in my sample grew up in households with an average of four children. Those with the greatest number of siblings gravitated toward the enterprising and social professions and those with the least number toward the artistic.[S15] Some of the reasons for this become clear when we examine the order of their birth.

Many assume that first-born children are more likely to become eminent. Anecdotal claims about the high proportion of first borns among famous and successful people are impressive.[10] Supposedly, over 50% of U.S. Presidents, 21 of the first 23 astronauts, and many Nobel Prize winners, corporate executives, college professors, and persons listed in *Who's Who in America* and *Men and Women in Science* are first borns.

Careful research studies also have been done on birth order. One large-scale study with 400,000 19-year-old Norwegian males showed a steady decline in intelligence level from the first to the last born, independent of family size and social class. Another study revealed similar results for 800,000 students who took the National Merit Scholarship Qualifying Test. Although they are highly controversial, findings of this sort need to be taken seriously, since they may contribute to the understanding of greatness.

Among the various studies in this area, one of the most imaginative is the report by Frank J. Sulloway on the influence of birth order on supporting innovative ideas in science.[11] Over the course of years, he gathered information on 2,784 scientists who expressed views about 28 different scientific controversies spanning the last 400 years, such as the Darwinian revolution (1859–1870), the Copernican revolution (1543–1609), relativity theory (1905–1911), quantum theory (1905–1911) and spontaneous generation (1800–1859). Birth order best predicted the scientists' opinions about radically innovative theories. Those born later consistently supported scientific theories that possessed liberal or radical leanings, while first borns initially only accepted the most conservative new theories, those that reaffirmed the social, religious, and political status quo. Sulloway explained this tendency by claiming that since first borns were sandwiched between parents and younger siblings, they occupied a unique place within the family constellation and, therefore, were likely to receive special treatment from parents. Often serving as surrogate parents for younger siblings, eldest children were likely to be more respectful toward parents and other authority figures, and therefore more conforming, conscientious, conventional, and religious. In contrast, later borns, who were less likely to identify closely with parents and figures of authority, tended to rebel against the authority of their elder siblings.[12]

There are other theories about why first borns and later borns differ so much.[13] Intrauterine or congenital factors could have an important bearing on the early development of first borns. First borns may be exposed to more trauma and damage during labor and delivery than later borns. Or they may have the advantage of a "richer uterine environment." One could argue that parents are more likely to be too protective and indulgent with first-born children and may interfere with their later self-sufficiency and sense of independence. As the focus of their parents' attention, only children may not merely have a greater opportunity than first and later borns to develop certain skills and conversational abilities; they may also tend toward self-centeredness and assume that the world revolves around them. Oldest children risk "dethronement" when younger siblings are born. They also are expected to assume more adult responsibilities.

Siblings also influence each other. Children with siblings develop different outlooks and aspirations than those without. It may be, as certain authors proposed, that the reason that the birth order of the child in the family influences intellectual levels during the early years is that the first born mainly interacts with mature adults while later borns have greater exposure to the immaturities of their older siblings.[14]

Finally, there are powerful historical and economic factors surrounding the importance of birth order. Primogeniture and lines of succession to the throne or inheritance of family businesses or other practices related to birth order are rooted in social tradition. Often, the status attributed to the first-born male may not only affect the way others treat him but also the way he eventually comes to view himself.

My sample of eminent persons offers an opportunity to clarify four issues of special interest. I address (1) whether, as others claim, first borns (including only children) are overrepresented among eminent persons; (2) whether only children or first borns are more likely than later borns to gravitate toward certain professions; (3) whether birth order affects the susceptibility to mental illness; and (4) whether birth order has any bearing on lifetime creative achievement.[15]

If there were an underrepresentation of first borns in my sample of eminent persons, any further examination of the relationship of birth status to achievement would be superfluous.[16] Among the eminent persons in my study, 14% are only children, 30% first borns, and 56% later borns, with women and men making up roughly the same proportions of each group. Since the selection of these persons, while unbiased, was not random, I could not statistically compare the rates of first borns and later borns to those for the general population, even if this information was available from appropriate census data. This left only one option: an estimate of whether the combination of only children and first borns were overrepresented in comparison to later borns within the sample itself for families of varying size.[17] For example, 100% of children could be expected to be first borns if they were only children, 50% if they came from two-children families, 33% if they came from three-children families, 25% if they came from four-children families, and so on. By comparing the actual frequencies with the expected frequencies of first borns and later borns for families of different size, it was possible to find out if the actual numbers of first borns in the sample were greater than expected by chance.

As it turns out, my analysis showed a definite overrepresentation of first borns among eminent persons,[S16] confirming observations by others about increased representation of first borns in various elite groups. But what does this overrepresentation mean? It may simply mean that the first borns came from smaller families than later borns (i.e., only children have no siblings, first borns average almost three, and later borns almost four) and, given equal resources in these families, first borns (including only children) had access to greater proportions of these resources, including the attention of their parents. This, in turn, may be advantageous for achieving eminence. Or it may mean that first-born status operates in as yet unknown ways.

The various findings show that only children were different in many ways from first borns with siblings, and first borns resembled later borns more than they did only children.[18,19] The most important results that bear on creative achievement, however, were those that turned out to be not statistically significant. Only children, first borns, and later borns did not differ in their social conformity, affiliativeness, avocational creative activities, or antagonism toward their fathers or persons in authority, characteristics that have been attributed to each of these birth-order categories by theorists in the past. This raises doubts about whether the tendencies of first borns and later borns to be original or to support radical views are actually different.

Birth order may have had no obvious effect on attitudes toward authority, but it did seem to have an impact on career choice, but only for males. The male only children were more likely to become actors, nonfiction writers, explorers, and musical performers (mainly the artistic types), while later borns were more likely to become soldiers, public officials, and social activists.[S19] Birth order, interestingly, did not influence the tendency of males to enter professions similar to those of their fathers.

Aside from the matter of career choice, various analyses also revealed that birth order conferred no special advantage in the originality of people's works or the extent of their creative achievements, and that held for men and women alike.

TRAITS, ATTRIBUTES, AND BEHAVIORS

So far we have discovered that the social backgrounds of people, the income levels and educational experiences of their parents, and the degree of social conformity and creative involvement their parents show have a large bearing on their choice of careers. Other factors also can affect career choice; these include health status, social behavior, innate talent, education, and other early life experiences.

Health

Many have suggested a link between physical frailty and the development of creative interests in children. Ill health not only limits a child's options for personal expression but also alters the relationship the child has to parents and peers. Many anecdotal accounts exist about the major role that ill health or physical debility plays during childhood in the later development of eminence. Some claim that genius represents a compensatory response to a childhood disability or deficiency; others claim that the mind flourishes when the body fails.[20] One study, for example, found that 26% of eminent persons were sickly as children but offered no information on whether this rate varied for different professions.[21] Although nothing is known about whether the eminent are more likely than members of the general public to have physical disabilities or suffer from major medical problems during childhood, we can at least establish whether those who entered certain professions were more likely than those who entered others to have more physical problems during their youths.

Among the eminent persons, about 10% had genetic, congenital, or acquired disabilities of one sort or another during their youths,[22] with the rate ranging from 21% in natural scientists and 15% in poets to 0% in sports figures.[S20] How their particular disabilities affected their personalities and career choices is difficult to say, but certain speculations are possible. The ways children react to these handicaps should vary, depending upon such factors as the attitudes of their parents, the resources and opportunities available to them, temperaments, and special talents and abilities. For some, a physical handicap can be psychologically devastating. For others, it may spur them on to success in other areas or cause them to overcompensate in certain ways. Such compensatory responses may have played a role in the careers of many of those with such speech impediments as lisping, stammering, or stuttering (including gifted orators, such as Aneurin Bevin and Winston Churchill and such masters of the English language as Truman Capote, Katherine Mansfield, Somerset Maugham, Delmore Schwartz, Emile Zola, Anatole France, and Thomas Wolfe) and in the careers of some of those with impaired hearing, including Thomas Edison, the inventor of the phonograph.

The ways that children with various visual difficulties, such as crossed eyes, drooped eyelids, blindness, severe nearsightedness, or red–green color-blindness responded to their disability are not always clear. Auguste Rodin's extreme nearsightedness probably contributed to the highly tactile nature of his sculptures. But it is difficult to say how the vision problems of other eminent people, such as Jean-Paul Sartre (inability to use his right eye), Susan B. Anthony (crossed eyes), or Henry Sloane Coffin (hereditary difficulty with one eyelid) affected their outlook and behavior.

Most of the children with developmental handicaps, notably dyslexia or lag in speaking, eventually overcame or compensated for their handicaps. Albert Einstein, who hardly talked as a child, showed no real problems in doing so after the age of 9. Although he suffered from dyslexia,

John Lennon became a superb lyricist and performer. Woodrow Wilson, who probably had dyslexia, went on to become a master of the English language.

About one-third of the handicaps involved congenital or acquired deformities of various kinds, such as severe curvature of the spine, hunched back, polio, or rickets. Jane Addams, for instance, had tuberculosis of the spine, which left her pigeon-toed and caused her to keep her head cocked to one side. F. Tennyson Jesse suffered from severe rickets. V. Khodasevich was born with six fingers on each hand. Ring Lardner had a deformed foot and wore a brace until age 11. Berthold Brecht and Irving Thalberg had congenital heart defects. Allen Dulles had a club foot. Claude Debussy had large bony protuberances on his forehead. Andy Warhol had albino skin. Because of crippling accidents, Toulouse-Lautrec had badly deformed and stunted legs. (See Appendix C for a complete listing of these disabilities.)

Other medical problems also affected these individuals. Unfortunately, since appropriate statistics were not available for the general population at the time I could not determine whether the rates of these problems in children who later become eminent were higher than those of the general population. About 10% had a prolonged period of illness of at least 6 months' duration, such as asthma, tuberculosis, heart condition, incapacitating allergies, a "weak disposition," or some other ill-defined physical problem, usually resulting in their missing school and in being regarding as "sickly." During childhood 8% had a serious, often life-threatening illness or accident. For example, at the age of 5 Tennessee Williams nearly died of diphtheria. His eyesight and kidneys were badly damaged, he could not walk and for 2 years pulled himself about on a small handcar. John Steinbeck developed pneumonia and pleurisy as a teenager, was comatose for days, and was confined to bed throughout the summer. After an emergency appendectomy at the age of 8, Evelyn Waugh could not walk, had to undergo "electric treatment," and was sent to a girl's school to recover. Andy Warhol contracted rheumatic fever and "St. Vitus' dance" at the age of 8. John Reed's severe kidney problems began during childhood. William O. Douglas had infantile paralysis as a child and was not expected to survive. Anton Chekhov developed peritonitis at the ages of 10 and 15. Randolph Bourne's spinal tuberculosis caused him to have a deformed back and stunted his growth. Wilfred Blunt almost died of pneumonia at the age of 9. Frida Kählo had polio. Berthold Brecht was born with a cardiac defect. And Edvard Munch, George Orwell, John Cheever, and Albert Camus suffered from tuberculosis.

How, then, did these various physical problems affect the later career choices and creative achievements of many in my sample? On this matter the findings are reasonably clear. The health status of children definitely had an effect on career choice. Not surprisingly, those who suffered from ill health as children tended to gravitate toward more "cerebral" professions, while those who enjoyed good health as children tended to gravitate toward professions that required physical stamina, robust health, and agility.[S21] Poets, fiction writers, and natural scientists (31 to 38%), for example, were far more likely than explorers, soldiers, musical performers, athletes, and social figures (9 to 11%) to be either handicapped, sickly, or seriously ill as children. As it happens, the results also revealed that the presence of prolonged health problems in youngsters can have salubrious effects on their later creative achievements. I address this issue in more detail later in the book.[23]

Social Behavior

Learned social behavior can influence how people adjust to or are accepted by various professions or social circles. Temperament, interpersonal skills, and personal abilities can place people at a competitive advantage for achieving success in one profession and at a disadvantage in another. For instance, those professions that demand public trust and interpersonal skills are more apt to draw people who are sociable than those who prefer to work alone. Likewise, professions that require social conformity are more apt to draw people who seem normal and stable than those who are moody or odd. These expectations would hardly be surprising if they were found to be true, but they have never been assessed in relation to the lives of eminent persons.

As it happens, what is generally the case turns out to apply to eminent persons as well. Enterprising and social types, such as famous companions, military officers, architects, and public officials (57 to 69%) were more likely than investigative and artistic types, such as social scientists, natural scientists, artists, and fiction writers (19 to 36%), to be sociable as youths. By "sociable," I mean that they got along well with other children, belonged to various clubs, bands, or organizations in school, and participated in other group activities.[S22] Fiction writers, poets, social scientists, and explorers (37 to 40%) were more likely to be moody, irascible, or emotional than public officials, natural scientists, sports figures, musical composers, businesspeople, and military officers (15 to 20%).[S22]

About 5% of the eminent people in my study were described in biographical sources as decidedly "odd," peculiar, weird, offbeat, or eccentric as children, and another 13% of them as equivocally so. Examples of this oddness are plentiful. Jean-Paul Sartre was cantankerous, irascible, and unpleasant toward peers. Many thought him "strange." He had an unconventional manner, often, for example, correcting his language professor with an attitude that flew in the face of the rigid hierarchies of European academic institutions. By the age of 13, Willa Cather cut her hair shorter than most boys, dressed in boy's clothes, and added a "Jr." or "M.D." after her name. As an adolescent, Carl Van Vechten grew one long "talon-like nail" on the little finger of his right hand and dressed unconventionally. The neighbors of Rita Hayworth thought that she could not speak English because she was so shy. Victoria Woodhull had the urge to teach and preach from an early age, gathering neighborhood children around her and crying for them to repent. When they lost interest, she quickly resorted to livid tales about Indian scalpings. Shirley Jackson was a restless and high-strung loner as a child and claimed to be clairvoyant. John Lennon learned to put himself into a trance by staring at his eyes in a mirror for an hour, and from an early age he believed himself to be a "mad genius." By the age of 10, Orson Welles developed a reputation as an oddball by smoking cigars and wearing makeup to appear older. Cecil Beaton dressed elegantly at school and wore makeup to increase his attractiveness. And Truman Capote, who was the class mascot and the butt of jokes, had many affected mannerisms and seemed peculiar to his peers.

Among the various professions, actors, fiction writers, nonfiction writers, and artists (7 to 12%) were more likely than businesspeople, explorers, social figures, or well-known companions (0%) to be thought odd or peculiar.[S22] The finding that the greatest proportion of odd or peculiar youths gravitated toward artistic occupations supports the general observation about the greater tolerance of these occupations for persons who do not act and appear "normal." While these overall rates were low, they nevertheless were statistically significant.

THE EDUCATIONAL PROCESS

Special Abilities

Precocity, or the achievement of advanced levels of mastery in a specific field at a relatively early age, can be critical for success in certain professions. Precocity or giftedness involves the possession of a special ability or talent in music (e.g., perfect pitch, composing skills, finger dexterity), art (e.g., color sense, draftsmanship), mathematics (e.g., computational ability), kinesthetic activities (e.g., physical agility, speed, coordination), language (e.g., photographic memory, an "ear" for dialect), or leadership, usually appearing before the age of 13 and not necessarily associated with general intelligence level. The rates of precocity reported in other large samples of eminent persons have ranged from 5 to 34%,[24] although the criteria used to make these judgments were not given. In my sample of eminent persons, 20% were precocious. The percentage is highest for musical composers (48%), followed next by musical entertainers (40%), physical scientists (31%), and poets (28%).[S23]

Although there are exceptions, the kinds of giftedness eminent people showed as children usually gave them distinct advantages for success in their particular fields. In music, these were perfect pitch, sight reading, the ability to play by ear, an incredible memory for melodies, an innate sense of rhythm, or a remarkable facility at playing an instrument. Gustav Mahler began composing before he mastered the scales on the keyboard, and gave his first concert at age 10. Rachmaninoff played complete pieces of music by ear at the age of 7. Leopold Stokowski conducted his first orchestra at age 12. Claude Debussy entered the Paris Conservatory at age 10. Marc Blitzstein played the piano by ear by the age of 3. John Barbirolli had a reputation as a prodigy cellist by age 12 and was drawn to conducting even earlier. By his mid-teens, Sidney Bechet was a working musician and a notable clarinetist. Bix Beiderbecke was written up as a 7-year-old musical wonder because of his ability to play any selection if he knew its tune, even though he never had taken a music lesson and did not know one key from another. At 5½ years of age, Pablo Casals sang well enough that he joined the church choir as a second soprano and often informed the other singers when they were off key. Glenn Gould displayed perfect pitch when he began piano lessons at the age of 3 and later could sight read and immediately memorize any piece. By the age of 5, Lorenz Hart began composing light verse and was gifted in rhyming.

For those who were to achieve greatness in comedy, singing, dance, or other physical performances, their precociousness usually involved remarkable physical skills, an extrordinary sense of rhythm or grace, exceptional singing ability, or an intangible "stage presence." Jackie Robinson, Babe Ruth, and Hobie Baker showed great physical agility as youngsters. Buster Keaton was the star of a family vaudeville act when he was 4. Charlie Chaplin showed comedic talent at an early age. Judy Garland had a great stage presence and was performing at the age of 2. Enrico Caruso had "a voice like an angel" from a very early age. Marilyn

Miller showed remarkable dance talent at age 4. Fred Astaire danced professionally at the age of 6.

For those who were to become artists, the precocity often showed itself in draftsmanship and an ability to draw from memory. Edward Hopper, Lucien Pissarro, Pierre-Auguste Renoir, Frederic Remington, James Abbott McNeill Whistler, Pablo Picasso, Alberto Giacometti, and others showed superior drawing skills as children.

Those who were to make their mark in fields such as politics, acting, science, philosophy, or writing, which required verbal skills or a broad-based knowledge, usually displayed precocity in the form of photographic memory, a facility for language, or reading at a very young age. With his phenomenal store of information, James Cain was a precocious "whiz kid" by third grade. At the age of 4, Hugo Black was reading fourth-grade readers with ease. Montgomery Clift wrote, produced, and acted in his first play at age 8. Alfred Lunt, Jr. was writing and producing plays at age 8 and received recognition as a performer at the age of 12. Lynn Fontanne was reciting Shakespeare with perfect diction by the age of 5. Cyril Burt began acquiring several languages at a very early age. Adolf Berle was hailed as an intellectual prodigy and entered Harvard at age 14. Leon Blum was quoting the classics by the age of 5. Mikhail Bulgakov wrote his first novel at the age of 7. At the age of 10, Judy Holliday was tested as having an IQ of 172. Carl Jung was reading Latin at the age of 6. Huey Long and Teddy Roosevelt had photographic memories. Rex Stout was reading at 18 months. Amy Semple McPherson could recite full passages from the Bible by the age of 5. J. R. Oppenheimer delivered a scientific paper to the New York Mineralogical Club during his early teens. Alfred Barr had a phenomenal memory. John Middleton Murray was doing quadratic equations and was the author of a treatise on Gothic architecture by the age of 7. Jean-Paul Sartre learned to read by the age of 3 and already was writing novels by the age of 7. Upton Sinclair had a photographic memory, sold a short story by age 14, and began supporting himself by writing by age 15. H. P. Lovecraft had an amazing memory and was reading by the age of 3, writing by the age of 4, and composing his first story by the age of 5 or 6. D'Annunzio could translate the most difficult Latin authors without trouble and memorize lengthy poems before age 10, and published his first collection of poetry to critical acclaim at 16. Edna St. Vincent Millay wrote her first poem at the age of 5, read Shakespeare before the age of 9 and Tennyson and Milton by age 12, had her first poem accepted by a national magazine at age 14, and had won several poetry awards by age 18.

Training

While giftedness is certainly advantageous for success in certain fields, it is not essential, as the vast majority of nonprecocious eminent people in my sample demonstrate. Even when it is present, it does not necessarily lead to great achievement. For their talent to flourish fully, gifted children need appropriate training and encouragement. They also need to be highly motivated to practice and learn.[25]

One of the early indicators of intellectual curiosity and an eagerness to learn is associated with reading. The various biographical sources reveal that 37% of the subjects loved to read in their youths. Not surprisingly, the greatest percentage of avid readers is found among those who were destined to produce books or articles—namely, those who became poets, fiction writers, and nonfiction writers, as well as social scientists and natural scientists (40 to 68%). Those headed toward careers in sports or business were least likely to be avid readers (16 to 19%).[S24]

During their youths, these eminent persons showed a wide range of educational experiences.[26] Only 2% had no formal education, 19% completed grade or elementary school, 24% completed high school, 13% completed technical or special school, 19% completed college, 18% completed graduate school, 2% received another form of education, and information was not available on the remainder. Up through high school or college, the artistic types (12%) were the most likely and the investigative types (3%) the least likely to have difficulties with their teachers.[S25] To some extent, these differences probably reflected the relative disinterest of the artistic types in formal education, as well as their greater degrees of moodiness.

Compared to other types, actors, famous companions, social figures, businesspeople, explorers, and musical entertainers were more likely to have had little formal education; fiction writers were more likely to have only completed high school; musical composers and artists were more likely to have attended special schools, such as music conservatories or art academies; poets, nonfiction writers, and social activists were more likely to have completed college; and natural scientists, public officials, and social scientists were more likely to have completed graduate studies.[S26] The Holland classification revealed that 57% of investigative types completed their graduate studies compared to 27% of social types, 27% of enterprising types, and 10% of artistic types.[S27] Although the average level of education differs significantly among the different professions and, naturally, is higher within those professions in which career advancement requires more education, the results also reveal that a college education is not necessary for eminence. Almost half of all eminent persons only managed to finish high school and about one-fifth only finished grade school or junior high school. This relative lack of emphasis on advanced schooling probably is not as much the case today as it was when these individuals grew up.

Obviously, attending school does not guarantee academic success. For those who went on to high school or college, only 20% consistently received superior grades. Natural scientists (56%) were most likely to receive superior grades, followed in turn by social scientists, public officials, social activists, and military officers (20 to 39%).

Many notable people were among those who performed poorly or below average academically. Errol Flynn frequently skipped school, and was expelled several times for truancy and fighting. Gary Cooper dropped out of high school several times and never managed to complete college. Steven Crane failed out of Syracuse University. John Lennon, perhaps because of his dyslexia, was a poor student and flunked all of his examinations at age 16. Paul Gauguin was a consistently poor student who rarely studied. Anatole France failed his baccalaureate exams several times and finally passed at the advanced age of 20. John Paul Getty received poor marks in high school, and then went on to an unsuccessful stint at a military academy. Leo Tolstoy failed to complete his studies at the University of St. Petersburg. James Jones earned mostly C's and D's in high school. Frank Lloyd Wright received low grades in school and was a recurrent dropout, and went on to do poorly while spending only three terms at the University of Wisconsin. Pablo Picasso had trouble with reading, writing and arithmetic in parochial school. P. G. Wodehouse came in 24th of 25 in the sixth-form classical exams. Henri Matisse failed the entrance exam to the *Ecole des Beaux-Arts* on his first try and only scored a 37 out of 100 on his second try. Eugene O'Neill dropped out of Princeton after 1 year for poor academic standing. George Orwell was a poor student at Eton and required tutorial assistance. Adlai Stevenson was not much of a student at Choate and Princeton, and failed after 2 years at Harvard Law School before eventually graduating from Northwestern in law.

In general, artistic types were most likely to get poor or below average grades.[S28] They also were least apt to win various academic honors or awards.[S29] This shows that success in the creative arts had little to do with academic achievement. A highly significant relationship between educational accomplishments and the extent of professional achievement exists only for those not in the creative arts, especially in fields that require advanced academic degrees.[S30]

Mentors

Mentors can also potentially be an important part of the educational process. The tradition of "mentoring" extends back to antiquity. In many disciplines, esteemed and trusted persons take younger apprentices under their wings, share their wisdom and knowledge with them, offer support and encouragement, and when possible, help them to advance in their careers. Camille Pissarro served as mentor to Cézanne and Gauguin. Louis Sullivan served as mentor and teacher to Frank Lloyd Wright. Bertrand Russell was the student of and, later, collaborator with Alfred North Whitehead. Early, Freud served as a mentor of sorts for Carl Jung and an array of other notable psychoanalysts. On a more general level, almost half of all Nobel laureates in science since 1925 studied under Nobel laureates themselves, indicating a type of selection process that tends to link masters with masters-to-be.[27] One intriguing study which measured intergenerational effects within Western civilization across 15 creative disciplines for 130 generations, showed that generations with very few creators were followed by similarly deficient generations, while generations with many outstanding creators were followed by similarly flourishing generations, suggesting that some sort of mentoring process had been at work.[28]

Among our eminent persons, almost one quarter had identifiable personal mentors of a sort. Perhaps because of educational tradition, investigative types were most likely to have had mentors, followed in turn by social, artistic, and enterprising types.[S31] We also should note that a reliance on mentors not only may have to do with traditional practices within certain fields but also with the attributes of persons in those fields as well. For those individuals who tend to be antagonistic toward authority, or whose work is mainly of a solitary nature, or who are inclined to be loners, the paternalistic nature of the novice–mentor or student–master relationship may not be psychologically acceptable. This may account at least potentially for why poets and fiction writers appear to rely so little on personal mentors.

CAREER CHOICE

It is hard to determine why people gravitate toward different professions. In different societies and at different times in history, people pursued their occupations because of birthright, divine inspiration, a "calling," family circumstances (farm, business), health, physical attributes, geography, socioeconomic factors, religion, gender, race, or necessity. In more recent times, choice has played an increasingly important role. Ideally, this choice involves people finding the right match between their personal abilities, aspirations, and resources, and fields that accommodate them.

When we examine the lives and accomplishments of the eminent people in our sample, the question seldom arises as to whether their career choice or life work constituted a suitable choice. They seem destined for their occupations and roles. Their occupational activities seem to repre-sent natural extensions of their personalities and abilities. Most eminent individuals thus appear to approach their professional roles naturally, with perhaps some digressions or detours along the way. When career shifts occur, they seem to be natural outgrowths of what happened before and of new opportunities that present themselves. There are no sudden revela-tions, epiphanies, or callings or long periods of existential reflection, after which these individuals make radical career changes. But since such impressions are the products of hindsight, even though they may be generally correct, they tend to obscure unique personal experiences that can have profound effects on the career choices of certain people.

Epiphanies and Callings

Sometimes mysterious factors seem to be at work that impel individuals in one direction or another, factors that appear to defy logical or scientific analysis. This is the case with "crystallizing experiences" that not only point individuals in certain career directions but also give them the motivation to pursue their goals.[29] These experiences or "callings" tend to change people's opinions about their domain of interest, their performance in it, and their views of themselves. Only some time later, rather than at the time of the experience, does an individual come to single it out as having crystallized his or her subsequent interests and activities. Some of these experiences occur at a very early age, while others occur later in life. Along the way, individuals may have "refining" experiences that increase their commitment to a particular field. Less than 5% of the eminent persons in my sample had epiphanies of this sort. Because experiences such as these are sometimes invoked to justify a belief in the divine nature of creative achievement or the role of destiny in greatness, I offer a sampling of examples.

Elizabeth Blackwell was moved by her dying friend's plea to devote herself to the care of suffering women by pursuing a career in medicine. The more she thought about that prospect, the more she was drawn to it, even though she was aware of the incredible obstacles she would face in becoming the first woman doctor. One evening, as she stood in the darkness by the window and looked out at the dim mountain outlines in the distance, she was overcome by dread of the future and a terrible doubt about the course she had taken. In despair, she silently cried out to God for guidance. Suddenly, she became aware of a powerful presence that flooded her soul with a brilliant light. All doubt about the future, all hesitation, fell away. She felt that she knew without any question that her course was in harmony with the divine Will. Fortified by this certainty, she felt able to withstand any hardships and endure any potential abuse from those inside and outside the medical profession.

The apocryphal legend about Augustus John claims that as a young man he hit his head on a rock while diving and emerged from the water a genius. Before his accident others regarded him as modestly talented, but afterward as a master draftsman and a superb painter.

Albert Szent-Györgyi decided to become a medical researcher at age 16 after "something" suddenly changed. He believed he had a special gift that would allow him to hear Nature's "voice" and translate that feeling into action.

Joseph Conrad said that he never imagined himself a writer until one day ashore when, for want of something to do, he found himself beginning the novel *Almayer's Folly*. Later, he went on to explain the necessity that impelled him to write was a hidden, obscure necessity, "a completely masked and unaccountable phenomenon. . . . I cannot trace it back to any mental or psychological cause which one could point out and hold to."

At the age of 11, Bertrand Russell began studying Euclid with his older brother as tutor. This turned out to be one of the great events of his life, "as dazzling as first love." He found that he had no difficulty mastering what his brother told him was a difficult proposition. For the first time he realized that he might have some intelligence. From that moment until he and Alfred North Whitehead finished *Principia Mathematica* when Russell was 38, mathematics was his chief source of happiness.

At age 4 or 5, Albert Einstein apparently experienced a "wonder" when his father gave him a simple magnetic pocket compass. This influenced him deeply for the remainder of his life. Einstein later went on to say that during all his years of inquiry, even before he made his discovery, "There was a feeling of direction, of going straight toward something definite."

Mary McCleod Bethune, who founded the first school for Negro girls, claimed that about the time she became concerned with the development of Negro women, she became ill and feverish, and in her delirious state, dreamed she was standing on the brink of the St. Johns River and had to cross over. No bridge or boat was in sight. As she puzzled over what to do, someone appeared and told her to look behind her. When she looked back, she saw a large army of young people coming after her. The man handed her a notebook and pencil and said, "All must pay to cross over. You are going to cross this river but, before you go, you must write down the names of all the young people you see in the distance." Shortly after she awakened, her pastor visited. She revealed her dream and asked him what it meant. He said, "You will build a great school and many thousands of young people will pass through your hand. Many years will be spared to lead you to them." Her pastor's interpretation was eventually proved true.

Dorothy Eady offers perhaps the most dramatic example of this kind of experience. When she was 3 years old, she fell down a flight of stairs, was knocked unconscious, and was mistakenly pronounced dead by a doctor. Soon after her accident, she began having recurring dreams of a huge building with columns and a garden filled with flowers and fruits. On awakening, she often would cry out, "I want to go home," but was unable to tell where that was. When she was 4, her parents took her to a museum, and when they came to the Egyptian exhibit, she broke free and began running crazily through the rooms, kissing the feet of all the statues, and later announcing to her parents, "Leave me . . . these are my people." When she was 7, she was thumbing through one of her father's magazines and suddenly became transfixed by a photograph of *The Temple of Sety the First at Abydos, Upper Egypt*, recognizing it as the building in her recurrent dreams and believing that she had once lived there in a previous incarnation. As she got older, she became more and more convinced that she had been an Egyptian princess over 3,000 years ago. Finally, at age 29, she abandoned her middle-class English background to marry an Egyptian and direct the search for the gardens connected to the Temple of Sety. She supposedly showed an uncanny ability to pinpoint where the excavators would find a line of tree roots. She finally settled in Egypt to become the Keeper of the Temple, a revered local figure, and an internationally recognized expert on hieroglyphics.

Many other examples exist. A religious experience inspired Malcolm X to proselytize. At age 17, after being out of school for 2 years due to illness, Robert Goddard, while in a tree, had a "fantasy" in which he saw a mechanical device whirling faster and faster into space. At that moment, his existence seemed purposeful and he rededicated himself to pursuing a career in science. While standing on a mountain top and watching the thunder clouds roll overhead, Dorothea Lange claimed to have had a mystical experience that convinced her to devote herself to photography. Paul Tillich, who went on to become a renowned theologian, claimed that his traditional conception of God collapsed and a completely new understanding arose one night in 1915 after witnessing the horrors of war.

My reason for describing these dramatic but relatively uncommon experiences is not to demonstrate the irrational sources for occupational choice or the spiritual basis for creative achievement. What these experiences illustrate is the reason for the zeal, conviction, and sense of destiny that many eminent people manifest in the pursuit of their goals. This zeal is not, however, any less evident in those who do not have epiphanies or crystallizing experiences. In their cases, we have to seek reasons for their professional fervor and unbounded confidence in more natural causes.

Age of First Notable Professional Accomplishment

Past research shows that the earlier individuals become productive in their careers, whether it is in mathematics, the investigative sciences, philosophy, classical music, the humanities, or the arts, the more contributions they make over the course of their lives. There is evidence that the peak productive age occurs at about 40 years, with the number of major scientists and creators rapidly rising to this peak from their mid-20s and then descending from it more slowly afterward, so that persons 40 years of age or younger produce about half of all contributions. One study, for example, found that the peak period at which 696 classical composers produced the most frequently heard melodies was from 33 to 43 years of age. The timing of this peak period, naturally, varies considerably among professions.[30]

Among the various professions, two to four times the percentage of artistic types (19%)—especially musical entertainers, actors, and musical composers—as compared to other types (4 to 9%) were likely to have had their first professional success before the age of 21.[S32] These early successes comprise publishing their first story or book, giving their first professional concert or theatrical performance, gaining their first elected office, winning their first professional competition, presenting their first scientific paper, giving their first public speech, achieving their first major business success, patenting their first invention, making their first discovery, having their first gallery exhibition, or designing their first building. The average ages at which artistic, social, investigative, and enterprising types achieved these initial successes were 24, 29, 30, and 31 years, respectively.[S33] Women as a group made their first professional accomplishments about 1 year later than men (28 versus 27 years old).

Examples of those who achieved early success are plentiful. Rita Hayworth danced professionally at age 12, was on screen at age 16, and acted in her first major film at age 20. At age 19, Langston Hughes published an essay, "The Negro Speaks of Rivers," in the *Literary Digest*. Both John McGraw and Babe Ruth signed professional baseball contracts before they were 19. At age 18, Nijinsky had his first major ballet success. Edith Piaf began performing professionally at age 15. At 14, Pablo Picasso painted the "Barefoot Girl" and "Beggar." By the age of 17, Sergei Prokofiev wrote his first symphony and piano pieces and made his first public debut. Sergei Rachmaninoff composed his famous *Prelude in C Sharp Minor* at the age of 20. Queen Victoria began her 63-year reign at 18. At the age of 19, Darryl Zanuck sold a story to Fox Film Company and a screenplay to Universal, and at age 20 began working as a gag writer for Charlie Chaplin.

What these assorted results suggest is that people are more likely to achieve early success in those professions that do not require any formal training or approval by professional credentialing boards: professions, such as the creative arts or sports, in which precocity, exceptional skill, and talent are so essential. They are less likely to do so in those professions, such as the natural or social sciences, jurisprudence, or politics, that require more experience or extensive, formal training to acquire knowledge and to perfect personal skills.

These, then, are some of the important factors operating on eminent persons during childhood, adolescence, and early adulthood. What seems clear so far is that individuals within the different professions already differ as youths in many important ways, and that these differences tend to be consistent and persistent. As suggested by the developmental theory of eminence, a powerful "organizing principle" appears to be at work, which not only shapes the environments in which these youths operate but also continues to shape them. Even before they enter the artistic, enterprising, investigative, and social professions, they appear to be developing into distinctly different types. What we have yet to establish is whether or not this differentiation continues into the later lives of these people and in what ways, if any, their careers further mold them.

CHAPTER FOUR

The Adult Years

I n his book, *Creating Minds*, Howard Gardner[1] analyzed the lives of seven extraordinary individuals, each selected to represent a different form of intelligence. The creative genius of Sigmund Freud supposedly lay in his linguistic and personal skills; of Albert Einstein, in his logical–spatial abilities; of Pablo Picasso, in his spatial, personal, and bodily sense; of Igor Stravinsky, in his musical and artistic abilities; of T. S. Eliot, in his linguistic and academic skills; of Martha Graham, in her bodily and linguistic abilities; and of Mahatma Gandhi, in his personal and linguistic skills. Despite these differences, the theme of social marginality pervaded their work. Einstein and Freud were Jews in antisemitic, German-speaking countries; Graham competed in a male-dominated field; Gandhi took on the British empire; and Stravinsky, Eliot, and Picasso produced many of their major works in countries not their own. Aside from their social marginality, all showed socially undesireable personality traits. Gardner claimed that these seven persons behaved like most creative geniuses, pursuing their own goals with a self-centered single-mindedness, displaying little regard for the approval or disapproval of others, and no reservations in promoting their own work. In the process, they used others to advance their professional work, dropping them once their usefulness was over. "The carnage around a great creator is not a pretty sight," Gardner concluded, "and this destructiveness occurs whether the individual is engaged in a solitary pursuit or ostensibly working for the betterment of humankind."

Although Gardner's opinions merit attention, they cannot substitute for scientific fact. Generalizations of this sort from so small and select a sample are risky since they indict all creative geniuses on the basis of a few, and because of the lack of a suitable control group, seriously misrepresent the situation. It is possible, for example, that the personal characteristics ascribed to these seven creative geniuses apply equally well to most ambitious people, even if they are not especially gifted.

Other stereotypes of eminent people are common. As children, creative scientists supposedly come from stable homes, enjoy school, experience poor health, read voraciously, be shy, and admire their fathers; as adults, they supposedly are independent, aesthetic, energetic, introverted, stable, self-sufficient, solitary, nonconformist, innovative, indifferent to religion, distant toward their parents, and more strongly committed to their work than to social and sexual activities.[2] Creative architects supposedly are open to new experiences, nonconformist, innovative, independent, aesthetic, energetic, and strongly committed to their work.[3] Creative writers are said to be independent, imaginative, aesthetic, and, along with artists, skeptical, unconventional, extroverted, and self-sufficient. Although they tend to be psychologically troubled, they have the psychological resources for dealing with their troubles.[4] As separate characteristics of people in specific fields these are intriguing claims, but when considered together, they lose their descriptive value. The characterizations of these different professional groups begin to sound alike, suggesting that they are less distinctive of particular professions than of successful or creative persons. To date, however, no studies have confirmed this to be so.

What can we say with relative certainty about the attributes of eminent people that might contribute to their specialness and distinguish one professional group from another? From the vast and often confusing literature, there are only several general observations about which most experts agree. While eminent persons are highly intelligent, beyond having I.Q.'s of over 120, no relationship exists between their actual intelligence level and the extent of their creativity.[5] Persons with high (but not the highest) intelligence who are very persistent will more likely achieve eminence than those with the highest degree of intelligence who are less persistent.[6] "Creators" differ from "leaders," and within the group of creators, scientists show attributes different from those of literary persons.[7] Needless to say, indications of future eminence are much easier to figure out retrospectively than to predict in advance.[8] These are important observations, but they tell us little about any personal characteristics that can distinguish members of a particular profession from those of another.

If we can put aside for the moment the distorting influence of social prejudice on career choice, we may assume that two complementary processes shape the kinds of personal attributes found in persons in different professions: (1) professions tend to be accommodating to or selective for personal traits in individuals which either aid or, at worst, do not interfere with their successful performance; and (2) most individuals, if they have the opportunity to do so, tend to be drawn to those professions in which they can best display their natural gifts and that appreciate or, at worst, do not penalize them for their personal characteristics. This assumption has certain implications. Those professions in which success depends largely upon interpersonal skills, personal influence, or public trust should be more accommodating of persons who are emotionally stable, sociable, affiliative, conventional, and "normal" than of those who are moody, solitary, and nonconformist. Those professions in which success depends upon making discoveries, instituting social change, challenging tradition, or extending intellectual frontiers should be more accommodating of persons who are irreverent, antagonistic toward established authority, moody, and eccentric than those who are socially conforming, conventional, and respectful of authority. Or from the perspective of the individual, those persons who are emotionally unstable, confrontational, unconventional, or nonaffiliative should find the creative arts more accommodating than other professions, such as public office or the military, which require public accountability and social acceptance. Those persons who are adventuresome, physically healthy, and willing to risk their lives should find certain professions, such as social activism, sports, exploration, or the military, more accommodating than the natural or social sciences, which rely largely on intellectual perseverance. These are some of the expectations. We now need to determine if they are true.

SOCIAL BEHAVIOR

Friends and Colleagues

It is truly a small world as far as eminent people are concerned. As the saying goes, birds of a feather flock together. It is astounding how many great people manage somehow to find one another. A powerful clustering tendency seems to be at work in all fields, which brings talented people together, not only after they are famous but often long before. Future Nobel laureates manage to train under Nobel laureates themselves. Struggling young writers, poets, musicians, and artists who eventually will succeed manage to meet in cafés, pubs, conservatories, or art academies. When famous, they continue their relations or gravitate toward other famous people, form friendships, share ideas and work, and correspond. Their gatherings represent "invisible colleges" in which they learn and share their views.

In the 1950s and turbulent 1960s, Jack Kerouac, Allen Ginsberg, and William Burroughs, among others, were part of the Beat movement, championing pacifism, reverence for nature, and the enhancement of personal consciousness. Known as the "Fugitives" because of their contributions to a magazine by that name, John Crowe Ransom, Robert Penn Warren, Allen Tate, and others became an influential group in American literature after World War I. By the 1920s, Langston Hughes, Jean Toomer, Richard Wright, and Zora Neale Hurston were all part of the Harlem Renaissance, which was a flowering of black culture. In the early 1900s, the English and American poets, Amy Lowell, Richard Aldington, and William Carlos Williams, joined Ezra Pound and T. E. Hulme and called themselves the Imagistes. Ezra Pound also discovered and helped launch the careers of Robert Frost, James Joyce, and T. S. Eliot.

In the late 19th Century, a group of French painters managed to coalesce—Pissarro, Degas, Manet, Cézanne, Monet, Renoir, and Alfred Sisley—and launch the impressionist movement. Delighting in witty repartèes, insults, and *bon mots*, celebrities such as Alexander Woollcott, Harpo Marx, Dorothy Parker, George S. Kaufman, Robert Sherwood, and Robert Benchley met regularly for lunch at the Algonquin Hotel in New York. Among the group of creative Hollywood writers and artists who were subpoenaed to appear before the House Committee on Un-American Activities were Dalton Trumbo, Ring Lardner, Jr., and an array of other notables. Known as "The Eight," Robert Henri and John Sloan were among a group of realistic painters in New York City in the late 19th and early 20th centuries. Others derisively referred to this group as the "ashcan school" because of its use of garbage cans and backyards as motifs for its paintings. In the early 1900s Virginia Woolf and her artist sister, Vanessa Bell, their husbands, the author Leonard Woolf and the art critic Clive Bell, along with the economist John Maynard Keynes, E. M. Forster, Lytton Strachey, Roger Fry, and Duncan Grant first assembled informally on Thursday evenings near London in Bloomsbury, and appropriately became known as the Bloomsbury group. Numerous other famous people met in bistroes and cafès on the Left Bank of the Seine to discuss philosophy, politics, and art or gathered on Saturday nights at Gertrude Stein's salon in Paris.

What do these clusterings tell us about these eminent people? Even though most of them are independent, self-sufficient, and used to working alone, they appear to have a great need to associate with others of their kind—people of comparable talent and intellect whose work and opinions they respect. Through contact with these people, they sharpen their wits, try out their ideas, display their works, and try to validate their own greatness. They seem to need these people as colleagues and friends, at least until they become well established in their fields and develop other personal agendas.

Social Acceptability

Those who work closely with others have less latitude to be moody than those who mainly work alone. As already noted, the roots of the behavior of eminent people extend back to their childhood. Among members of the various professions, poets, fiction writers, artists, musical composers, and musical entertainers (48 to 59%)[S1]—largely the artistic types—continue to be more likely than soldiers, politicians, and social scientists (22 to 24%) to be "moody," volatile, irascible, or highly temperamental.[S1] People who are accountable to the public are also more likely to show socially approved behavior than those who are not. Greater percentages of people in the social (61%) and enterprising (59%) professions tend to be gregarious, friendly, and sociable than those in the investigative (39%) and artistic (45%) professions.[9] Affiliative behavior also reflects sociability. Social activists, public officials, social scientists, and architects, in particular, are more likely than actors, musical entertainers, artists, poets, and explorers (mainly, the artistic types) to belong to and participate actively in various professional, civic, religious, social, and other organizations.[S1] The fact that all of these social behaviors have roots in childhood suggests that they are not a reflection of vocational expectations alone.

The case of Hugo La Fayette Black serves to illustrate this kind of sociability, which, although it helped him in his career, almost ruined it for him as well. Raised in a strict religious household, Black excelled in school and went on to become a lawyer and then a Senator, before being appointed by President F. D. Roosevelt to the United States Supreme Court. Being very affiliative, he belonged to the Baptist church, Masons, Newspaper Club, Odd Fellows, Pretorians, Knights of Pythius, Birmingham Country Club, American Legion, and assorted other groups. However, when word leaked out after his appointment to the Court that he also was once a member of the Ku Klux Klan, people began clamoring for his resignation. He managed to weather this storm and, surprising many, went on to become a great liberal Supreme Court Justice, laying the foundations for many landmark civil rights decisions, such as Brown versus the Board of Education.

Social Conformity versus "Differentness"

As a military man and politician, Dwight D. Eisenhower exemplifies the general social conformity and certain of the other social behaviors found in the enterprising types. His origins were humble. Neither of his parents were especially creative. His mother was an intelligent, outgoing woman and his father a strict disciplinarian who ran a failing business. An average student at West Point, Eisenhower was sociable, friendly and well-liked. He showed little interest in art, music, or literature but was very involved in sports and the outdoors, patterns that, in this study, tend to be more associated with enterprising types. Enterprising types, for example, are over twice as likely as artistic types to display great interest in athletic activities, and they are less likely than artistic and social types to have creative hobbies or interests.[51] With this background, it is not surprising that Eisenhower respected authority, including that of his parents, that he always followed orders, even when he disagreed with them, and that he was very socially conforming. This conformity probably accounted for his attitude as President of Columbia University that exceptional scholars held little value if they were not first exceptional Americans, an attitude which greatly embarrassed his faculty.

Identifying social nonconformity is a bit more complicated. Since the boundaries between social nonconformity and eccentricity are often blurred, I decided to use the more embracing idea of "differentness" to capture the commonality of both. Eccentricity denotes the extent to which people display oddities, peculiarities, idiosyncrasies, or otherwise unusual behavior that deviates from the norm; it may be innate, learned, or deliberately cultivated.[10] Whether it is the result of predisposition, design, or principle, nonconformity indicates a deviation from mainstream social views, the adoption of unconventional positions or the rejection of traditional codes of dress, beliefs, or public behavior. Sometimes it is difficult to distinguish these behaviors from social obtuseness. What others sometimes forgive in celebrities or well-known persons as eccentricities or nonconformity, they may interpret in others as outspokenness, tactlessness, crassness, rudeness, impulsiveness, inconsiderateness, or crudity. Since many eminent persons display such behavior at some point in their lives, we shall reserve the term "different" only for those who behave eccentrically, quirkily, or unconventionally almost as a way of life or a characteristic mode of response.

Andy Warhol serves as a prototype for this attribute of differentness, as well as for many other features of artistic types. Coming from an uneducated, working-class family, Warhol's early exposure to art came from his mother who, perhaps inspiring his later work, painted designs on utensils and flowers on cans. When he was 8 years old, Andy developed rheumatic fever and St. Vitus dance. His mother reacted to his illness by becoming overprotective and giving him enemas to keep him healthy. Sometimes when they were together, he and she would draw for hours. As a youth, he was shy, effeminate, and "odd," with his long white hair and slight figure. In high school, although he excelled in art classes, he was otherwise an unexceptional student, and did not belong to any clubs or participate in sports. As an adult, he was moody and yet gregarious, and loved to put on outrageous and fashionable parties. Although he already had gained serious attention as an artist from his serial images, his notoriety exploded after an assassination attempt by a deranged woman actress. Exulting in his fame, he played up his nonconformity, dressing shockingly and being open about his homosexuality. To accentuate his appearance, he initially wore a silver blond wig, changed the way he spoke, at times mumbling incoherently, and exaggerated his effeminate, dancer's walk. Later, he began wearing dark glasses, tight black jeans over panty hose, and high-heeled boots. As some observed, his greatest invention appeared to be himself.

Among our eminent individuals, 28% showed "differentness" of this sort as a characteristic mode of response or way of life. Artists, musical performers, social activists, poets, and fiction writers (34 to 49%) were more likely than soldiers, public officials, composers, and natural scientists (9 to 18%) to be different.[51] Many of these people were the same ones who, as children, acted odd or weird.

Because this "differentness" appears to be so bound up with the creative arts (although not exclusively so), we may wonder about its relationship to the creative process, about how much thumbing one's nose at social convention may be a central aspect of challenging established tradition. Surprisingly enough, as statistical analyses show, such behavior turns out to bear no relationship to originality, productivity, or lifetime creative achievement. I examine this relationship more closely later. I merely document here some of the forms this differentness takes.

W. H. Auden showed little regard for others. At dinner parties and gatherings, he often not only wore dirty, outlandish, or baggy clothes but also would wolf down his food, put his cigars out where he pleased, or play the piano in the face of others' objections. James Gordon Bennett, Jr., famous for his eccentricities, once rode through Paris with a donkey beside him. A sign around the donkey's neck proclaimed that it was the only intelligent American in Paris. He also raced carriages through the streets, urinated in the parlor at his pre-wedding party, and claimed to worship owls. Harry Crosby wore black fingernail polish, had crosses tattooed on the bottom of his feet, and enjoyed dropping water bombs from hotel balconies onto passers-by. Glenn Gould wore scarves, mufflers, and gloves even on hot days, and hated to be touched by anyone except a masseuse. Charles Laughton dressed in untidy clothes, neglected his personal hygiene, seldom looked anyone in the eye, and often stood or laid down in front of a painting for hours. Leo Tolstoy tried to give up his property in later life, became a vegetarian, knitted his own clothes, and espoused revolutionary ideas attacking both the church and the military. Isadore Duncan wore a tunic and sandals all the time as street clothes and showed a defiant rebelliousness, insisting on making pro-Communist speeches in the United States even after she was warned that she would be forbidden to give performances again. Theodore Roethke insisted on sleeping with numerous blankets no matter what the weather, so that at night he perspired profusely and had to change pajamas several times. As a result, it was not unusual for him to put 20 pairs of pajamas in his laundry by the end of the week.

Often, this unconventional and sometimes outrageous behavior was clearly meant to shock. In one trial, Lenny Bruce not only refused to take the oath when placed on the witness stand but, when defending himself, asked prospective jurors, "Do you ever masturbate?" Tallulah Bankhead, who supposedly had over 5,000 lovers, walked around naked at parties regularly and often carried on conversations while sitting on the toilet. William March, who always dressed conservatively in expensive clothes and appeared to be the epitome of the Southern gentleman, delighted in embarrassing and shocking people by detailing in his most exaggerated Southern accent his Freudian analyses of their behavior or asking questions like, "Have you ever made love to a corpse?" Dorothy Parker, known for her mordant wit, went to theaters unchaperoned, smoked in public, took irreverent positions on most issues, and supposedly had sex once in public. Janis Joplin flouted convention with her provocative advocacy of sexual freedom and drugs. Frida Kählo dressed in flamboyant, mostly Mexican outfits and delighted in making embarrassing sexual remarks in public and at social gatherings. Jim Morrison espoused chaos and disorder, and in many ways was the ultimate nonconformist generally gravitating toward the seamier side of life. He wore the same pair of leather pants until they reeked and at the height of his popularity stayed at a $10-per-night motel. Sylvia Ashton-Warner often behaved outrageously, once inviting a minister to her house and greeting him with every expletive she knew. On another occasion she placed her feet on the table in such a position that her male guest could see up her dress and asked him what he thought of legalized prostitution. She also supposedly danced nude in her yard, and sometimes invited people for dinner and served nothing at all.

RELATIONSHIPS TO ESTABLISHED AUTHORITY

To a large extent, we should expect that people who do not conform to social standards will not tolerate well the opinions of those in positions of authority that differ from their own. This tendency for individuals to chafe under the constraints of established authority should be more marked in those professions that rely on novelty, innovation, and discovery than in those in which the perpetuation of tradition is important. As indirect measures of this tendency, we can examine how individuals within the different professions respond to different forms of established authority. These forms involve their relationships with their personal gods, their relationships with their parents, their relationships with superiors or employers, and their relationships with society and the law. We may assume that those who are more socially marginal should be more rebellious in all of these areas.

As an archetypal rebel, Augustus John demonstrated these tendencies well. His mother had a talent for art and played the piano and his father, a successful solicitor, composed organ music and enjoyed photography, so that Augustus learned to appreciate art at an early age. In time he came to despise his proper, conformist, solidly middle-class background. He was a moody, mutinous student in grade school and left high school at age 16 after a bad incident with a teacher. In art school, he met and married a fellow student, who bore four children and died giving birth to the fifth. His marriage did not, however, prevent him from having numerous mistresses and affairs and producing at least five illegitimate children. Even with his tendency for melancholia and fondness for drink, John was always a very prolific painter. He became a living legend for many, although this was perhaps less due to his avant-garde art than for his outlandish dress and imposing presence. John did in fact make an art out of his nonconformity, carefully keeping his shoes unpolished, wearing secondhand gold earrings and a black silk scarf with a silver brooch, sporting a hat with a gypsy design, neglecting to shave, and punctuating this striking look with unpredictable comments. He became a symbol of social rebellion through his irreligious views, lack of mentors, hatred for patron–artist dealings, and automatic antagonism toward anyone in a fatherly or authoritarian role. Despite his renown, he seemed to have a problem with his identity, claiming, "I have no character. . . . I am just a legend. I'm not a real person."

Religious Beliefs and Practices

As with Augustus John, we may assume that the religious beliefs of people reflect the extent to which they seek social support for their views. In countries in which the vast majority of people attend church or espouse religious beliefs, those who are atheists or agnostics risk social censure. Because of this, we should anticipate that the professions with higher percentages of irreligious persons should be those that tolerate nonconformity, that favor scientific proof over accepted belief, and that foster solitary activity. In contrast, those professions with higher percentages of religious persons should be those that emphasize conformity, encourage traditional beliefs, and foster group activity. Surprisingly, other than some indication that eminent scientists tend to be irreligious,[11] little information has previously been systematically gathered about the religious views of eminent persons within the different professions.

Among the eminent individuals in my sample, 8% are atheists, 21% are agnostics, 11% hold unconventional religious beliefs such as Swedenborgianism, transcendentalism, Tolstoyism, occultism, or their own spiritual views, 25% are believers who do not attend church, 7% attend church irregularly and 28% attend church regularly. These percentages reveal a higher percentage of nonbelievers among the eminent than among those in a recent survey on over 4,000 Americans, in which only 8% described themselves as atheists or agnostics.[12] Among the various professions, musical composition, art, the social sciences, and the natural sciences include the highest percentage of atheists (11 to 15%). Nonfiction, art, fiction, and the natural sciences include the highest percentage of agnostics (25 to 38%). Poetry, the natural sciences, and fiction contain the highest percentages of individuals with idiosyncratic beliefs (17 to 22%). And public office, the military, social figures, and social activism have the greatest percentages of persons who attend church regularly (42 to 60%). The Holland classification of occupations clarifies this situation. Among the four professional types, the investigative types (12%) are about three times as likely as the enterprising types (4%) to hold atheistic beliefs; artistic types (25%) and investigative types (20%) are more likely than the other types (15%) to hold agnostic beliefs; investigative types (17%) and artistic types (14%) are more than two to three times as likely as enterpris-ing (5%) or social types (5%) to hold idiosyncratic beliefs; and enterprising types (45%) and social types (43%) are over twice as likely as artistic types (19%) and investigative types (17%) to attend church regularly. The four occupational types are comparable in their rates of not going to church and irregular church attendance.[S2]

Relationships with Authority Figures

Besides the church, there are other important forms of established author-ity to which individuals are exposed. From birth on, most persons have to deal with parental authority and, if they have to work for others, with supervisors and employers. For some such as Dwight Eisenhower, who respected his parents and cherished his service under Douglas MacArthur, these relationships are gratifying and rewarding; for others such as Augus-tus John, who despised his father, fought with his teachers, and resented all forms of authority, they are difficult and rankling. Although responses of this nature tend to be highly individualized, certain kinds of responses seem more likely to be associated with certain occupational types.

   The results, in brief, reveal that during their adult years, about twice as many artistic types (24%) as other types have distant, antagonistic relationships with their mothers, and that almost twice as many inves-tigative types (25%) and artistic types (30%)—especially fiction writers, poets, musical entertainers, and actors—as enterprising types (17%) or social types (12%) remain antagonistic toward their fathers.[S3] Although it is more difficult to determine the quality of their relationships with supervisors, employers, superiors, or other authority figures during their adult lives, it is possible to identify characteristic patterns of response toward nonparental figures whose decisions can have harmful or benefi-cial effects on their careers. Of the 590 individuals on whom this information was available, 6% percent maintain close relationships, 67% have unremarkable relationships, and 27% are antagonistic toward peo-ple with potential authority over them. Enterprising types (15%)—mainly military officers and businesspeople—are less likely to have antagonistic relationships, while social types and artistic types (31 to 36%)—mainly social activists, artists, sports figures, actors, and fiction writers—are more likely to have them.[S3]

   In general, all these findings are consistent with expectations. Artistic types, with their tendencies to be temperamental and nonconforming, are more likely than enterprising types, with their tendencies to be sociable and conforming, to have frictions with authority figures, including their parents. Within the social types, social activists in particular are more likely than enterprising and investigative types to come into conflict with people in authority. Investigative types, although they are often alienated from their fathers, are less apt than artistic or social types to have difficulties with their superiors or employers, perhaps because of their even temperaments or because of the necessity to get along with authority figures in order to advance in their careers.

Encounters with the Law

Besides religious, parental and work-related forms of authority, many of those in my sample had encounters with social and legal forms of authority as well. A certain number of legal difficulties people have may be related to the very nature of their professions, but they may also bring some of these difficulties upon themselves. Businesspeople, directors and actors, and architects, who rely heavily on contract negotiations, may be expected to sue or to be sued simply as a matter of course. Others such as social activists, who directly challenge the law, may show a greater likelihood of being prosecuted, imprisoned, or even killed in more repressive regimes. There are others who, because of their litigious or provocative natures, may be more inclined to initiate or invite law suits. The eminent persons in the sample confirmed these expectations.

About 15% of eminent persons were defendants and 7% were plaintiffs in a major civil suit. Statistics are not available on how these rates compare to those for the public at large. As a group, businesspeople are most likely to sue and be sued.[53] Of a more serious legal nature, 10% of the entire sample went to jail or received suspended sentences or had to pay fines for civil or criminal matters. The greatest percentages of individuals affected were sports figures, musical entertainers, social activists, and members of the theater community (16 to 37%).[53] Some examples illustrate these legal problems.

Ty Cobb was arrested on a couple of occasions on assault and battery charges, and in 1912 was suspended from baseball for attacking a fan. Hart Crane was arrested once on assault and battery charges and later for sexual relations with a minor. Jack London was arrested for vagrancy and brawling in a bar. Malcolm X was arrested for larceny in Michigan and burglary in Massachusetts. Edvard Munch was arrested for fighting in a café. Enrico Caruso was convicted of molesting a woman. Bill Tilden, the tennis star, was arrested at least twice for sexual transactions with a minor. Joseph

Pulitzer was arraigned on a charge of assault with intent to kill. Alan Turing was convicted of "homosexual offenses" and "treated" with female hormones. Truman Capote was convicted for drunk driving on at least two occasions and received a contempt of court citation for ignoring a subpoena. Jim Morrison was arrested for petty larceny as a student and, in 1969 alone, had 29 paternity suits filed against him. Lenny Bruce was arrested several times on obscenity and drug charges. Charlie Parker was arrested once for nicking a cab driver with a knife and another time for nonpayment of child support. Ben Reitman was arrested for vagrancy over 40 times in the United States and other countries. During Prohibition, Barney Oldfield was put in jail so often for various offenses that Harvey Firestone had a man on duty at the police station each Saturday evening whose sole job it was to bail out Oldfield before the press arrived. And Sam Spiegel, the movie producer, received a 9-month sentence for passing a bad check and was deported to Poland, was arrested again for passing bad checks in London and Los Angeles, was arrested once again in Mexico for embezzlement, and then was arrested again for being an illegal alien.

There are other kinds of serious legal difficulties or personal dangers people are exposed to or sometimes even court by virtue of the nature of their work. Such is often the case for those who challenge social tradition, try to overthrow existing governments, or seek to expand individual rights. Emma Goldman serves as a prototype for this kind of social activist. As a child, her rebelliousness, by her own account, caused her religious teacher to tell the class that she was a terrible child who would grow into a worse woman, that she had no respect for her elders or for authority, and that she would end in the gallows. Feeling rejected by her father, she married at age 17 in order to leave home and then left her marriage at age 20 to embark on her activist career. After the Haymarket Square executions, she had an epiphany that convinced her of the evils of government and the necessity for anarchy. She then went on to organize the first International Anarchist Congress and devoted herself to various radical causes. A compelling and tireless speaker, she lectured over 300 times in 1 year alone on topics ranging from birth control to family planning and free love. Because of her views and activities, she served many jail sentences, once for inciting a riot, once for anticonscription work, and once for supposedly inspiring a young man to attempt to assassinate President McKinley. Eventually, the U.S. government deported her to the Soviet Union as an undesirable alien. None of her arrests nor her eventual deportation were completely unexpected, since such harassment by governmental authorities went with the activist life.

In my sample of eminent persons, 10% were either persecuted, excommunicated, jailed, or exiled because of political or social actions during some point in their lives. Social activists (46%) were almost twice as likely as poets (21%) and three times as likely as social scientists (14%), the next two highest groups, to be punished for such "crimes," some of which were due to the temper of the times: the fight for civil rights, the actions of the House Un-American Activities Committee, and other social causes.[53] Margaret Sanger was arrested for picketing on behalf of birth control. Carrie Nation was arrested often for assault and destruction of property while waging her campaign against drinking. Dashiell Hammett, Lillian Hellman, and Dalton Trumbo were harassed by the House Un-American Activities Committee during the McCarthy era. After World War II Ezra Pound was charged with treason, propaganda, and aiding and abetting an enemy. Upton Sinclair was arrested for illegal picketing with coal miners. Bertrand Russell was convicted in 1915 for writing a leaflet against conscription, and was imprisoned for 2 months for inciting the public to civil disobedience when he advocated nuclear disarmament in 1960. Dietrich Boenhoffer was arrested by the Gestapo and eventually hanged for his involvement in an attempt to kill Hitler. Samuel Gompers was arrested often for organizing strikes and various labor-related activities. And Martin Luther King, Jr., was arrested often on charges stemming from his civil rights work.

INTIMATE RELATIONSHIPS

Sexual Orientation

Before this study, little systematic information was available about the relationship between the sexual orientations and the career choices of eminent persons. The results show that there definitely is one.

For the purposes of classification, those individuals are termed heterosexual who confined their sexual relationships exclusively to members of the opposite sex (or at least for whom there was no evidence to the contrary). Those individuals are considered homosexual who confined their sexual relationships exclusively to members of the same sex (or at least for whom there was no evidence to the contrary). Bisexual individuals had relationships with persons of both the same and opposite sex (despite whatever preferences they may have had). Hyposexual individuals were sexually abstinent or ascetic, giving few signs of having had romantic or sexual involvements with members of the opposite sex or having so rare or infrequent encounters that these played insignificant roles in their lives. The cause for this low level of sexual interest or involvement is unclear. It could reflect disinterest in, aversion toward, or inhibitions about sex, suppressed homosexual inclinations, an overriding preoccupation with work, or simply the lack of suitable, socially acceptable opportunities for any romantic or sexual relationship.

The life of Nikola Tesla demonstrates well what I call "hyposexuality." An eccentric and outspoken genius, who constructed the first induction motor and invented the alternating current electrical system, Tesla seemed indifferent to women, never courted or married, gave no evidence of being homosexual, and presumably remained sexually abstinent, claiming that a wife would hamper his inventiveness. This also seemed to be the case for both of the Wright brothers, who invented the 3-D system of airplane control.

The 1948 Kinsey Report estimated the rate of homosexual behavior (including bisexuality) to be 10%. More recent surveys estimate the rate to be between 1 and 5%.[13] Within my sample of eminent persons, 83% are heterosexual, 5% homosexual, 6% bisexual, and 6% hyposexual, when those with the unknown sexual orientations are excluded from the calculations. Some intriguing differences emerge when gender is taken into account. While about 5% of both women and men are homosexual, women show a fourfold increase in bisexuality (12% versus 3%) and a twofold increase in hyposexuality (10% versus 5%) compared to men.[54]

There are marked differences in sexual orientation among the various professions. Poets, fiction writers, companions, and social figures are more likely than others to be homosexual (10 to 14%). Musical entertainers, fiction writers, poets, artists, architects, and members of the theater are more likely to be bisexual (9 to 13%). Social scientists, natural scientists, and social activists are more likely to be hyposexual (13 to 17%). And explorers, businesspeople, military officers, public officials, companions, and sports figures show the highest rates of heterosexuality (89 to 100%). In summary, then, the results show that the creative arts professions attract higher proportions of homosexuals and bisexuals, the sciences attract (or promote) a higher proportion of sexually abstemious persons, and the enterprising professions, such as politics, business, and the military, attract the highest proportions of heterosexuals.[55] As for gender differences, greater proportions of women than men, despite their professions, display bisexual behavior or are sexually abstinent.

The Marital Situation

Although the vast majority of eminent persons marry (84% in the sample), we still know little about this area of their lives.[14] Presumably, the spouses they chose to marry, their fidelity to them, their decision to divorce, and the size of their families indicate something important about them since such decisions reflect their values. They also offer a glimpse of the world these people live in when they are not engaged in work.

When we examine the various findings, a general picture begins to emerge. As a rule, certain types of people not only gravitate toward certain kinds of professions, but they gravitate toward certain kinds of spouses and construct family lives that fit them as well. Therefore, we should not be surprised to find that the enterprising types (93%), mainly military officers, public officials, and businesspeople, are most likely to marry, and investigative types (76%), who often are loners, are least likely.[S6] At the one extreme, actors, famous companions, and musical entertainers average about two marriages per person, and at the other extreme, artists, explorers, social scientists, and poets average about one.[S7] Naturally, the number of marriages is a good indicator of the number of divorces. About 36% of those who marry divorce at least once, a rate generally higher than that for the general population.[15] As might be expected, the artistic types (42%), especially musical entertainers and actors, have the highest divorce rates, and the enterprising types (22%), especially public officials and military officers, have the lowest.[S6–S8]

Information about marital fidelity is difficult to uncover and, naturally, is likely to be underreported, especially when people manage to conduct their affairs discretely or secretively. Still, it is remarkable how much of this information can be found in the various biographical sources. The available information reveals that about 38% of married eminent persons have had at least one documented extramarital affair. Consistent with expectations, those in the artistic professions (43%), especially theater, poetry, musical composition, and fiction, are more likely to be unfaithful to their spouses than those in the investigative professions (25%).[S6] While roughly equal proportions of eminent men and women marry, women are far more likely to divorce than men (49% versus 32%) and to have extramarital affairs (45% versus 36%).[S9] These surprising findings may partly be due to the fact that most of the women in the study were in the artistic rather than the more conventional professions; women are more likely to have extramarital affairs if they are in the artistic professions than in others (56% versus 20 to 36%).

Men who are actors or adventurers have the highest rates of marital infidelity (56 to 63%).

A general rule about intimate relationships thus holds true. At one end of the continuum, the enterprising types, who tend to get along well with others and conform to social expectations, are more likely to have stable marriages and remain faithful to their spouses, or at least to show great discretion in their affairs. At the other end, the artistic types, who are more moody and nonconforming, are more likely to get divorced and to be unfaithful.

What now can we say about the first spouses eminent persons choose to marry, usually before achieving the full extent of their fame? Overall, the occupational activities and other characteristics of these spouses appear to follow logically from the value systems that tend to accompany the different professional types. With some exceptions, the general rule is that individuals tend to marry persons with similar or complementary interests, who are most likely to suit their practical and professional needs. Consistent with this rule, we find that enterprising types, mostly men with traditional value systems, are more likely than other types to marry spouses who are homemakers (75% versus 41 to 51%); artistic types are more likely than other types to marry spouses who also work in the creative arts (33% versus 5 to 19%); and investigative types and social types are about twice as likely as other types to marry spouses who work in one of the applied professions (about 25% versus about 12%).[S10,S11]

Among these spouses, 58% showed marked involvement in art, music, poetry, photography, or other creative media. Understandably, artistic types are over twice as likely as enterprising and investigative types to marry spouses with marked creative interests (73% versus about 30%).[S6] More moody and emotionally disturbed themselves, artistic and social types are also more likely than enterprising and investigative types to marry spouses who suffer either from alcoholism, substance abuse, severe depression, major mood swings, psychosis, severe anxiety, severe personality problems, or other psychiatric conditions (13% versus 5 to 9%).[S12] As we shall see later, this is partly a case of like attracting like.

These are the statistics. They say little about the quality of the marital relationships of eminent people in general. To learn more about these relationships, we need to rely on impressions gathered from anecdotal accounts. The most consistent, if unsurprising, impression gathered from these accounts is that women who marry eminent men have to take a back seat to their work, while men who marry eminent women have to allow them time and freedom to pursue their work, giving them what Virginia

Woolf said women needed in order to achieve: financial security and a "room of one's own." Unless the marriage lets them do what they feel compelled to do, it will not last. This fact explains at least in part why husbands and wives who are both eminent have difficulty maintaining a marriage. Remarkably, in my large sample, there are almost no exceptions to this observation.

Children

Although only 62% of all eminent persons have children, men are far more likely than women to do so (66% versus 49%). This probably reflects how much more difficult it is for women to become eminent when they also have the responsibilities of child rearing. In general, businesspeople, public officials, explorers, and military officers (70 to 81%) are more likely than poets, musical entertainers, social scientists, sports figures, artists, and fiction writers (49 to 56%) to have children.[S6]

The average number of children among eminent persons is about two, with a range from zero to 15 children.[16] Businesspeople, famous companions, public officials, architects, explorers, and social activists average about two to three times the number of children as poets, sports figures, and musical performers.[S13]

Not surprisingly, many children pursue careers similar to their eminent parents. About 42% of the individuals with children have at least one child over 21 years of age in a similar or related profession. Actors, public officials, natural scientists, artists, architects, and nonfiction writers are most likely to have at least one child in a similar or related profession (50 to 67%).[S14] About 44% of all eminent persons have at least one child with strong creative interests. Actors, architects, artists, poets, and nonfiction writers (60 to 75%)—that is, artistic types—are more likely than other professionals to have children involved in art, music, writing, theater, or other expressive media. So, it seems, just as members of the creative arts are more likely than those in other professions to have parents with creative interests, they are more likely than those in other professions to have children with creative interests, too.

What can we say about the children of eminent people in general? We know that they have many advantages. They usually are well off financially; they tend to travel; they are often raised in exciting households and meet many exciting visitors. They tend to be exposed to all the major issues of the day and learn about art, music, and culture, and to have the benefits of fine educations. If they choose to follow in their parents' footsteps, they have all kinds of connections and opportunities open to them. Most important, they have mothers or fathers whose accomplishments they can be proud of.

Yet these children also suffer. While there is no evidence that eminent persons are less caring or loving than other parents, they have other interests that command their attention. Because of their all-consuming commitment to their work, these parents may show *de facto* emotional neglect, causing the children to vie for their attention and approval. But perhaps this is the way it is in most households with at least one ambitious, success-oriented parent. What perhaps distinguishes the households of the eminent from others is that no matter what these children accomplish, their famous parents often cast shadows so long that most of their children are kept from realizing their own potentials and finding their own places in the world. Many of these children believe they come up short or, when they do succeed, suspect it is because of their famous parents. It is not that a lot of these children do not become successful in various pursuits. But with their favored backgrounds we should expect even greater accomplishments from them. Except for a few Hollywood stars, virtually no children of eminent people in my sample achieved eminence in their own right.

Perhaps of more serious concern was the emotional toll that having an eminent parent had on children. Although information on these children is sketchy and unavailable on most of those who are still alive, some disturbing trends seem evident. For all of their exceptional achievements, fame, and awards, 20 of these eminent persons have had at least one child take his or her life and more than 80 so far have had children with serious mental problems. This incomplete information suggests that the lifetime rates of mental illness for these children will be exceptionally high.

All of Robert Frost's children, for example, tried unsuccessfully to be writers or actors. Of the five who lived past childhood, one daughter had a "nervous breakdown," another daughter was committed to the state mental hospital, and one son suffered from depression and eventually committed suicide. One of Albert Einstein's children was diagnosed as schizophrenic. Ambrose Bierce had two sons who also pursued careers in journalism. The oldest son committed suicide at 16 and the youngest died of alcoholism at 27. Two of John Barrymore's children, Diana and John, Jr., not only pursued acting careers but, like their father, were alcoholics. Diana also took her life at the age of 37. Thomas Edison also had two children who became alcoholics, one of whom committed suicide. Alfred Stieglitz's daughter became psychotic after giving birth to a child and spent the rest of her life in a mental institution. Mark Twain's daughter, Clara, had a "nervous breakdown." Arnold Toynbee's son committed suicide after flunking out of school. One of Eugene O'Neill's sons, Eugene, Jr., a brilliant classicist, was an alcoholic and eventually committed suicide. His other son, Shane, a mediocre actor, abused alcohol and drugs. James Joyce's daughter, a talented woman who unsuccessfully pursued careers in singing, art, and dance, had to be admitted to an asylum for schizophrenia. Karen Horney, the psychiatrist, had two daughters who suffered from emotional problems. Thomas Mann's son, also a writer, committed suicide. Among the captains of the auto industry, Horace Dodge, John Dodge, John Ford, and Edsel Ford, all had children who became alcoholics. Of Ernest Hemingway's four children, one drank heavily and one had a "mental breakdown."

These examples are sufficient to show the kinds of problems found in these children. Many of these children unsuccessfully pursued careers similar to those of their eminent parents. What precise role their relative failures played in their mental problems is hard to determine, but I suspect that it played some. Although it is advantageous in many obvious ways for children to have parents who are very successful, in more subtle ways it can be a terrible burden as well.

MALADY AND MORTALITY

As with any sample of people, a certain portion of eminent persons may be expected to suffer from serious, chronic, life-threatening or debilitating medical illnesses of at least 6 months' duration. Because of lore that certain chronic illnesses may contribute to creativity, especially among people in the creative arts, I documented their potential existence in individuals before the age of 50, as well as after the age of 50 when the rates of these illnesses would be expected to be higher (excluding all illnesses developing during the year before their deaths). These chronic illnesses included endocrine (e.g., diabetes, thyroid), cardiovascular (e.g., hypertension, heart trouble); gastrointestinal (e.g., liver dysfunction, gastric ulcer); pulmonary (e.g., emphysema, asthma); infectious (e.g., tuberculosis, malaria); neurological (e.g., seizures, paralyses, dementia); oncologic (e.g., cancer); orthopedic (e.g., slipped disc, bone disease, severe arthritis); and other disorders.

Earlier studies on eminent persons report rates of chronic medical illness, varying from 10 to 25%.[17] For my entire sample, 30% suffered from one or more of these chronic illnesses before age 50, and 36% after age 50. Artistic types, especially composers and fiction writers, are more likely than enterprising types, especially businesspeople and military officers, to have a chronic illness before the age of 50 (34% versus 20%).[S15] After age 50, differences in the rates of chronic illness among the various professions become smaller.

The situation with Frida Kählo, the artist, or John Barrymore, the actor, are illustrative of the kinds of physical problems many of these individuals have to endure even as they create. At the age of 18, because of an accident, Kählo was skewered on a metal handrail that entered her left side and came out her vagina. Despite periodic surgeries, body casts, steel corsets, bone fusions and weight apparatuses, she never fully recovered from the accident that fractured several vertebrae, her pelvis, collar bone, right leg, and several ribs and left her in chronic pain for the remainder of her relatively short life. In the case of Barrymore, most of his chronic illnesses—bleeding duodenal ulcers, cirrhosis of the liver, blood clots, gout, eczema, and a heart attack—seemed direct or indirect consequences of his raging alcoholism, which also contributed to the ruin of his career.

Since the health of people differs significantly for those in different vocations, it should come as no surprise that their life spans do as well. This partly reflects the hazards of their vocations and the means by which they die. In the sample, almost 9% died by accidental or incidental means, over 4% by suicide, about 85% by natural means, and the remainder from unknown causes.[S15] Architects, politicians, nonfiction writers, companions, social figures, natural scientists, entrepreneurs, and artists are most likely to die of old age, disease, or natural means (90 to 100%). Not surprisingly, members of those vocations that court the greatest physical risks, such as explorers and adventurers, social activists, soldiers, and athletes, have the highest rates of premature, violent death (16 to 44%) (see Appendix D).

Within my sample, the number of assassinations and murders is striking. Leon Trotsky, Martin Luther King, Jr., Carlos Tresca, Lord Mountbatten, Harvey Milk, Rosa Luxemborg, Malcolm X, Jean Juares, Huey Long, Allard K. Lowenstein, Archduke Franz Ferdinand, Rasputin, and Robert and John F. Kennedy were assassinated. Marvin Gaye, Robert Johnson, Marc Blitzstein, Dian Fosse, Joseph Orten, Pier Paolo Pasolini, and Kit Lambert were murdered. Almost all of these people either were in high-risk professions, made powerful enemies, were personally provocative, or took controversial stands. For some, the circumstances of their deaths made them martyrs.

With certain groups of individuals being more likely than others to develop chronic medical illnesses or to die prematurely, we should not be surprised to find that longevity rates differ substantially among the professions. Explorers or adventurers, musical performers, poets, and sports figures had the shortest life spans (average age = 51 to 60 years) and architects, famous companions, social figures, and social scientists had the longest (average age = 74 to 77 years).[S16] Of course, some part of these differences was attributable to the gender composition of these different professions, women being more prevalent in certain professions and tending to outlive men.

Alma Schindler Mahler-Werfel exemplifies the tendency for famous companions to outlive their eminent spouses. A beautiful woman, with no great talent other than her irresistible charm, she attached herself to several creative geniuses and then resented them for their narcissism. Her first serious flirtation was with Gustav Klimt. At the age of 22 she married Gustav Mahler, who died 9 years later. She then began a passionate affair with Oskar Kokoshka, the painter, poet, and playwright, who was so enamored of her that he took a life-size doll made to look like her everywhere he went. While she was still involved with Kokoshka, she married the great architect Walter Gropius, originator of Bauhaus. Her third marriage was with Franz Werfel, the poet, who died when she was 67. Over this period, she experienced the death of three of her children, which she believed to be a punishment for her many indiscretions.

These are the major characteristics associated with the various professional types. What they show is that any observations about eminent people in general, such as those having to do with certain undesireable personality traits, obscure the many differences existing among them. The kinds of traits common among certain occupational types may be uncommon among other types. What is especially impressive is that these distinguishing characteristics are not limited to one area but cover almost every aspect of their adult lives, including their social behavior, religious practices, encounters with the law, sexual orientations, selection of mates, fidelity during marriage, physical health, cause of death, and longevity. These are important differences, if not in their nature then certainly in their sheer numbers and scope. They challenge us to sharpen our focus more.

REDUCING COMPLEXITY

How do we make sense out of the bewildering array of findings spanning the youth and adult years of eminent persons, and get beyond the shadowy impressions developed so far about the general differences among them? What we need is a way to pare down the large number of specific characteristics we have been discussing to a handful of more general ones. That should allow us, then, to learn how the different professional categories fare on these more general characteristics. Factor analysis offers a way to do this. Essentially, the purpose of factor analysis is to simplify the description and understanding of complex phenomena by identifying a relatively small number of underlying, nonobservable factors that can be used to represent relationships among sets of many interrelated, observable variables. For example, if we have five separate variables—weight, height, verbal ability, mathematical ability, and reading comprehension—a factor analysis might identify two underlying factors, body build (weight, height) and general intelligence (verbal ability, mathematical ability, reading comprehension) to account for them all. Then, instead of using the original five variables, we could use the two factor scores, each representing a more meaningful measure, to compare different groups.

To reduce complexity, I ran an *exploratory* factor analysis, using a four-factor solution on 48 separate variables, covering the entire life span of persons, to determine whether meaningful sets of attributes existed. The results, which mainly serve as *conceptual guides*, revealed that they did.[S17] The first factor comprised aspects of social adjustment, the second of personal well-being, the third of upbringing, and the fourth of mating. Each of these factors significantly distinguished members within certain professions from those within others, but the same professions were not always involved. As demonstrated below, they offer a better way to conceptualize many of the specific findings we noted before.

The first factor, *social adjustment*, is mostly concerned with social behavior. Those who are more socially "marginal"—in particular, actors and musical entertainers, and to a lesser extent, fiction writers, artists, and poets (mainly the artistic types)—tend to be socially alienated and have continuing conflicts with authority. As youths, they are less educated, do less well academically, accrue fewer academic honors, and are less likely to have mentors. As adults, they are moody, nonconforming, and eccentric. They avoid joining various organizations and tend to be irreligious. They have strained relations with their mothers and fathers, are antagonistic toward those in authority, and often have trouble with the law.

In contrast, those who are more socially "centered," mainly the investigative and enterprising types—in particular, natural scientists, social scientists, public officials, and military officers—tend to be more socially well adjusted, get along well with others, and appear respectful of authority. As youths, they are better educated, do better academically, win more honors, and are more likely to have mentors. As adults, they are even-tempered, more

athletically than aesthetically inclined, relatively conforming and conventional, belong to many social, religious, professional, or political organizations, and operate in the social mainstream. They have close relationships
with their mothers and fathers, are respectful to superiors and others in
positions of authority, and tend to be law abiding and religious.

The second factor concerns primarily *personal well-being*, including
physical health and general behavior. Toward one extreme are those who
engage in creative work—in particular, poets, fiction writers, natural
scientists, and social scientists (mainly the investigative and artistic types).
As youths, they are more likely to be physically disabled, to be "sickly," and
to have weathered a major, life-threatening illness. They tend to be
precocious children who love to read, seem peculiar to others, and mostly
keep to themselves. Other students tend to tease them, and they have
frequent conflicts with their teachers. As adults, they spend much of their
time in their laboratories, studios, or studies or in other solitary pursuits.
They are more inclined to be atheists or agnostics or to have unorthodox
religious views. They also suffer from various chronic medical illnesses
throughout the course of their lives.

At the other extreme are those who appear normal and well-adjusted—
in particular, social figures, businesspeople, social activists, and politicians
(mainly the social and enterprising types). As youths, they tend to be
even-tempered, "normal" looking, sociable, and bright but not necessarily
precocious. They are accepted by their classmates and get along well with
their teachers. They have no physical disabilities and enjoy good health. As
adults, they participate in many social functions, interact well with others,
and attend church regularly. As they grow older, they are reasonably healthy
and are not as likely to suffer from chronic medical illnesses.

The third factor involves *upbringing*. At one extreme are those who
are born with many social advantages: mainly well-known hosts and
hostesses, patrons, art collectors, and connoisseurs, and the lovers and
mates of famous people. Women are strongly represented among these
individuals. They generally come from the upper social strata and have
successful and wealthy fathers. Often Protestant, they possess strong aesthetic interests, and come from urban settings.

At the other extreme are those who are born more socially disadvantaged: mostly the artistic types (especially musical entertainers, composers,
and actors) and social activists and sports figures. Mainly non-Protestant,
they come from lower-class backgrounds, and have more unsuccessful and
poorer fathers. They tend to be raised in small towns or rural areas. During
their lifetimes, they are more apt to be prosecuted for political or social

reasons or encounter other legal difficulties. Despite their social disadvantages, greater proportions of them experience their first major professional success before the age of 21.

The fourth factor, *mating*, mostly deals with sex, romance, and marriage, as well as longevity. At one extreme are the actors and entrepreneurs (mainly the enterprising types), who are mostly heterosexual, marry more often, divorce more often, and have more extramarital affairs. They also tend to die by natural means and to live longer.

At the other extreme are the poets, social activists, social scientists, and artists. They have a greater representation of homosexuals or bisexuals and, perhaps partly because of this, are not as likely to marry, divorce, or have extramarital affairs. They also are more likely to die of suicide or accidents and, consequently, have shorter life spans.

These assorted results offer strong support for the existence of professional types. What needs to be emphasized, however, is that the notion of professional types only refers to the general characteristics of entire occupational groups, not to the specific characteristics of the individual members. This is an important distinction. It means that it is possible for certain professional types to be defined by attributes that a minority of its members possess, if the percentage is greater than those for comparison types (e.g., 40% versus 20%), even though these different types may share many attributes in common. These results also reveal the multidimensional nature of differences among professional types. Members of certain professions may differ from those of others on one dimension, from others on a second dimension, yet others on a third dimension, and so on. Professional types, therefore, become progressively better defined when many reference groups are used. All this points up the dangers in using stereotypes and prototypes to portray professional types.

There is another important lesson to be learned from these various results. Although many youthful attributes of these individuals continue into adulthood—that is, moody, unsociable, and "odd" children tend to become moody, unsociable, and eccentric adults[S18]—the development of a professional role is anything but a static process. Once established in their respective careers, individuals appear to have certain special life experiences as well—legal entanglements, exposure to mentors, extramarital affairs, divorces, chronic illnesses, conflicts with authority figures, or homosexual relations—that appear to become part of the fabric of their lives and serve to consolidate their professional identities even further.

CHAPTER FIVE

Impediments to Eminence

*I*n the late 1920s, Robert E. Park introduced the notion of "marginal" people whose fate it was to live on the borderline between two cultures.[1] These people are cultural hybrids, never quite willing to break with their past traditions and never quite accepted into the society in which they seek to find a place. Given their ambiguous position in society, they develop distinctive personality characteristics. Idealistic, cosmopolitan, and rootless, they acquire a wider vision, a keener intelligence, and a more detached and rational perspective. But this is at the cost of a spiritual instability, heightened self-consciousness, restlessness, and a vague sense of mental ill-being. In their roles as "outsiders" or "strangers," they often serve as catalysts for social progress and cultural ferment.

This intriguing notion suggests that certain kinds of people, with characteristics markedly different from those we have examined so far, tend to be associated with social innovation and growth. These are people who somehow manage to make their mark despite existing in an alien, even hostile culture. In a sense, they belong and they do not belong. They are a part of the cultures in which they live, yet stand apart from them. They are simultaneously accepted and rejected. Never fully integrated into their societies, they are participant observers. As members of their societies, they challenge the very basis of its mores and values, eliciting either persecution and repression or eventual accommodation and acceptance.

Historically, artists, writers, actors, and musicians have operated on the social fringe, appreciated by a certain segment of the populace for their creativity and vision, but frowned upon for their life-styles and deviant values. As our own findings already reveal, a substantial portion of the artistic types function at the social periphery as outsiders. Nonconformist, avant-garde, rebellious loners, they challenge the status quo and promote social change.

However, the notion of social marginality extends beyond professional boundaries. It includes any groups of people who are caught between two cultures, not quite fitting in the one and not quite accepted in the other. Many minority or disadvantaged groups qualify as being socially marginal. For example, women who try to compete in male-dominated professions, Jewish persons who seek acceptance in a Christian culture, blacks who expect equality in a white society, and homosexuals who proclaim their sexual normality in a predominantly heterosexual community all exist on the social periphery. If the supposed relationship between social marginality and cultural progress holds true, it is a paradox that those who are most alienated from society should be among society's greatest benefactors.

It is difficult enough for anybody to achieve eminence, let alone greatness, even with the advantages of social status, wealth, cultured parents, and a fine education. Imagine what it must be like for people who not only may lack these advantages but are actively discriminated against and prevented from achieving. Even today, certain professions still seem to select not only for people with the right kind of skills and credentials but also for the "right" kinds of people. The "right" kinds of people often have excluded women, blacks, Jews, and homosexuals. Despite these prohibitions and prejudices, many socially disadvantaged individuals have found suitable occupational outlets for their extraordinary abilities, and some even have managed to do so within professions inhospitable toward them.

While it is easy to overlook the creative achievements of any single disadvantaged group in our sample, largely because any single group represents a small fraction of the total, it is difficult to overlook them all. A composite of all those who are not whites, Christians, heterosexuals, or males represents almost half the entire sample.

Besides the broader question of whether being socially disadvantaged represents an impediment to eminence and creative achievement, several other issues also arise. These address whether members of socially marginal groups gravitate toward certain professions more than others, whether they make unique professional contributions because of their "differentness," and whether they suffer more emotionally because of the social and vocational obstacles they face. My findings shed light on each of these issues.

GROUP FEATURES

Gender

Although women make up roughly half the general population, they accounted for about one-quarter of my sample of eminent persons. Not surprisingly, compared to men, women had the greatest opportunities to achieve fame as the wives or lovers of distinguished men (94%) or as social figures (73%), playing the role of hostess, collector, philanthropist, or patroness of the arts. Other fields that appeared to accommodate them included social activism (41%), theater (37%), musical entertainment (40%), architecture or design (30%), and writing (25 to 28%). Very few achieved prominence through business, public office, the military, musical composition, or the natural sciences (0 to 8%). Overall, they had above their average representation in the social (35%) and artistic (27%) professions and below their average representation in the investigative (21%) and enterprising (10%) ones.[51]

Compared to men, these women came from wealthier and higher social class backgrounds. Their parents were more likely to be divorced or separated, and their mothers or siblings were more likely to be emotionally disturbed. They had less formal education, received fewer academic awards, and had fewer professional accomplishments. They also were less athletic than men and belonged to fewer social organizations. While their marriage rates were similar, they were more likely to divorce and to have substantially fewer children. They also were more inclined to be bisexual or homosexual and to lead more unconventional lives.[52]

The notion that eminent women led more unconventional lives than eminent men might seem surprising, given the social constraints on women, especially before the mid-20th century. But when we examine the lives of these extraordinary women, the reasons for their nonconformity become clear. Very few of them could have achieved what they did if they had conformed to traditional female roles. The very process of becoming eminent was selective for those who could overcome those social obstacles or restrictions that kept them at a competitive disadvantage with men.

For these women, their lack of conventionality took many forms. Emma Goldman left her husband and parents to pursue a life dedicated to political action. She defied the morals of her day by living communally with her lover and several friends. Karen Horney, the psychoanalyst, proclaimed that "there is nothing more unbearable than the thought of disappearing quietly in the great mass of the average, nothing more fatal than the reproach of being told that one is a nice, friendly average person." She acted out this conviction with her flamboyant clothes, her nonconformist professional views, and her predilection for affairs. Vita Sackville-West enjoyed cross-dressing, impersonating men and, even while she maintained a conventional, married life with a husband and two sons, had sexual affairs on the side. Already known for what were considered her "eccentric" ways, she managed to shock people even more by eloping with another married woman to the continent. Simone de Beauvoir maintained a life-long, open relationship with Jean-Paul Sartre. As a writer, lesbian, and patroness of the arts, Gertrude Stein exemplified the Parisian bohemian lifestyle of the early 20th century.

There are many theories about why women have been so underrepresented within certain professions and why their creative achievements have been fewer than those of men.[2] Although I do not necessarily subscribe to any of these theories, I mention them to show their diversity.

According to biology-based theories, men hold an "advantage" over women because of their superior mathematical–logical–spatial abilities, their left-brain dominance, their higher androgen levels, and their greater aggressiveness, competitiveness, or physical prowess. Women also have been said not to be as motivated as men toward creative achievement because they can satisfy their biological urge for creativity through procreation.

Psychological theories largely emphasize that women have been trained not to succeed and compete in a "man's world." Since they are psychologically conditioned by an environment that values nonassertive, insecure, conforming, "feminine," and family-oriented attitudes in women, they come to place a different premium on different tasks and competencies, favoring those that are more socially appropriate for women and avoiding those that place them in direct competition with men.

Social theories emphasize the powerful role expectations for women: the primacy of the family, their subjection to their fathers and husbands, and their personal fulfillment through their children's and spouses' careers. Given these expectations, women have not had suitable educational opportunities to compete successfully with men, or when they have had them, they were not as likely to find work environments that were suitably receptive to their skills. The lack of suitable role models or mentors put them at an even greater disadvantage. Women were simply not supposed to be successful. The classical mythological rendering of this role restriction can be found in the Muses, who, although responsible for all creativity in the arts and sciences, were supposed to inspire men to great deeds rather than accomplishing them themselves.

The 40-year outcome study at Stanford on over 1,500 gifted children, 671 girls and 847 boys, with IQs equal to or greater than 135, dramatically illustrates the power of these gender-based stereotypes.[3] Most men at mid-life achieved prominence in professional and managerial occupations, becoming successful scientists, writers, artists, lawyers, physicians, or psychologists. The women, in contrast, mostly ended up in traditional female occupations. About 50% were full-time housewives. Of those working full-time, 21% were teachers in elementary or secondary school, 20% were secretaries, 8% were social workers, and 8% were librarians or nurses. Although these women as children possessed an intelligence and professional potential comparable to men, only 8% became executives, 9% writers, artists, or musicians, 7% academicians, and 5% physicians, lawyers, or psychologists. This phenomenon represents the "homogenization" of American women,[4] a social process in which women are socialized to pursue the same roles despite their individual aptitudes, talents, or abilities.

Germaine Greer, in her important book, *The Obstacle Race*, made a powerful case for social structure as the major influence on female artistic accomplishments.[5] Adopting a historical perspective on this topic, she documented many obstacles that confronted women artists over the centuries. Until the late 19th and early 20th centuries, almost all female artists had a close personal connection with a dominant male artist—usually their fathers, but often their lovers or masters—from whose influence they found it hard to liberate themselves. Moreover, life for unmarried female artists was not easy, especially if they did not have the financial or moral support of their families. Even when they did, they usually were not admitted into the male-dominated academies to obtain the education and training necessary for an artistic career. As late as the 1850s and, in some parts of the Western world, the early 1900s, women artists were not allowed to work with nudes.[6] Women artists were at a great disadvantage, since they were expected to confine their paintings to portraiture, landscapes, and still lifes or to indulge in primitivism and naive art (an art form that borrows the "peasant" perspective, which is suposedly the result of ignorance and lack of formal training).

What pertains in art most likely holds true in architecture, mathematics, physics, politics, and a host of other male-dominated professions. Given these formidable obstacles to success, it becomes as appropriate to ask how many women managed to achieve what they did as it does to ask why the amount of their accomplishments has not been as great as that for men.

Professional discrimination of this sort assumes other forms and other consequences when directed toward blacks, Jews, or homosexuals. It is not necessary to document the long history of persecution and the job discrimination these groups have had to endure, ranging from legal impediments to entry into certain professions (e.g., gays in the military), to quota systems for educational institutions and training programs (e.g., former quotas for Jewish persons in Ivy League schools), to outright segregation (e.g., inability of blacks to enter certain white institutions). Exposure to prejudice and bias such as this is bound to affect the recipients and influence their choice of professional careers. It also is bound to contribute to their sense of social alienation, which certain authors regard as important for innovation and creativity.

Race

Blacks made up only 4% of my entire sample—about one-third to two-fifths of their percentage for the population at large in the United States between the years 1890 and 1990.[7] They were proportionately represented or overrepresented only in sports (26%), the musical entertainment industry (30%), the natural sciences (5%), and musical composition (4%). Almost no blacks had become famous enough as architects, artists, entrepreneurs, explorers, military officers, expository writers, or poets to have had biographies written about them and then reviewed in the *New York Times Book Review*, suggesting either that hardly any entered these professions or that if they did, their opportunities for professional fame were limited. The Holland classification highlighted the professional inclinations of blacks. The highest percentages were in the social type occupations (9%), next highest in the artistic (4%) and investigative type occupations (4%), and the lowest in the enterprising type occupations (1%).[51]

In their personal lives, eminent blacks differed from whites in several important ways. Their fathers were more likely to work at lower level jobs, to be more poorly educated, and to make less money. Their mothers were less likely to be homemakers and more likely to work at unskilled jobs. Their parents were less likely to remain married. And although blacks were less likely than whites to go to college or graduate school, they were over twice as likely to have had their first professional success before they were 20.[53] This is likely due in part to the nature of the entertainment and sports professions.

Religion

Unlike gender or race, religion seemed to have a different impact on representation within the various professions. Since Catholicism or Protestantism was the dominant religion within almost all the Western countries in this sample, only Judaism was a minority faith, and of all the religions represented here, it was the one most consistently persecuted throughout the ages. For the purposes of this survey, individuals were classified according to their parents' religious affiliation, whether the individuals as adults professed this faith or not. No attempt was made to distinguish among the different Catholic religions (i.e., Roman, Greek Orthodox, Russian Orthodox), various Protestant denominations (i.e., Baptist, Methodist, Lutheran, Episcopalian, etc.) or between reform and Orthodox Judaism. Instances in which information about the parents' religious affiliation was unknown or unconventional or in which mixed marriages existed were not included in the analyses.

Most of the past studies on the relationship of religion to achievement focused mainly on science. In a study of Nobel laureates, one researcher found that Jewish persons made up 19% of the 286 Nobelists of all nationalities named up to 1972, a percentage many times greater than their representation in their various countries of origin.[8] Of the American laureates, 72% were Protestant, 1% were Catholic, and 27% were Jewish, although Jewish persons comprised only about 3% of the U. S. population. Among the American Nobel laureates who had won awards in the biological sciences, excluding medicine, 39% were Jewish, 54% Protestant, and 7% Catholic. Among those who had won awards in the biological sciences, including medicine, 29% were Jewish, 61% Protestant, and 10% Catholic. Among those who had won awards in chemistry, 11% were Jewish, 84% Protestant, and 5% Catholic. And among those who had received awards in physics, 41% were Jewish, 59% were Protestant, and 0% were Catholic.

How can we interpret these findings? The number of Jewish persons among the Nobel laureates may partly reflect their predilection for fields such as molecular biology, virology, microbiology, biochemistry and medicine that are eligible for the Nobel Prize, than those such as botany, zoology, or agriculture which are not.[9] By way of comparison, a study of 60,000 academics at colleges and universities throughout the United States found that 14% of physicists, 8% of chemists, 21% of biochemists, 13% of sociologists, and 17% of psychologists had Jewish social origins.

In my sample of eminent persons, about 15% came from Jewish backgrounds (a proportionately greater percentage than that for the U.S.

population and for most of the other countries represented), 20% from Catholic backgrounds, 57% from Protestant backgrounds, and 8% from other backgrounds.. As anticipated, significant differences existed for these different religious groups in their representation among the 18 general professions. Except for exploration and sports, Jewish persons were over-represented in all professions, and particularly in business (36%), social activism (29%), the social sciences (19%), musical composition (15%), art (14%), nonfiction writing (14%), and architecture or design (13%).[51]

In more personal matters, Jewish persons were more likely than Catholics or Protestants to be raised in urban settings, to come from lower social class backgrounds, and to have more poorly educated and less successful fathers with few creative interests.[10] This probably reflected the more recent immigrant status of many of their parents. Along with Protestants, they were more likely to do well academically and complete college and graduate school. Perhaps because of the careers they chose, which required more training, they were less likely than Catholics or Protestants to achieve their first professional success before the age of 20.[54]

Sexual Orientation

The situation for gays and lesbians seems superficially different from that of other disadvantaged groups. Since others cannot easily identify them by their gender, skin pigmentation, physical features, or names as socially undesirable, homosexuals should not suffer overt professional discrimination unless they are forced to or choose to reveal their sexual orientation. If they choose to conceal their sexual orientation and suppress any overt behavior sometimes associated with it, they theoretically should have as much access to any of the professions as heterosexuals. To some extent, then, any overrepresentation or underrepresentation in one profession or another should reflect its relative appeal for these particular individuals and the opportunity it affords them to express their particular gifts.

Examination of the results revealed significant differences in the distribution of homosexuals (including bisexuals) among the 18 general professions. Although 11% of the entire sample was homosexual or bisexual—a figure that roughly corresponded to that in the 1948 Kinsey Report[11] but was much greater than the 1% to 4% estimates in more recent surveys[12]—they were proportionately overrepresented among poets (24%), fiction writers (21%), artists (15%), and musical entertainers (15%), and underrepresented among military officers, explorers, public officials, natural scientists, businesspeople, social scientists, social activists, and expository writers (0 to 6%). With the Holland classification, a clearer picture emerged of the distribution of homosexuals and bisexuals among the various occupations. Among the artistic types, 15% were represented, 7% among the social types, 3% among the enterprising types, and 5% among the investigative types.[51]

In other aspects of their lives, homosexuals and bisexuals showed marked differences from heterosexuals. While they had comparable social backgrounds and educational experiences, they were more likely to come from broken homes, to have had conflicts with fellow students at school, and to have had their first professional success before they were 21 years old.[55]

What can we say about the impact of social discrimination on the professional choices, mental health, and accomplishments of eminent people?

As to whether certain disadvantaged groups were more likely to gravitate toward certain professions than others, the results showed this to be so, although they did not always establish whether this was because of design or necessity. The problem was that it was difficult to sort out the relative influence of social selection and self-selection for a professional career.[12] Take the case of science, for example, a field in which women, blacks, and homosexuals were underrepresented. Since advanced degrees are necessary for advancement in science, it means something different if there is an adequate pool of qualified, minority candidates with Ph.D.s to choose from than if no adequate pool exists. If there is not an adequate pool, then social, familial, and perhaps psychological factors, operating on people from a very early age, are probably responsible for the underrepresentation. If there is an adequate pool, then a more overt form of discrimination is probably at work.

This point needs elaboration. Take the case of women whose representation in science has been far less than men. Of the 866 members of the National Academy, only eight were women, and of the 281 scientists who received the Nobel Prize, only five were women.[13] What about the pool of candidates from which these women came? While women received 40% of the baccalaureate degrees in the United States, they received 32% of the master's degrees, and interestingly, only 11% of the doctorate degrees by 1960. While this discrepancy seems to be lessening over time, as of the late 1970s, only about 12% of science Ph.D.s in the United States were women.

As for whether sexual discrimination existed in science once women obtained their Ph.D.s, the results remain inconclusive. Although one study, which examined a matched sample of about 500 men and women scientists who were academically employed in chemistry, biology, or psychology departments, concluded that they were treated similarly by the reward system in science, it also noted that women received less professional recognition.[14] Many more studies along these lines in many more fields need to be done before this issue can be settled.

The difficulties in evaluating whether blacks are systematically discriminated against in science are perhaps even more severe. The central problem is that there have been few blacks with doctorates in science, a prerequisite for academic advancement and usually for grant support. In one survey of 63 doctoral programs,[15] the results showed that less than 1% of all Ph.D.s awarded between 1964 and 1968 went to black Americans. Even today, blacks continue to receive a disproportionately low percentage of science Ph.D.s conferred in any given year. Although failures in the educational system and professional discrimination may partly account for the relative paucity of blacks in science, complex social forces operating on blacks from a very early age probably are also at work.

Unfortunately, it is hard to explain why homosexuals are underrepresented in the sciences in comparison to other professions. Perhaps the sciences happened to hold less attraction for the particular eminent homosexuals in my sample. Or perhaps there was something about being homosexual that made people incline toward the more expressive or creative professions. In any event, while overt discrimination toward homosexuals appeared to exist in many fields, such as the military or public office, it was difficult to document its existence in science.

The available statistics also offer little support for the belief that Jewish persons have been systematically discriminated against in the sciences, especially after World War II. A prior study on this matter found no evidence of discrimination against Jewish persons in the American scientific community, since religion had no relationship to scientific output and since Jewish persons were more likely to be recognized for their work than non-Jews.[16] Information was lacking about whether a similar situation applied to Jewish persons in the arts and other professions.

As for the question of whether socially stigmatized individuals experienced more mental and physical difficulties than their counterparts, the answer is unequivocally "yes." In almost all instances, these socially disadvantaged or marginal groups were adversely affected in either their emotional health, longevity, or relations with society.[S2–S5] In virtually no instance did any of these socially disadvantaged groups fare better than their less stigmatized peers. Although women lived longer than men, they were more likely to experience severe anxiety, have adjustment disorders, abuse drugs, and have unspecified mental problems. Higher percentages also attempted suicide and received some form of mental health care. Blacks were more likely than whites to abuse drugs and attempt suicide. They also had dramatically shorter life spans, living about 11 years less.

Compared to heterosexuals, homosexuals were more likely to suffer from anxiety, adjustment problems, alcoholism, drug abuse, anxiety, and depression, and to receive some form of mental health treatment for their problems. They were more likely to die by suicide or accident, and their life span was also considerably less—about 7 years. While Jewish persons did not have significantly higher rates of mental illness than Catholics or Protestants, they did receive more mental health care. However, the appearance of a predilection for receiving mental health care may perhaps have been inflated by the tendency of certain Jewish psychiatrists or psychoanalysts, such as Anna Freud, Helena Deutsch, Victor Tausk, Wilhelm Reich, Otto Rank, and Melanie Klein, to be psychoanalyzed as part of their training.

Besides experiencing adverse psychological or physical effects, these socially marginal groups, as expected, were more socially alienated as well. Eminent women tended to be less affiliative, more eccentric, and more nonconforming than men. Blacks experienced more social friction than whites, especially in the form of legal difficulties. Jewish persons were more likely to reject formal religion and be prosecuted for their political or social views. And homosexuals were more likely than heterosexuals to be nonconforming, nonaffilative, and eccentric.

THE IMPACT OF SOCIAL MARGINALITY ON CREATIVE ACTIVITY

So far we have noted the profound effects of social marginality on various aspects of people's lives. What about its impact on the lifetime creative achievements of these individuals? The findings on this matter are mixed. Among all these marginal groups, women appear to be the most disadvantaged, the magnitude of their overall creative achievements being significantly less than that of men. Many of the potential reasons for this already have been discussed. As for the other groups, essentially no significant differences in the extent of lifetime professional accomplishments exist between whites and blacks, Christians and Jews, or heterosexuals and gays. In other words, despite the overrepresentation or underrepresentation of these socially marginal groups in various professions, no evidence exists that their alienated status gives them any special creative advantage.

The unique differences between socially marginal and nonmarginal groups have more to do with the kinds of professions they choose and the nature of their causes than with the magnitude of their creative achievements. In fact, as the notion of social marginality implies, these individuals serve as a ferment for cultural change, causing their societies to accommodate their special needs. To shed light on this matter, we need to examine these groups separately, since each group seems to respond in distinctive ways.

Of the 243 eminent women studied, about 12% made women's issues a major focus of their work and activities. Of these women, a number achieved some degree of posthumous fame by being the first of their gender to become prominent in a particular field and then devoting themselves to women's causes. Elizabeth Blackwell, for instance, managed to become the first woman doctor in the modern era, despite being refused admittance to medical schools in Philadelphia and New York. Upon completion of her training in Europe, after being unable to obtain a medical position in a hospital or clinic, she finally opened her own dispensary, staffed entirely by women. Later, she returned to London and helped found the London School of Medicine for Women. Amelia Earhart became famous as the first woman to fly over the Atlantic and, later, for her active efforts to open aviation to women and end male domination of that new field. Nancy Astor, an outspoken advocate for women's rights, was the first woman to sit in the British House of Commons. Lucy Sprague Mitchell was the first woman faculty member at the University of California at Berkeley and eventually became the first Dean of Women. Jeannette Rankin, the first woman member of the U.S. Congress (1917–1919, 1941–1943), was a pacifist and crusader for women's rights. Victoria Woodhull was the first woman to run for the U.S. Presidency.

Other than establishing many "firsts," women also made their mark through social activism, organizational activities, writings, and various other works for the betterment of women. One important issue had to do with the right of women to control what happened to their own bodies. Margaret Sanger believed that every woman had the right to plan the size of her family and devoted herself to removing the legal barriers against contraception and birth control. Although she was indicted for mailing material advocating birth control and later served 30 days in the workhouse for opening the first U.S. birth control clinic, she continued to write many books and articles on this topic and founded the American Birth Control

League. Josephine Butler worked toward abolishing the 1964 Contagious Disease Act that forced prostitutes to be involuntarily examined for suspected venereal diseases and detained in certified government hospitals. She published many pamphlets on social injustices, education for women, and double standards in sexual morality.

Other important issues had to do with the right to vote and own property. Julia Ward Howe, who wrote the lyrics for *The Battle Hymn of the Republic*, was president of the New England Women Suffrage Association. Susan Anthony actively campaigned for the right of women to control their own property, to have guardianship of their children in case of divorce, and to vote. Hannah Sheehy-Skeffington, who spent 2 months in prison for protesting against the exclusion of women from the Home Rule Bill and who later went on a hunger strike in sympathy with English suffragists who had been denied political equality, helped to found the militant Irish Women's Franchise League in 1908. Others championing the political equality of women were Carrie Chapman Catt, who played a key role in causing the adoption of the 19th Amendment (suffrage) in 1920; Elizabeth Cady Stanton, who fought against legal restrictions and discriminations against women; and Jane Addams, who argued for an 8-hour working day for women and supported women's suffrage. Other contributions to the women's movement had to do with defining the special needs of women. Helene Deutsch was one of the first women analyzed by Freud, the second woman admitted to the Vienna Psychoana- lytic Society, and author of the two-volume work, *The Psychology of Women*. Simone de Beauvoir, who founded the League for Women's Rights, wrote the seminal work on gender inequality, *The Second Sex*. Julia Morgan, one of the first women to be admitted to the American Institute of Architects and perhaps best known for overseeing the 20-year building program at San Simeon for the Hearst family, became committed to architectural projects associated with the early development of American women's movements, such as women's residence halls and community clubhouses. Although many other eminent women were not counted among those who were actively and specifically involved in women's issues, we should note that many of them, especially the artists and writers, were sympathetic to these issues or actively involved in left-wing politics, racial equality, or other human rights struggles.

The situation with race was somewhat different. Of the 40 eminent blacks in the study, about 68% made racial issues a major focus of their work. As with women who achieved firsts in certain fields, some blacks became famous by being uniquely situated to break the race barrier. Hattie

McDaniel, for example, was the first black actress to win an Oscar. Jackie Robinson was the first black to play professional baseball, and became an outspoken advocate for civil rights.

Other blacks gained fame for their creative contributions to a distinctive style of music, which expressed certain aspects of the black experience. The *Encyclopedia Americana* describes "jazz" as an "improvisational, Afro-American musical idiom that developed in the United States during the 20th century" and the "blues" as a vocal and instrumental jazz style of black American origin. Among the blacks in my sample, jazz and blues musicians were well represented. Some great performers or composers included Louis Armstrong, Josephine Baker, John Coltrane, Duke Ellington, Alberta Hunter, Robert Johnson, Bessie Smith, Fats Waller, and Dinah Washington.

Social activism represented another professional vehicle for black concerns. The efforts of Martin Luther King, Jr. on behalf of civil rights and racial equality and Malcolm X regarding black power and independence are legendary. Perhaps less known today are the achievements of others. Booker T. Washington founded Tuskegee Institute in 1881, was an advisor of Presidents, and was the leading black political patronage broker of his day. Marcus Garvey organized the first important black nationalist movement in the United States, based in New York's Harlem. The goals of the Universal Negro Improvement Association that he founded were to promote unity among blacks throughout the world by instilling in them a pride of race, and to build a black-run Negro nation in Africa. William Henry Hastie was a distinguished black jurist and pioneer in civil rights legislation. He was involved in landmark cases on equal pay for black school teachers, equal educational opportunities for blacks at the graduate level, and antisegregation in interstate commerce, he was also a catalyst for racial integration of the armed forces. Charles Hamilton Houston, also a civil rights lawyer, was the architect of the NAACP legal program against racial segregation and laid the groundwork for all subsequent civil rights litigation. George A. Wiley was a black chemist who resigned from a notable career to work for the Congress of Racial Equality and who helped found the National Welfare Rights Organization.

Others fought for racial equality in other ways. Langston Hughes, especially through the powerful medium of his poetry, portrayed blacks with great sensitivity and skill. Mary McLeod Bethune founded Bethune-Cookman College for Negro girls in 1904, directed the Division of Negro Affairs of the National Youth Administration from 1936 to 1943, and, among other offices, served as a special advisor on minority affairs to

President Roosevelt. Monroe Nathan Work edited nine editions of the Negro Year Book, organized 17 Negro health weeks, produced a massive bibliography of blacks in Africa and America, and made many other contributions to black advancement. Zora Neal Hurston was the foremost writer on Afro-American folklore. Franz Fanon, a psychoanalyst and social philosopher, became known for his theory that some neuroses were socially generated and for his writings promoting the national liberation of colonial people. James Baldwin, through his powerful essays, novels, and plays, became an important interpreter of black–white relations in the United States and a spokesman for the civil rights movement.

Being Jewish appeared to have a different impact on the professional activities and personal commitments of people than being female or black. Of the 127 Jewish individuals in the study, 16% (about two-thirds of whom were ardent Zionists) were actively involved in Jewish matters in their work. This number did not include those who had a broader interest in leftist or general human rights causes. Among those whose life work centered on the betterment of Jewish persons were David Ben-Gurion, Chaim Weizmann, and Theodor Herzl, all of whom were instrumental in the creation of Israel. Henrietta Szold, also active in Zionist causes, wrote articles for the Anglo-Jewish press and was a founder of Hadassah, the Women's Zionist Organization of America; she also became the first woman member of the World Zionist Organization. Isaac Mayer Wise was the founder of reform Judaism in the United States, and his son, Jonah Bondi Wise, headed the Central Synagogue in New York, created the popular Message of Israel weekly radio program, and was prominent in Jewish affairs.

There were other outlets as well for Jewish concerns. Martin Buber, a world-famous Hebrew scholar and philosopher, wrote several books on Judaism and Hasidic life and helped to found the Hebrew University. Harry S. Wolfson was a professor of Hebrew literature and philosophy at Harvard and wrote many articles in these areas of study. Trained as a philosopher, Hannah Arendt wrote various works dealing with antisemitism and the persecution of the Jews, the best known of which were *The Origins of Totalitarianism* and *Eichmann in Jerusalem*.

Finally, we need to look at the effect of sexual orientation on professional work. Of the 105 homosexuals or bisexuals in the study, only 13% explicitly addressed homosexual themes in their work or formally worked for the betterment of other homosexuals. Except for Harvey Milk, the assassinated Supervisor of San Francisco, almost all of the other eminent persons whose work explicitly reflected their homosexuality were writers.

Marcel Proust explored the homosexual world in his *Remembrances of Things Past*. J. R. Ackerley wrote openly of his homosexuality in *My Father and Myself*. Truman Capote's first novel, *Other Voices, Other Rooms*, told of a young boy's discovery of his homosexuality. Jean Cocteau published *Confessions of a Homosexual* anonymously. Rainer Werner Fassbinder, the German film maker, theater director, and screen writer, pursued homosexual themes in many of his films. After E. M. Forster's death, his early novel, *Maurice*, which explored the effects of homosexuality on coming of age, was published. Federico Garcia Lorca explored personal struggles with homosexuality in his poetry. André Gide was violently attacked for his defense of homosexuality in *Corydon*. Djuna Barnes arranged for her lesbian *Ladies Almanack* to be published posthumously. And Tennessee Williams dealt with homosexuality in a veiled way in his play, *Cat on a Hot Tin Roof*.

What becomes immediately apparent from these observations is that despite some overlapping general concerns about human rights and equal opportunities for all persons, each of these four socially stigmatized groups has its own separate agenda. Within the sample, special women's issues involved the right to vote, the right to use birth control, and the right to work in male-dominated occupations. Special black issues involved civil rights, equal opportunity and, for some, the expression of the black experience through jazz and the blues. For Jewish persons, these special issues involved the preservation of the Jewish experience, the creation of Israel, and the pursuit of the Zionist cause. For gays and lesbians, special issues were less clear but suggested an emphasis on a better understanding and acceptance of homosexuality by members of society.

Within their professional work and personal lives, blacks seemed most profoundly affected by their social stigmatization, with most of them actively involved in issues or experiences special to them, compared to far lower percentages for the other groups. Although this dramatic difference might be interpreted in many ways, it probably reflected the greater professional obstacles and social disadvantages that blacks faced, which likewise contributed to their being so underrepresented among the eminent.

The situation was entirely different for homosexuals. Unlike the militancy and social activism shown by blacks and members of the other socially stigmatized groups on behalf of their colleagues, and that shown by gay organizations today, virtually no eminent homosexuals in the study formally participated in organizations that expressed the naturalness of homosexuality, petitioned against discriminatory practices, or openly sought greater public acceptance and understanding. With notable exceptions, those individuals identified as addressing special homosexual issues usually did so by allusion or, if writers, mostly within the context of fiction. When they engaged in more frank discussions, several did so by publishing their books anonymously or posthumously, as was perfectly understandable given the intolerant attitudes of society and the temper of the times, both which dictated more secretive life styles.

While these observations make it clear that social marginality can shape the professional interests and personal activities of people,[16] we also should note that this does not necessarily hold for the vast majority of eminent women, homosexuals, Jewish persons, and a sizable portion of blacks. Although they may be sympathetic and sensitized to many special issues affecting them and other members of their groups, they go about their work and daily lives, like anyone else, with no special focus on their minority status. As with other eminent people, their work is all-consuming and, along with family and social obligations, they have time for little else. What recognition they seek is for themselves as individuals and not as exemplary representatives of their gender, race, creed or sexual orientation. Fortunately, the social and professional gains made by other members of their socially disadvantaged groups pave the way for them better to realize their goals.

CHAPTER SIX

The Measure of Achievement

How do we objectively measure the creative achievements of people? Where along the continuum of importance, for example, should we position Edison's development of the light bulb compared to Jung's psychological system that illuminated human nature? How should we compare the originality of Einstein's theory of relativity to Margaret Mead's writings on cultural relativity? Are the biochemical discoveries of Szent-Györgyi of greater value to Western society than Kafka's portrayal of social alienation, Virginia Woolf's insights into the illusory nature of the self, Frida Kählo's artistic renderings of her personal pain, Duke Ellington's jazz compositions, or even the cartoon fantasy world created by Walt Disney? These are not idle questions. Without a way to compare the relative accomplishments of people, there can be no science of eminence.

In the past, a variety of approaches have been used to measure the relative standing of people within their fields. These included using "experts" to judge the importance or significance of peoples' works, counting the number of lines assigned to people in encyclopedias, gauging the extent to which the works of various people are represented in anthologies, or counting the number of articles, compositions, patents, or artistic productions attributed to people or the number of references to them in the literature.

Although useful, these approaches beg the question by leaving the judgment of relative creative achievement to others (i.e., encyclopedia editors, peers, reference sources) whose own criteria for eminence remain unknown. Also, the use of indirect measures of eminence, such as the number of lines assigned to people in standard encyclopedias or the number of references to them in the literature, ignores the importance of including such attributes as originality, versatility, contemporary or posthumous fame, influence over others, technical skill, or productivity as essential features of eminence. Approaches of this sort also are not appropriate when applied to people like athletes, singers, actors, and dancers who, because of the nature of their professions, are not likely to be included in standard encyclopedias or reference works. Most important, none of these approaches offers the same yardstick to measure the relative eminence of people, irrespective of their professions. As a result, they do not allow direct comparisons, for instance, of the relative eminence of a composer to a writer or an explorer to a politician.

To remedy these lacks, I undertook some time ago to develop a broad-based instrument, known as the *Creative Achievement Scale*, which could serve as a measure of relative eminence[1] (see Appendix E). This scale consists of 11 items, differing in relative importance. The "major" items include posthumous recognition, the universality of the contribution, the anticipation of social needs, influence over others, originality, and the extent of innovative accomplishments over the person's adult lifetime. The "intermediate" items include versatility, productivity, and contemporary fame. The "minor" items include professional competence and non-vocational creative pursuits. Naturally, because of the nature of these items, some degree of overlap among them is inevitable.

Since these items represent the building blocks for eminence, they need to be described in some detail. We also need to know how our distinguished persons fared on them.

THE ELEMENTS OF EMINENCE

Posthumous Recognition

Perhaps the foremost indicator of relative eminence is the extent to which people are remembered after their deaths. Unlike the fickleness and evanescence of contemporary fame, posthumous reputation, once established, sometimes persists for centuries.[2] People who were famous centuries ago, such as Aristotle, Caesar, Napoleon, Leonardo da Vinci, or Michelangelo, continue to be famous, as can be seen from the amount of space allotted to them in standard encyclopedias.

What contributes to posthumous renown is not mysterious. Generally, people whose achievements, creations, or names remain known at least one full generation after their deaths (the criterion I used to establish posthumous fame) have achieved something of lasting importance—launched political, religious, scientific, or social movements still in existence, changed the character of nations, accomplished phenomenal athletic feats, made momentous discoveries, produced works that are collected in major museums, composed music with lasting appeal, produced writings or movies or given performances that have become the standard by which to measure others, established philanthropic organizations that continue to exert worldwide influence, or had monuments, parks, institutions, and national holidays named after them because of their extraordinary achievements.

Among the people in my study, close to one-quarter achieved maximum posthumous recognition of this sort. Musical composers, physical scientists and inventors, artists, fiction writers, and architects—the investigative types and the artistic types—commanded the greatest posthumous fame.[51] Examples of those who have gained a foothold on "reputational immortality" include composers such as Béla Bartók, Claude Debussy, Antonín Dvořák, Edward Elgar, Edvard Grieg, Gustav Mahler, Sergei Rachmaninoff, Maurice Ravel, Igor Stravinsky, Richard Strauss, Duke Ellington, George Gershwin, Cole Porter, and Kurt Weill; scientists such as Harvey Cushing, Alexander Graham Bell, Thomas Edison, Alexander Fleming, Niels Bohr, and Marie Curie; artists such as Mary Cassatt, Diego Rivera, Paul Cézanne, Pablo Picasso, Edgar Degas, Marcel Duchamp, Edward Hopper, Gustav Klimt, Edvard Munch, Georgia O'Keeffe, Jackson Pollock, Pierre August Renoir, John Singer Sargent, James Whistler, and Henri Matisse; writers such as Thomas Hardy, Jean Cocteau, James Joyce, William Faulkner, F. Scott Fitzgerald, André Gide, Ernest Hemingway, Henrik Ibsen, Marcel Proust, Rudyard Kipling, George Bernard Shaw, Leo Tolstoy, Thomas Wolfe, and William Butler Yeats; and assorted others from political, business, and other arenas such as Frank Lloyd Wright, John F. Kennedy, Winston Churchill, Franklin Delano Roosevelt, Andrew Carnegie, and John D. Rockefeller, Jr.

The high name recognition of these people should be sufficient to illustrate the relative timeless quality of their fame. But often, as happens when people are viewed through the prism of posthumous fame, a subtle transformation takes place. Some undergo a centaurlike fusion with their works. They become cultural icons, shorthand, multimedia representations of that for which they have become famous. When people come to represent important symbols for certain ethnic or religious groups, written references to them begin to take on the quality of hagiographies. The myth comes to represent the greater truth. They undergo a social sanctification process, and like patron saints, tend to symbolize some special quality or feat. Thus Marilyn Monroe became a symbol of innocent sexuality. James

Dean represented troubled, rebellious youth. Albert Einstein and his equation $E = MC^2$ become inseparable. Martin Luther King, Jr. symbolizes the struggle for civil rights. Others, especially celebrities, take on Olympian personal qualities, with exaggerated virtues or faults. Sometimes their failings come to characterize them (e.g., Herbert Hoover and the Depression). Once people are accepted into this cultural pantheon of heroes, not only their accomplishments but social, political, religious, or scientific forces determine if their legacies will be perpetuated and for how long.

Universality of Contributions

Another important dimension of exceptional achievement has to do with the extent to which people produce inventions, ideas, or works that have broad human application or embody universal values or ideals. Maximum "universality" indicates that a work or performance represents a general standard of beauty or truth, offers a fundamental understanding of humans or nature, or possesses classical or multicultural appeal. Evidence of this exists when writings are translated into other languages, works of art are exhibited in museums in many countries, the contributions of individuals usually affect all media of expression within their particular fields or disciplines, entertainers are invited on multinational tours, inventions, discoveries, or products enjoy worldwide use, and the social, political, religious, or aesthetic movements initiated by individuals transcend national boundaries.

The discoveries of Thomas Alva Edison, for example, qualify as having universal use. Although he offered no new vision of the universe, he made two great discoveries in the "invention factory" he founded in Menlo Park, New Jersey. The idea for his first invention, the phonograph, came to him while he was trying to improve a telegraph repeater. Once, when working with the repeater, a tape gave off a light, rhythmical noise that sounded like indistinct human speech. What would happen, he wondered, if he connected a telephone diaphragm instead of the telegraph arm to the embossing needle? Could he record in the tape the vibrations of the human voice, which then could be played back? After a series of experiments, he finally hit on the idea of using tinfoil instead of tape, and in a demonstration later to a small group, recited the memorable words, "Mary had a little lamb," which he then, to their amazement, played back. He later went on to even greater renown and fortune by making the commercial use of the incandescent lamp a reality (which, contrary to popular myth, he did not invent). Unlike other rival inventors at the time, who used low-resistance wires and rods, Edison believed that the key to an efficient lighting system was a lamp with a high-resistance "filament." After thousands of experiments in search of such a filament, he finally found a lamp that burned for 40 hours with carbonized thread.

Among our eminent persons, 14% produced works or products with this kind of momentous impact, worldwide use, or universal appeal. These persons mostly came from professions whose media of expression could transcend the limitations of language or cultural barriers. The means for communicating with a worldwide audience was a universal language, not primarily based on words, expressed through music, art, architectural design, mathematics, science, invention, and assorted commercial products. Because of this, musical composers and natural scientists, whose works could be used and appreciated by all people, were more likely than military officers, social activists, politicians, or businesspeople, whose activities and goals had more national, regional, ethnic, or special group focus, to produce works with this kind of universal appeal.[51]

Setting New Directions

Some people are able to rise above the limitations of their societies or eras by setting new directions, anticipating social needs, creating new fields, developing new products, or demonstrating particular foresight through science fiction, economic forecasts, musical trends, architecture, experimental theater, or other media of expression. Because their works, creations or ideas are often radical or revolutionary in nature, they tend to arouse controversy, rejection, antipathy, or apathy from their colleagues or society at large. Because of this, there is a lag time of variable duration between the introduction of their ideas and their eventual acceptance.

It is possible, of course, to set new directions without arousing antagonism, but this is more likely to occur with modifications of or gradual changes in existing paradigms than with the introduction of entirely new paradigms. Shifts in traditional ways of thinking, believing, behaving, or experiencing the world, such as the shift from representational to nonrepresentational art, from tonal to atonal music, from a causal to a probabilistic universe, or from the innocence of childhood to the existence of infantile sexuality, seem to generate automatic resistance. It is the discontinuity in understanding, the necessity of making a major conceptual adjustment, that seems to be so emotionally and psychologically jarring for people. People seem least willing to accept new views when they have a personal stake in old views, especially when the new views offer no immediate advantage. By adopting radically new views or innovations, people implicitly acknowledge that their past professional judgment or behavior may have been based on false or deficient premises. This is something many people are unwilling to concede, especially if their past successes were predicated on these older views. Social acceptance of these ideas usually occurs as the older generations die off and the younger generations grow up with such ideas already established.[3]

Among our eminent persons, over one-third showed an ability to transcend the limitations of their professions, their societies, or their times to a substantial degree. Trend-setters of this sort—most notably natural scientists, musical composers, artists, poets, and social scientists—were understandably most likely to be found in those professions associated with the process of discovery or innovation.[S1]

Examples of the social or professional resistance toward the trend-setting contributions of pioneers are plentiful. Alexander Fleming's 1922 paper on lysozyme and his 1928 discovery of the antibiotic actions of the penicillin mold were met by pervasive apathy among his colleagues. In fact, from 1922 on he was nominated 14 times to become a Fellow of the Royal Society and was turned down each time, until he won the Nobel Prize in 1945. Although Nikola Tesla, the Serbian inventor of the rotating magnetic field, foresaw robots, advanced aircraft, wireless radio, broadcasting, and forecast radar he was not taken seriously at the time. Sigmund Freud's early observations on childhood sexual abuse as the cause of hysteria were met with ridicule and derision by his colleagues. Niels Bohr's doctoral thesis on the structure of the atom, which later won him a Nobel Prize, was turned down earlier by the University. The audience reacted angrily to Igor Stravinsky's opening night performance of his pioneer work, *The Rite of Spring*. Alfred Kinsey was attacked initially by both the public and his fellow scientists for his trailblazing work on human sexuality. Arnold Schoenberg's introduction of the atonal system and 12-note scale incensed music critics and musicians. Martin Luther King, Jr. generated widespread antagonism during his civil rights struggles and eventually was assassinated for his beliefs. Pablo Picasso's early Cubist paintings met with tremendous resistance, with contemporary critics denouncing them as worthless, barbaric, and the work of a madman. For many years, many of Joseph Lister's colleagues resisted his advocacy of antisepsis during surgery. Similar examples are plentiful, demonstrating that people who introduce new methods or advocate new ideas that threaten to disrupt, overthrow, or radically change the traditional paradigms within their professions are likely to endure hostility, resistance, and even persecution by their colleagues or the societies in which they live.

Influence on Other Professionals

An important element of eminence involves the extent to which individuals influence contemporary and future colleagues or the public at large. Those with maximum influence do so through international leadership, diplomacy, expertise, or innovation in their fields, serving as presidents of prestigious organizations or as editors of important journals. As prominent leaders or celebrities, they have access to large, devoted audiences. They have many imitators and attract many followers, disciples, or adherents. Classes, lecture time, biographies, articles, and dissertations are devoted to them and their works. Highly respected in their fields, they win the highest honors and awards: the Nobel Prize, the Pulitzer Prize, Knighthood, or Dame Commander of the British Empire, the Lasker Award, Oscars, Gold Medals, Lifetime Distinguished Achievement Awards from various organizations, Presidential Medals, Orders of Merit awards, Lenin Peace Prizes, invitations to deliver prestigious lectures, election to the Hall of Fame, honorary memberships into select societies, Keys to the City, election to the highest professional or social offices, honorary doctorates, profiles in national magazines, major retrospective exhibitions at the Museum of Modern Art or at the Louvre, and the naming of public buildings, parks, roads, and holidays after them.

In his later years and after his death, Carl Jung possessed this kind of ever-widening influence. A disciple of Freud's who later became an apostate, he developed an entire system of analytical psychology, which continues to attract many followers and to influence modern psychological thought. Jung's genius was to draw from many different sources—psychology, mythology, religion, and art—trying to isolate a common psychological thread connecting all ethnicities and all generations. He did this with his theory of a basic collective unconscious shared by all people, which finds its expression in the emotionally charged symbols, themes, and images—what he called primordial archetypes—that emerged spontaneously in dreams, myths, fantasies, and delusions. These major archetypes, which were limited in number, involved the great themes of birth, death, power, rebirth, the hero, the child and the demon, among others. Jung also formulated the notion of the psychological bisexuality of humans, with each person possessing a different balance between the masculine archetype, the *animus*, and the feminine archetype, the *anima*. He regarded other complementary opposites, such as introversion and extroversion, as existing in humans as well. Self-realization and psychological health came about only through a creative synthesis of these opposing elements. These views were original enough and differed substantially enough from established psychoanalysis to attract many adherents throughout the world. Today, as with psychoanalysis, there are numerous Jungian institutes, which train practitioners in the theory and practice of analytic psychology.

Among our eminent persons, about one-fifth exerted maximum influence of this sort on their contemporaries and future generations. Even though people who wielded such great influence on their colleagues could be found in almost all professions, they were more likely to come from the ranks of the natural scientists, musical composers, architects, and musical entertainers—again, people who worked in professions whose media of expression transcended national language barriers or whose products were potentially accessible to all.[51]

Originality

One of the most important dimensions of creative achievement involves innovation or originality. But innovation or originality can vary in degree and importance. Although their own work is not distinctive or original, some people achieve eminence by their ingenuity or diligence in implementing the basic ideas of others or of their times. Others who are more innovative make accomplishments within the context of tradition but with a new twist or perspective. While representing progress or an extension of what existed before (e.g., setting a new record), their accomplishments offer no major changes in perception, understanding, or behavior. Others, who display an even higher level of innovation or originality, produce works that modify basic principles, concepts, or theories, or change a component of a whole system rather than the entire system itself. At the highest level of innovation or originality, people create original products that are qualitatively different from what existed before. They employ ingenious strategies to solve previously insoluble problems, or make major discoveries that represent watershed events in the development of a discipline. The works or accomplishments of these individuals represent scientific, artistic, or conceptual breakthroughs that revolutionize an entire field, open new frontiers, establish new disciplines, create new genres, or radically alter interpretations of human nature or reality.

Among our eminent persons, about one-fourth showed these highest levels of originality. Natural scientists, followed next by musical composers, architects, artists, and poets, were those most likely to make major discoveries, show the greatest originality, or extend the frontiers of their fields.[51]

It is ironic that Alexander Graham Bell, who started his career at a school for deaf mutes in Boston and who, until his death, regarded himself as a teacher of the deaf, should have created an instrument that the deaf could not use and that alienated them even more from society. Long before Bell made his discovery, the groundwork for the telephone already had been laid. Scientists already knew about electromagnetism: that electric currents generated electric fields around themselves. They also knew about induction: that a magnetic field changing in strength or position could generate a current in a circuit. It was Bell's genius to recognize that the varying sound of the human voice could be made to alter the intensity of an electrical current, which then could be reproduced in speech. This was the fundamental principle underlying his invention of the telephone.

The biochemical achievements of Albert Szent-Györgyi were impressive in an entirely different way. With his discovery of 4-carbon fumaric acid, he laid the foundation for the discovery of the Krebs cycle. He received a Nobel Prize for his work on Vitamin C and the nature of cellular metabolism. He postulated the existence of Vitamin P as necessary for the maintenance of the capillary structure. He discovered the protein actin and explained its role, along with myosin and ATP, in muscle movement. Besides "fathering" the field of modern muscle physiology, he also pioneered an original way of looking at the cancer problem and the nature of life itself.

Alan Turing described a universal machine capable of modeling the process of computation. It would consist of no more than a continuous tape divided into cells. The machine would be capable of moving the tape to the right or the left, to print the numbers 0 or 1, to stop the tape, and to erase. On the basis of this universal machine, Turing was able to prove that there were noncomputable functions and that predicate logic was undecidable.

Duke Ellington, perhaps the greatest jazz composer, violated traditional rules and broke new ground in his classical compositions. His inclination to break rules, according to certain critics, was almost a matter of temperament rather than a rational process and characterized much of his work. If he suspected, for instance, that traditionally one was not supposed to use parallel fifths, he would immediately find a way of using them; or if he learned that major sevenths must always rise, he would write a tune in which the line descended from the major seventh. He did not even formally plan most of his compositions before he came to the studio, creating them extemporaneously.

When people manifest this degree of originality or inspiration, it is little wonder that some attribute almost divine powers to them. People who break out of traditional thought patterns and ways of interpreting reality achieve what should be impossible. Later I comment on the qualities of mind, personality attributes, and life experiences necessary for certain gifted people to make these momentous breakthroughs.

Extent of Innovative Accomplishments

People need not confine their creations, trend-setting works, masterpieces, innovations, discoveries, or great deeds to one field or discipline. Those who have a broad-based, Renaissance genius capable of crossing intellectual domains may make original or novel achievements in several fields during their lifetimes. Had they not become eminent in one field, they likely would have become eminent in another.

Among our eminent persons, about 1% made innovative or original contributions of this sort in three or more separate fields; 7% in two separate fields; 62% in one field; and 30% in no field. Investigative and artistic types—mainly architects, followed next by natural scientists, social scientists, poets, artists, and musical composers—were those who made the most varied original contributions.[51]

The breadth of achievements for certain of these individuals was phenomenal. Churchill was not only a great statesman, but a superb essayist and historian. Harvey Cushing was one of the founders of neurosurgery, an outstanding scientist, and an author of several "classics" on the history of medicine and surgery, many of which he illustrated himself. Albert Schweitzer was a famous missionary physician, a philosopher, and theologian of some renown, as well as a concert performer and composer. Noel Coward was an outstanding playwright, actor, composer, novelist, and director. Percy Crosby was not only a noted cartoonist, the creator of Skippy, but published widely in fiction, poetry, philosophy, politics, as well as literary and art criticism.

Numerous other individuals made substantial contributions in at least two fields. Fred Astaire was a dancer and actor; Albert Camus a writer and philosopher; Charlie Chaplin an entertainer, director, and playwright; Claude Debussy a composer and pianist; Walt Disney a cartoonist and entrepreneur; Albert Einstein a physicist and philosopher; John Huston an actor and director; Cole Porter a composer and entertainer; Paul Robeson a singer, actor, and talented athlete; James Thurber a cartoonist and writer;

Leo Tolstoy a novelist, philosopher, and religious leader; and Andy Warhol an artist and film director.

While these limited examples show that people may express their genius in many areas, they shed no light on the potential plasticity or adaptability of geniuses who have made their mark in only one domain. What would have happened if, for some reason, certain persons had been thwarted in expressing their particular gifts? Would they have found some other way to achieve eminence or greatness? Suppose, for example, Claude Debussy had been deaf, Georgia O'Keeffe blind, Leo Tolstoy dyslexic, or Martin Luther King, Jr. white. Or suppose they were born in different cultures and had no opportunity to pursue the fields in which they made their mark. What would their lives and accomplishments have been? This is, of course, an impossible question to answer, but it allows me to make an important point.

According to a leading theorist on creativity, at least three conditions are necessary for optimal achievement.[4] People must possess *domain-relevant skills*. These include formal knowledge about a domain such as art, music, or science, and the appropriate technical skill to be proficient in that domain. People who acquire this level of knowledge and skill require appropriate formal and informal education for the development of their innate cognitive abilities or perceptual and motor skills. People also must possess *creativity-relevant skills*. These include an appropriate cognitive style capable of generating novel ideas and a work style that allows for their expression. Appropriate cognitive and work styles depend upon experience in the generation of ideas and certain personality characteristics, such as self-discipline, perseverance, and nonconformity. And last, people must possess the proper *task motivation*. The reasons for performing a particular task or creating a new work must be appropriate, driven more by inner necessity than by conformity to social expectations.

This formulation is helpful, since it shows the complexity of factors involved in creative works. We can assume, then, that extraordinary people such as Tolstoy, O'Keeffe, Debussy, or King could be expected to make extraordinary achievements in completely different fields only if all the conditions for achievement were met. Success requires more than creativity, knowledge, or perseverance: it requires certain fortuitous circumstances as well. Francis Galton's claim that true genius cannot be denied only seems to hold if no serious impediments exist, if nothing prevents this genius from being expressed, and if society comes to appreciate it.

Versatility

Versatility (i.e., the degree to which individuals are active in more than one field or employ two or more media of expression) is related to but not identical with the extent of innovative achievement. This particular characteristic has less to do with originality than with competency, proficiency, skill, or even intense interest in different fields. In distinction to the broad-based genius that is necessary for achieving breakthroughs in different fields, versatility mainly refers to multiple talents, not to how great these talents are. It is possible, then, for people to be highly versatile or multitalented without necessarily making any original contributions.

Some years ago, Ralph K. White studied the versatility of a sample of 300 geniuses.[5] Employing the extensive biographical material compiled by Catherine Cox, he rated each person on the ability shown in 23 different fields. The results revealed that most of these individuals showed more than ordinary ability in five to ten fields. Nonfiction writers, leaders, and philosophers were the most versatile; scholars, religious leaders, scientists, poets, mathematicians, novelists, and dramatists were next; soldiers and artists after them; and musicians were the least versatile. He also found that certain of these abilities clustered together. Science, mathematics, medicine, invention and handiwork, and perhaps art formed one tight cluster. Poetry, fiction, drama, and perhaps nonfiction formed another; philosophy, social theory, history, and languages another; politics, warfare, and business another. Although the author expected to find a general aesthetic cluster, he found none. Poets seemed more like novelists or essayists than like musicians or artists; artists seemed more like scientists than like poets or musicians; and musicians were anomalous.

In our sample of eminent persons, 10% showed competency or proficiency in three or more separate fields (or two or more different media within at least one of two fields); 28% in two separate fields; 43% in two or more related media of expression within a particular field; and 19% in only one medium or none at all. Architects and designers showed the greatest versatility, followed next by natural scientists, fiction writers, musical composers, and artists.[S1]

Examples of persons with tremendous versatility were plentiful. John Held, Jr. was not only a proficient cartoonist and illustrator, but wrote fiction, made block prints, created bronzes, painted water colors, wrote children's stories, comic plays, and essays, and designed jewelry and doll furniture. John Huston was a director, writer, and actor. T. E. Lawrence led a legendary life as a scholar, soldier, and archeologist. Beryl Markham was an outstanding horse trainer in Kenya, a writer, and a pilot. Simone de Beauvoir was a novelist, philosopher, and political activist. Marc Blitzstein was a composer, playwright, lyricist, and librettist for his own works. J. B. S. Haldane, who did pioneer scientific work on respiratory mechanisms, was a brilliant biochemist, geneticist, physiologist, mathematician, and political activist as well. Bertrand Russell was a philosopher, mathematician, and social activist. George Santayana was a philosopher, poet, and literary critic. Orson Welles, an originator of the *film noir* genre and the perpetrator of the infamous 1938 radio broadcast about the invasion from Mars, was an actor, broadcaster, director, scriptwriter, and producer. Oscar Wilde excelled as a novelist, playwright, essayist, and poet. Alfred North Whitehead made important contributions to philosophy and mathematics. Alexander Woollcott, an original member of the famed Algonquin Club, was a talented journalist, drama critic, actor, playwright, world traveler, and radio broadcaster. Elsie De Wolfe, the backer of Cole Porter's first musical, the sponsor of Cecil Beaton's first show in New York, and one of the best dressed actresses on Broadway, was a director, businesswoman, actress, and the nation's first interior decorator. William Butler Yeats, the Irish poet, was also a playwright, novelist, essayist, and statesman. And Mark Twain was a novelist, essayist, and entertainer.

What these assorted observations suggest is that outstanding achievement in one field or with one medium of expression need not preclude interest or competence in another. Versatile people have broad-based talents and interests that are not so easily confined by the artificial boundaries of certain fields. Presumably, they resort to a variety of media of expression because no one medium satisfies them entirely or because having achieved mastery in one area, they feel challenged to seek it in others.

Although I concentrate here for obvious reasons on vocational activities, many eminent people also express their enormous creativity and ability in their leisure-time activities. One anecdotal study, for example, documented the high proportion of painters, sketchers, etchers, architects, photographers, weavers, cloth makers, woodworkers, metal workers, craftspeople, musicians, poets, dramatists, and fiction writers in a group of outstanding scientists, many of whom were Nobel laureates.[6] Within my sample of eminent persons, 60% engaged in a variety of creative hobbies.[51] Two of the more unusual creative hobbies were shown by noted scientists. Alexander Fleming, the discoverer of penicillin, took microorganisms that developed colors, smeared them on a petri dish, incubated them, and then, in a day or so, created "germ paintings" of all sorts. Besides conducting scientific experiments on peanuts and other crops, George Washington Carver used paints made from clays to paint over 70 pictures.

These nonvocational interests are not necessarily divorced from these people's professional accomplishments and lives. Just as peoples' work can become an extension of them, so also their hobbies. The creative nature of their hobbies may also be reflected in their work. The notion that avocational activities may have an important bearing on vocational creativity and achievement receives support from recent research.[7] Within a group of 40 scientists, including four Nobel laureates, various hobbies not only were significantly related to various modes of creative thinking but to scientific success as well. For example, the visual arts, including painting, drawing, and photography, along with certain musical hobbies, including composing, singing, and playing an instrument, were associated with using visual images while problem solving. Collecting art was specifically related to the use of abstractions during problem solving, while sculpting was specifically related to imageless, nonverbal thought and kinesthetic thinking. Creative writing and poetry were related to the use of visualized symbols during problem solving. Whether these specific hobbies facilitated specific modes of creative thinking in scientists or whether these specific modes of thought stimulated interest in certain kinds of hobbies could not be established by this study. But what the study did show was that the most successful scientists used these specific modes of thought in problem solving and engaged in these specific hobbies. Among these individuals, avocations, styles of thinking, and scientific success were integrally linked.

The reason that these observations are so intriguing is that they confirm the usefulness of the concept of "networks of enterprise"[8]—the implicit structure that people use to order their needs, perceptions, and activities—as a way of interpreting human behavior. Successful scientists are likely to use successful networks of enterprise in which all elements are connected with others. They are apt to view their hobbies not only as necessary for being cultured but as valuable forms of training for problem solving. This successful integration of important elements in the networks of high-ranking scientists is different from what happens in low-ranking ones. Many low-ranking scientists engage in as wide a range of activities as high-ranking ones, but unlike them, they lack a unifying focus or global perception of knowledge that integrates their perceptions and activities. Because of this, the elements within their networks compete with each other for their attention. As a result, for these scientists, hobbies detract from rather than enhance their creativity and problem solving.

Productivity

For many, productivity represents the hallmark of eminence,[9] and with good reason. Many famous artists, composers, writers, and scientists display a prodigious output. Productivity also represents a practical and objective criterion for eminence, since it can be counted and measured. But as attractive as this criterion is, it has certain drawbacks. The limited productivity of some, such as Niels Bohr, Franz Kafka, Marcel Duchamp, or Stephen Crane, shows that it is not always a good predictor of eminence. Productivity also does not assure quality. Many extremely productive people produce nothing of lasting merit. Productivity also differs across professions and, in some professions, is without exact measure. For example, how do we equate the number of paintings produced by an artist with the musical compositions of a classical composer, the novels by a writer, the buildings designed and built by an architect, or the performances of an actor or entertainer? How do we assess the relative productivity of a businessperson, a soldier, a politician, an athlete, a social activist, or an explorer?

Yet if the criterion of productivity is to have wide application and be an important dimension of professional achievement, we need to be able to extend its definition to activities customarily not included. Politicians should perhaps get credit for the number of their speeches or the bills they initiated and got passed. Entertainers and actors should be credited with the extent to which they vary their performances or play different roles or make different films. What this indicates is the need to judge the relative productivity of persons within the context or constraints of their fields.

For our purposes, then, productivity refers to the amount rather than quality of a person's professional output over an ordinary lifetime and need not be original or innovative. It can only be judged by the standards for productivity with a particular field. Athletes and dancers, who rely on physical agility, for example, have a shorter time frame for their accomplishments than, say, writers, composers, or actors. Because productivity becomes equivalent to the entire body of works over an ordinary lifetime, it likely will be influenced by longevity or certain age or expressive constraints operating within certain professions, assuming other factors to be equal. People who commit suicide or die at an early age are obviously less likely to have a prodigious output than those with a normal life span. Although equally driven and persevering, other individuals, such as politicians, soldiers, or entrepreneurs, who produce no personal, expressive works but rely mainly on other people for advice or to carry out their policies, can be assumed to show less personal productivity than those in professions that require individual expression or personal works.

Among our eminent persons, 31% displayed a prodigious output over the course of their lives; 35% produced an average body of work; 31% produced a small output, sometimes being limited in their productivity by prolonged illnesses, career changes, low motivation, writing blocks, hospitalization, imprisonment, premature deaths or other factors; and 3% had few if any works. Architects, composers, social scientists, natural scientists, nonfiction writers, artists, fiction writers, and musical entertainers—namely, the investigative types and artistic types[S1]—were more likely than other professionals to be prolific.

Special mention should be made of the fact that the exceptional productivity of almost one-third of our people represented truly phenomenal output. This supported observations by others that geniuses not only were highly ambitious and driven people but capable of prodigious amounts of work. Not all the work produced by great people is necessarily great, however. Some may be of mediocre or even poor quality. In the long list of examples below I make no judgment about the quality of this output. I also am not qualified to judge redundancy, repetition, and recurring themes within these works and how many of them are truly original. By deliberately giving many examples, I simply wish to dramatize the prominence of this feature.

The great composers appear to be a particularly prolific group. Bela Bartok, the Hungarian composer and pianist, produced over 100 works from 1904 to 1945. Duke Ellington created about 1,200 jazz compositions. Jerome Kern composed melodies for over 1,000 songs. Sergei Prokofiev, the Russian composer and pianist, wrote eight ballets, incidental music for four dramatic productions, eight film scores, 10 symphonies, nine concertos, about 20 suites, about 15 musical scores for instrumental ensembles, about 30 vocal symphonic musical compositions and cantatas, and about 20 sonatas and other piano works. Igor Stravinsky produced about 30 theoretical works, 34 orchestral works, 17 choral works, 25 vocal works, 15 piano works, 20 instrumental works and two arrangements of other composers' works. He also wrote two books, coauthored six books on commentaries and views, along with conducting orchestras and giving concerts. Arnold Schoenberg produced at least 50 opuses and about 10 books, in addition to a number of screenplays, a book of poetry, four collections of short stories, two novels, and his memoirs.

In their own way, the writers, playwrights, and poets were equally as prolific, although it was difficult to compare the amount of effort required for verbal compositions with that for musical compositions. W. H. Auden, the British–American poet, who became a dominant voice in 20th-century English verse, published at least 43 books or collections of prose and verse, as well as other writings. Vladimir Nabokov, during his first 2 decades of exile from Russia alone, published eight novels, two novellas, about 50 short stories, over 100 poems, four plays, several translations, and dozens of chess problems and crossword puzzles, besides teaching and avidly pursuing his hobbies in chess and lepidopterology. Tennessee Williams wrote 25 full-length plays, over 40 short plays, dozens of screenplays, two novels, one novella, over 60 short stories, over 100 poems, and an opera libretto. Jean-Paul Sartre wrote about 50 books, including novels, plays, collections of essays, and assorted other writing. Besides his being an actor, world traveler, radio broadcaster, and the drama critic for the New York Times, Alexander Woollcott found time to write over 20 books and anthologies, hundreds of magazine articles, and thousands of radio programs and theatrical reviews. Upton Sinclair wrote over 80 books. John Buchan, who served as British Governor-General for Canada and held many political posts, wrote over 50 books, including novels, collections of essays, biographies and histories. Agatha Christie wrote over 75 novels, many successful plays, and a book of poetry. John Middleton Murry, the English writer, published 60 books.

Art is another area where productivity becomes evident. However, because of the nature of the medium of expression and the inclinations of the artist, the length of time it takes to produce a work of art may vary greatly, from minutes (as in the case of many of Picasso's line drawings) to months. Paul Cézanne produced over 1,000 paintings, watercolors, and drawings. Jacob Camille Pissarro, a founder and leader of the Impressionist movement, produced at least 1,300 oil paintings, 190 gouaches, 102 pastels, and 55 fans, besides many watercolors, drawings, and at least 200 prints. During his short lifetime of 36 years, Henri Toulouse-Lautrec produced about 600 paintings, 330 lithographs, 31 posters, nine dry points and three monotypes, as well as thousands of drawings and sketches. Francis Picabia, the dadaist and cubist, produced over 400 paintings and lithographs, over 50 books, over 130 articles on art and related subjects, besides creating sceneries, sets, and costumes for several films. Pierre Auguste Renoir produced 720 paintings. John Singer Sargent painted over 600 portraits and over 2,500 other works.

Work output of this magnitude is not only found in the arts. Many of the natural and social scientists display it as well. Luther Burbank, the horticulturist, developed over 800 new varieties of fruits, flowers, ornamentals, vegetables, grains, grasses, and forage plants. Emile Durkheim, the sociologist, wrote 13 books and over 600 articles and reviews. Bill Lear, the aviator, inventor, and businessman, patented over 150 inventions and designs in electronics and aerodynamics. Arnold J. Toynbee published over 40 titles, including his monumental 12-volume work *The Study of History*. Ruth Benedict, the anthropologist, published over 60 works. John Dewey, the philosopher, writer, and social activist, wrote over 40 books, as well as 160 articles. Bertrand Russell, the philosopher, mathematician, and social activist, wrote about 50 books and numerous articles. John Ruskin, the art historian and essayist, produced 39 volumes of collected works. Robert Goddard, the astronautical scientist, secured over 200 patents during his lifetime, covering basic inventions in the field of rockets, guided missiles, and space exploration, and had another 131 patents issued after his death.

As impressive as this output is, the Herculean productivity of certain of these individuals is mind- boggling and deserves special emphasis. Thomas Alva Edison had 1,093 patents, an average of about one a week for over 20 years. Pablo Picasso, whose estimated works number over 20,000, produced 165 paintings in 1969 to 1970 alone. Le Corbusier produced 57 buildings, about 1,400 sets of plans, and over 50 books. Phenomenally productive writers sometimes required several identities to take credit for their many works. Georges Simenon, the creator of Inspector Maigret and perhaps the most prolific major novelist the world has ever known, published 220 books under his own name, another 200 shorter novels under 17 different pseudonyms, and more than a thousand articles and stories. Frederick Faust, best known for his novels about the West written under his alias, Max Brand, and the creation of his character Dr. Kildare, was also remarkably productive. Although he was prematurely killed in action during World War II at the age of 52, he published over 30 million words, the equivalent of about 400 novels, under 19 pseudonyms. A bibliography of his short stories alone, which number in the hundreds, fills over 20 pages. As indicative of his phenomenal abilities, we also should take note that in one 13-day stretch he set a personal record, and maybe a world record, of turning out 190,000 publishable words in the form of two long serials and a novelette—the equivalent of one book in every 4⅓ days.

There are some lessons to be drawn from these many examples. Obviously, what productivity of this sort suggests is that eminence does not come easily. These individuals work at it and keep working at it even after they have become relatively well-known. From the amount of work they produce, it is amazing that they have time for anything else.

Although many people need to produce a large body of work to come up with the few precious nuggets that will insure their place in history, productivity can also be a double-edged sword. After a while, people who produce too much may not be taken as seriously by their colleagues or the public at large, especially when certain patterns and themes keep reappearing in their works. These people walk a fine line between getting peoples' attention and turning them off. Rather than being viewed as prolific, they risk being viewed as hacks, which is partly why certain writers publish books under different names.

While productivity seems a necessary condition for eminence in certain fields, it is not a sufficient one. Many noneminent people may be equally as productive. What distinguishes the work of eminent and noneminent people is its relative importance and variety. This was clearly shown to be the case in a predictive study of scientific eminence.[10] The results revealed that scientists who published a series of five or more "high-impact" papers by the age of 45 along with simultaneous research involvement in several areas went on to produce high-impact papers in their late 50s and 60s, whereas the other scientists did not. A "high-impact" paper meant an article that colleagues cited 10 or more times over 15 years. Less than 1% of the papers achieved this distinction.

Contemporary Fame

Fame can be fickle and accidental, a consequence of good fortune, fashion, and circumstance. It can disappear as quickly as it arises. A writer with a bestseller may not produce another successful novel. A famous politician may lose an election due to events not under his control or fall out of favor in the wake of a scandal. An economic crisis may force an entrepreneur to go bankrupt. The popularity of actors and directors may plummet after their involvement with several flops.

While fame or celebrity status during people's lifetimes may not always be essential for achieving posthumous recognition, especially when their reputations are enhanced by the manner of their death, it does not hurt. Although only a small portion of celebrities, stars, and well-known people achieves lasting fame, nearly all eminent individuals have been famous during their lives.[11] Generally, the more famous people are during their lifetimes, the more famous they are likely to be after their deaths.

For the purposes of my study, fame was based on the extent to which the works, products, or performances of people during their lifetimes were admired, accepted by, or known to members of their own professions and/or the public. The degree of fame, celebrity status, or public acclaim roughly corresponded to the extent to which individuals had immediate name recognition, had their writings translated into other languages, had disciples and followers, had their works collected and exhibited in prestigious museums, or had their discoveries, products, or performances widely used, appreciated, or admired. Among our eminent people, about one-fourth achieved worldwide fame of this sort. Musical composers, natural scientists, musical entertainers, and architects—people whose media of expression were not bound by the limitations of language—were most likely to enjoy this status.

Although people gained contemporary fame or celebrity status in many ways, certain routes were more common than others. One common route to fame involved performing feats that captured the public imagination. Charles Lindbergh became an international hero after flying alone across the Atlantic, as did Beryl Markham after crossing in the other direction. Harry Houdini attracted huge crowds and extensive media coverage for his daring escape challenges and magic performances. Ernest Henry Shackleton gained fame when he headed a dangerous expedition to Antarctica.

Others gained attention for living near-legendary lives. The personal adventures of Ernest Hemingway rivaled those of any of his fictional characters. F. Scott Fitzgerald, along with his talented and unstable wife, Zelda, led a glamorous life marked by tragedy. Ezra Pound gained international renown not only for his poetry but for his treasonous activities during World War II. Barney Oldfield's achievements in car racing were almost dwarfed by his many misadventures.

Another common route to fame concerned the development of widely used products. Henry Ford became famous after his development of the Model-T car. Sigmund Freud gained fame because of the broad use of psychoanalysis as a method of treating neuroses. Alexander Fleming became famous for his discovery of penicillin. Alfred Hitchcock became famous for his suspense films. Walt Disney's name became associated with his popular cartoon characters.

Others became famous by attracting large followings. This was most likely to be the case with successful politicians, such as Winston Churchill or Franklin Delano Roosevelt, social activists, such as Martin Luther King, Jr., Emma Goldman, or Margaret Sanger, or founders of new religious or social movements, such as Mary Baker Eddy, the originator of Christian Science, or Carry Nation, the colorful, ax-wielding leader of the temperance movement. Those who are in the entertainment industry, who exploit the mass media, or who otherwise receive great public exposure also have good opportunities to achieve lifetime fame.

Finally, some became famous through associations with other well-known people. This association could come about through marriage or love affairs with them, through being their biological relative, through handling or critiquing their works, or through being their patrons or adversaries. In my sample of eminent people, this was the way that many spouses and lovers, hostesses, museum curators, and art and music critics gained renown.

Skill

Another aspect of professional achievement concerns the technical competence or skill people display in their works or creations. "Skill" refers to any special ability or facility with music, memory, mimicry, interpersonal encounters, mathematics, physical agility, color, drawing, spatial sense, mechanical ingenuity, writing, and so on, usually but not necessarily noted by the time the person is in his or her late teens. Skill or facility, however, need not be associated with innovation, creativity, or originality.

Among our eminent persons, less than 10% showed virtuosity, mastery, or "genius" in at least one special area. This type of virtuosity was mostly found in musical composers, musical entertainers, athletes, natural scientists, and social scientists.[51] In addition, about one-third had "exceptional" talents in a given area or medium of expression, or were experts in a special technique. Almost all of the remainder were "competent" craftspeople in their fields or media of expression, although they showed no exceptional natural talents, facilities, or skills.

Examples are necessary to illustrate certain of these virtuoso abilities. Enrico Caruso, the great tenor, could exert great anatomical control over his body. He developed a chest expansion of 9 inches and could put an egg in his mouth and close his lips without puffing his cheeks. Rex Stout began reading at 18 months. By the age of 7 he was one-fifth of the way through his father's library of over 1,000 books, and by the age of 11 he finished them. He also was considered a mathematical prodigy by age 10. Picasso's painting abilities were so extraordinary by age 14 that his father, a competent artist himself, turned his brushes over to him and gave up painting. Scriabin began composing in his early teens; his *Etude in C-minor*, composed at age 15, is still considered a masterpiece. Orson Welles was speaking in "polished sentences" by age 2 and acted in the Chicago Opera Company's production of *Madame Butterfly* at age 3. Leopold Stokowski conducted his first orchestra at age 12. Marc Blitzstein played the piano by ear at age 3, showed perfect pitch at age 5, gave his first public performance at age 7, and produced incredible compositions at age 13. Frederick Lindemann was a mathematical genius and lightning calculator as a child. He had an incredible memory and facility for figures and could memorize a page of them and add them up to thirty decimal places. Fred Astaire danced professionally at age 6. John Held, Jr., produced remarkable watercolors at age 8 and published cartoons by age 14. Gustav Mahler was regarded as a virtuoso at the piano by age 10.

Sometimes, these extraordinary abilities take unusual forms. Because of his photographic memory, which could store entire logarithmic tables that he could call up when needed, Nikola Tesla could invent and even pretest things in his imagination. He could change the construction, make improvements, operate the device in his mind, and perfect it without ever actually creating it. Only when he was sure he had corrected any problems did he put the device into concrete form. Often, he would experience inexplicable flashes of light when a new idea opened possibilities to him. He claimed that in the many years he conducted mental experiments, there was never an instance when the actual experiment, performed later, failed to conform to what he figured out beforehand from the available theoretical and practical data.

Glenn Gould had the remarkable capacity to process sounds in highly unusual ways. He could read magazines while talking on the phone and could learn a Beethoven score while carrying on a conversation. He liked to play two radios simultaneously, the FM to hear the music and the AM to hear the news. When he was in a hurry to learn a new score, he would run a vacuum cleaner or listen to any loud noise. Besides listening to and memorizing several things at once, Gould could hear with incredible precision. Sound engineers were once amazed to discover that he could differentiate between playbacks from two different digital recording systems with identical technical specifications. With his remarkable powers of concentration, he also could play chess blindfolded, even when participating in several games simultaneously.

Arnold Toynbee, the great historian, claimed to be able to experience mystical encounters with the past. On January 10, 1912, while contemplating the site of an ancient battle, he vividly "saw" in his mind's eye how the Romans had defeated the Macedonians there in 197 B.C. Three months later, in Crete, he envisioned the Turkish victory of 1669 when he caught sight of an abandoned Venetian villa. Another time, while visiting a remote site, he "fell again into the deep trough of Time" on seeing abandoned bronze cannons littering the site. There were other "transports" as well, infinitely brief but very poignant moments that, he believed, allowed him to achieve "a momentary communion with the actors in a particular historic event."

Although the possession of exceptional abilities such as these seems advantageous, especially in certain professions, it is important to note that almost two-thirds of our people managed to become eminent without them. Though this probably reflected the nature of their professions or fields, it also showed that far more than innate, extraordinary gifts are necessary for eminence. Even without any virtuoso talent or exceptional intelligence, many people managed to become eminent by capitalizing on whatever abilities they possessed and the circumstances that came their way.

LIFETIME CREATIVE ACHIEVEMENT

We can draw three conclusions from the observations so far. One is that lifetime creative achievement represents a complex phenomenon that includes many separate but interrelated components. Another is that the members of different professions fare better on certain of these components than on others. Yet another is that members of the artistic and investigative professions consistently do better on every component of creative achievement than those in the social or enterprising ones.

Since it is too unwieldy to categorize people by their standings on each of these separate components, we need a single, composite measure that takes all of them into account. The *Creative Achievement Scale*, with demonstrated reliability and validity, serves this purpose well. What is especially remarkable is that total scores on this scale assigned to eminent persons correlate highly with the actual number of lines allotted to them in both the *Encyclopaedia Britannica* and the *Encyclopedia Americana*. Since the amount of space allotted to people in these standard references is a measure of their relative eminence, regardless of their professions, then the total scores on this scale, which correlate highly with this amount of space, represent a measure of eminence as well. We can assume, then, that the higher the creative achievement of people, the greater their eminence or greatness.

When we compare the lifetime achievements of members of the different professions, we find, understandably, that musical composers, natural scientists, architects, artists, fiction writers, social scientists, poets, musical performers, actors and directors, and nonfiction writers rank highest and famous companions, social figures, explorers and adventurers, sports figures, military officers, athletes, and businesspeople rank lowest (see Figure 6.1).[52] These findings essentially show that while members of the various creative arts professions, as a whole, display greater creative achievement over the entirety of their lives than members of most other professions, they do not have a monopoly on it. Natural scientists, in fact, rank next to highest among all the professional groups, and social scientists or academicians rank higher than nonfiction writers, musical performers, poets, and members of the theater. This suggests that it is not so much the attributes of innovativeness or originality that distinguish members of the creative arts from those engaged in scientific and academic pursuits, but rather the formal requirements of their vocations. Those in the creative arts appear to rely more on personalized, stylistic, or private media of expression, while those in the natural and social sciences appear to rely more on impersonal, consensual, and public media of expression.

However, as the eminence of many politicians, social activists, entrepreneurs, explorers, and others bears witness, creative activity is not the only route to fame or greatness. Aside from the importance of making novel or unique contributions, individuals in fields other than the arts and sciences may require special personal qualities for success. Explorers or military officers, for example, need to be courageous or undertake bold initiatives; politicians need to understand the temper of the times and show

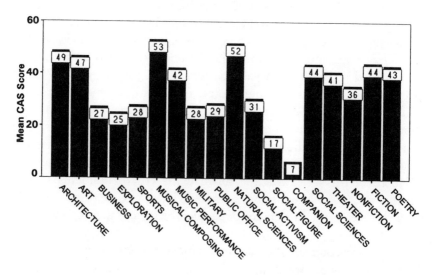

Figure 6.1. Creative Achievement Scale (CAS) scores.

great leadership abilities; entrepreneurs need to anticipate social needs, take risks, and know how to market products; and social activists need a strong sense of mission and purpose to endure the personal dangers of their activities. Because Western culture places different premiums on different kinds of professional accomplishments, the relative stature of persons in certain fields may be far less when compared to that of eminent people in general than when compared to that of people within their own fields.

So far, then, we have shown that the relative eminence of people can be measured by their creative achievements. Members of certain professions, as whole, show different degrees of creative achievement than those in other professions. Although this is hardly surprising, it is still important to demonstrate. If members of certain professions show greater creative achievements than those in other professions, we should not be surprised to find that they differ in their susceptibility to mental illness as well.

CHAPTER SEVEN

Mental Illness within the Professions

According to a tale by Sophocles, a snake bit Philoctetes after he came into possession of a miraculous bow that never missed its target. Because of the stench and ugliness of his wound, his fellow warriors banished him to Lemnos. Now, an outcast, he silently endured his anguish alone. A modern reading of the legend argues that his lingering pain, emotional agony, and social alienation was the personal price he had to pay for possessing this magical bow.[1]

Despite the message of this tale, the notion that people should have to endure mental suffering for their extraordinary gifts is not as fanciful as it first seems. In a penetrating analysis of this subject, Ruth Richards describes three biological models of ways in which sickness and health may be intertwined from an evolutionary standpoint. These models have to do with acquired immunity, compensatory advantage, and outmoded genetic blueprints.[2]

The *acquired immunity* model comes from the observation that certain people may gain a biological advantage after being exposed to certain diseases by acquiring a resistance to more virulent forms of these diseases in the future. This has been the rationale in the past for using attenuated viruses for certain vaccines or deliberately exposing children at an early age to chicken pox or mumps in order for them to avoid the potentially more serious consequences of these diseases during their adulthood. Thus getting sick, at least mildly so, can be a way of staying well in the future. Extrapolating to the psychological sphere, we can find an analogue of acquired immunity in the resistance of many great individuals to personal adversity or their courage in the face of danger. For certain people, their past exposure to troubled childhoods, emotional deprivation, broken homes, physical disability, or the early death of parents, instead of incapacitating them, may provide them with a "psychic immunity" to extreme stress later in life. It is as though they have been "fire-tested" and "kiln-hardened" by what they have had to endure. This may make them better able to go against the odds or confront difficult situations that others tend to avoid.

The *compensatory model* indicates that the presence of certain diseases in individuals may give them an increased resistance to other diseases. This is clearly seen in sickle-cell disease. While the person who inherits the disease from both parents develops a serious anemia with the risk of early death, the larger number of sickle-cell carriers who inherit the trait from only one parent develop only a mild anemia but show a positive compensatory advantage in their resistance to malaria. In the psychological sphere, manic–depressive illness seems an appropriate analogue. Not only does this illness have a strong genetic component, but it is often found in well-known creative persons. There also appears to be evidence that the normal relatives of bipolar persons, who are more likely to possess the trait for this disorder, are more creative than those of certain control groups. As for the nature of the compensatory advantage, it could comprise the fluent ideas, rapid thoughts, mental playfulness, and elevated mood commonly found in milder forms of mania. Persons with mania also may have greater access to the "mental edge of chaos," which provides a fertile source for new ideas and insights. Though incapacitating to most, this disease, especially in its milder forms, may give some of those afflicted an advantage over others in their creativity and work output.

The *outmoded genetic blueprint model* notes that those species that adapt best to changing environmental conditions tend to be most successful from an evolutionary perspective in perpetuating themselves. Those that do not tend to become extinct. Their genetic blueprints, which once were adequate for survival, now become outmoded. On an analogous basis, we may presume that certain psychological disorders in the past became extinct because they served no socially adaptive purpose and that certain of the ones that survived offered more advantages to the affected individuals and society as a whole. With some stretch of the imagination, we can view persons genetically predisposed to alcoholism or drug use, who experience alterations in consciousness while intoxicated, as engaging in trial-and-error experiments with different perceptions of reality. While almost all of the insights gleaned by chemical means prove trivial and useless, certain rare individuals may be able to rise above their addictions and capitalize on certain of their novel perceptions in their writing, art, or music for the enrichment of others. Because of these potential benefits, disorders of this nature may have some evolutionary advantage within a changing society while others, such as neurasthenia or catatonia, may not.

Although intriguing, speculations of this sort are justified only if it has been established that mental illness is common among the eminent. To date, this has yet to be established. Except for the results of more recent studies on writers and artists, including my own on women writers, the past studies on eminent persons, although plagued by serious methodological flaws, reported very low rates of mental illness, ranging from 2 to 10%, and none of these studies gave precise breakdowns about the rates and types of mental illness found in people within different professions. I plan here to remedy this lack.

The first task was to identify certain clusters of psychiatric symptoms and signs, known as "syndromes," in eminent people over the course of their lives. The criteria used to identify these different syndromes corresponded in general to Glossary descriptions in the *Ninth Revision of the International Classification of Disease*.[3] Given the nature of the data and continual changes in psychiatric diagnoses, the identification of stable patterns of psychopathology at different times provided a better reflection of the emotional disturbances people experienced during their lives than any single lifetime psychiatric diagnosis.[4] In a sense, this descriptive approach was consistent with the growing recognition of multiple psychiatric disorders (or of comorbidity) existing simultaneously or over time within many individuals.[5] With this approach, people could suffer from two or three separate psychiatric syndromes simultaneously, such as depression, alcoholism, and drug abuse, or suffer from them at different times in their lives, without the assumption that these syndromes shared a common cause.

Because this syndromatic approach was central to the classification of psychopathology, some clarification seems necessary about how it was applied. Howard Hughes, among others, offers a good example. The following is an excerpt from the special instructions he gave his staff for removing his hearing aid cord from the cabinet where it was kept:

> First use six or eight thicknesses of Kleenex pulled one at a time from the slot in touching the door knob to open the door to the bathroom. The door is to be left open so there will be no need to touch anything when leaving the bathroom. The same sheaf of Kleenex may be employed to turn on the spigots so as to obtain a good force of warm water. This Kleenex is then to be disposed of. . . . The hands are to be washed with extreme care, far more thoroughly than they have ever been washed before, taking great pains that the hands do not touch the sides of the bowl, the spigots, or anything in the process.

Howard Hughes' preoccupation with his health came to dominate his life. He required his aides to wear gloves when handing him objects and to write messages to him rather than spread germs by communicating verbally. He had his doors and windows sealed with tape to avoid dirt and refused to touch doorknobs. (This cluster of behaviors was coded as an obsessive-compulsive condition, representing one of the anxiety disorders.) At times, when constipated, he would spend up to 26 hours in the bathroom. Sometimes he would urinate on the floor but would not let the help clean it up, preferring instead to spread towels on the floor. The slightest change in his physical condition could throw him into a panic, and he took all sorts of pills to protect himself from germs and disease. (This cluster of behaviors was coded as hypochondriasis, representing one of the somatic disorders).

Even with these problems, he usually could rouse himself sufficiently to conduct his business affairs. But Hughes demonstrated other severe psychopathologies as well. During his second "nervous breakdown," he became psychotic, babbling incoherently, having tantrums, and urinating against the bathroom door. He then completely withdrew from the outside world. He devoted much of his time viewing motion pictures from his chair in a "germ-free zone" and spent hours cleaning his phone with Kleenex. He began spending more time in his bed, rarely bathed and let his finger nails and toe nails grow abnormally long. (This cluster of behaviors was coded as a psychosis.) He eventually emerged from this state but as time progressed began relying more on codeine (he had been using narcotics ever since a plane crash many years before) and was taking up to ten 10-milligram Valiums a day. (This cluster of behaviors was coded as a drug-related problem.) Although his physical and psychological condition continued to deteriorate, he still on occasion could pull himself together and surprise everyone with his grasp of business affairs.

Truman Capote experienced different constellations of emotional problems over the course of his life. From childhood, he suffered from "free floating anxiety," along with claustrophobia and a fear of abandonment. He described the hyperanxiety as "the mean reds" and said that he never was free of them. (This cluster of symptoms and behaviors was coded as an anxiety disorder.) Although he used alcohol and pills as a teenager, he kept his consumption under control until his 40s, when he became addicted to various tranquilizers and mood-altering drugs, such as barbiturates and later Valium. (This cluster of behaviors was coded as a drug-related problem.) By his 50s his drinking was out of control, causing him to attend Alcoholics Anonymous and to admit himself to various clinics to be treated for his uncontrolled drinking. (This cluster of behaviors was coded as an alcohol-related problem.) Several years later he saw two psychiatrists for severe depression and was contemplating suicide. "Every morning I wake up and in about two minutes I'm weeping," he said. "I just cry and cry. And every night the same thing happens. I take a pill, go to bed . . . and suddenly I start to cry. There's just so much pain somebody can endure. How can I carry it around all the time?" (This cluster of behaviors was coded as depression.) A few years later he was paralyzed by anxiety and the fear of dying. He began taking lots of Tuinal, continued to snort cocaine, and then after a period of more controlled drinking, began using cocaine heavily and had many hospitalizations for alcoholism and delirium tremens.

Delmore Schwartz, a former editor of the *Partisan Review* and the most widely anthologized poet of his time, experienced a different pattern of problems. In his 30s, he had his most serious and persistent episode of depression. He had trouble teaching classes, gradually became more disheveled and untidy, avoided people, felt gloomy and despondent, and became suspicious of everyone. (This cluster of behaviors was coded as depression.) But as inevitably happened after a depressive period, Schwartz's mood began to rise until it evolved into a full-blown manic episode. During these times he was talkative, emotionally volatile, hyperactive, sleepless, grandiose, tactless, socially inappropriate, and sometimes frankly delusional. Once, for instance, the police arrived to find him standing naked in the middle of the room with a lamp in his hand. (This cluster of behaviors was coded as mania.) For years, he also had been consuming massive amounts of alcohol and had great difficulty controlling his drinking. (This, along with other evidence of excessive drinking, was coded as an alcohol-related problem.) He had become dependent on barbiturates and amphetamines as well. His Dexedrine intake, which increased when he was depressed or countering the effects of sleeping pills, got to the point where he was swallowing them like candy, taking as many as 20 pills a day. (This cluster of behaviors was coded as a drug-related problem.) This naturally aggravated his mania and worsened his violent rages and suspiciousness.

These examples show the usefulness of a syndromatic approach to the classification of psychopathology. While a single diagnosis may be sufficient to account for the emotional problems in a large portion of people, it does not do justice to the range of different problems others experience over the course of their lives. In these instances, the identification of multiple disorders becomes necessary.

In addition to finding a method to determine psychopathology, we also need to know rates for the general population. To place these findings within an epidemiological context, we can use the results of the

Epidemiological Catchment Area (ECA) survey, a monumental study involving interviews at five different sites with about 20,000 individuals who typified the entire United States population.[6] For many reasons, the results from the ECA survey cannot be compared directly with mine. They can, however, provide a yardstick of sorts for gauging the relative extent of mental illness among these eminent people.[7]

What also needs to be recognized is that differences in sampling methods, diagnostic criteria, and population groups can result in wide disparities in the lifetime rates of mental disorders. The results of past epidemiological surveys illustrate this. In the Stirling County study,[8] the lifetime prevalence for *any* psychiatric disorder defined by the first edition of the *Diagnostic and Statistical Manual* of the American Psychiatric Association (1952) was 57%. Although the Midtown Manhattan study[9] did not determine the presence of specific mental disorders, it found that 23% of the sample population had significant psychiatric impairment and over 80% had some mild impairment. The results of the ECA study revealed a more conservative lifetime prevalence of 32% for *any* psychiatric disorder. With the present study, I made allowance for a certain degree of diagnostic uncertainty based on the available biographical information by identifying the presence of certain syndromes as "definite" or "probable." "Strict" criteria applied to the "definite" presence of a specific syndrome, and more "permissive" criteria included the "probable" presence as well. Although the more permissive criteria did not offer as much diagnostic certainty as the more strict criteria, they allowed lower thresholds for identification of specific syndromes, and as a result, seemed better suited for characterizing the extent and kind of emotional difficulties eminent people experienced over the years. That, after all, was what I wanted to document.[10]

One immediate problem had to do with whether members of certain professions were more susceptible than others to various *emotional disorders* and, if so, at what periods in their lives. The ECA study reported the prevalence for *any* mental illness to be 37% below age 30, 39% between age 30 and 44, 27% between age 45 and 64, and 21% over age 65. My study offered rates for somewhat different periods: before the age of 13, between ages 13 and 20, between ages 21 and 40, between ages 41 and 60, and after age 61. The rates based on more permissive criteria are much higher than those for the ECA study, while the rates based on more strict criteria are about the same.[S1]

Although we can find suggestive differences among professional types in their rates of mental illness during their childhoods, clear differences emerge once they become adolescents. Among teenagers, the prevalence of *any* mental illness is 18% (12% with strict criteria only). Those destined to become poets, musical performers, and fiction writers (29 to 34%) show higher rates than those who become businesspeople, soldiers, sports figures, explorers, politicians, social figures, and architects (3 to 9%).

Some of the emotional problems noted during the childhoods of the former group were quite severe. Ian Fleming began experiencing moodiness and periods of "black depression" at age 7. Rita Hayworth, who was abused and neglected at an early age, developed paralyzing shyness, almost muteness, as a child. Carry Nation was prey to visions, mostly of snakes, as a child, and at age 12 suffered from "moody and introspective fits." Boris Pasternak, who was hypersensitive and fearful as a child, said he was close to suicide between ages 6 and 8. Hank Williams was drinking heavily by age 11. Louise Brooks, the actress and dancer, was sexually molested at age 9, and by age 14 was drinking heavily. Before puberty, Mary Baker Eddy supposedly suffered from auditory hallucinations and paroxysms of anxiety; the doctor diagnosed her as having "hysteria mingled with bad temper." Andrè Gide suffered from fits of depression, unnamed fears, and "attacks of hysteria" as a child. From age 8 on, August Strindberg threatened suicide often. Andy Warhol supposedly had three "nervous breakdowns" as a child.

Once individuals become adults, the prevalence of psychopathology rises dramatically to 51% (39% for strict criteria only) between the ages of 21 and 40, and then begins to level off to 55% (40% with strict criteria) from ages 41 to 60, and to 44% (31% with strict criteria) from the age of 61 on. By this time, not only poets, fiction writers, and musical performers show high rates of severe emotional disorders (70 to 77%) but artists, composers, nonfiction writers, actors, and directors and, interestingly, athletes (59 to 68%) as well. Natural scientists, politicians, architects, and businesspeople show much lower rates in comparison (18 to 29%).

SPECIFIC FORMS OF MENTAL ILLNESS

Now that we have established that different types of professionals show different rates of mental illness at different periods in their lives, we can examine the lifetime prevalence of specific psychiatric syndromes and, by means of life table or "survival" analyses, the comparative ages at which members within the different professions are more likely to succumb to them.[11] Since these assorted findings will prove critical to our later assessment of the link between mental illness and creative achievement, I have taken the liberty of presenting them in some detail. I also offer examples when necessary to illustrate the kind of problems I am talking about.

Alcohol-Related Problems

Besides indications of physical addiction, such as intense craving for alcohol, uncontrolled drinking, and signs of alcohol withdrawal, the criteria used to establish the existence of alcohol dependence or alcohol abuse included evidence of the following problems related to compulsive, excessive, or continuous drinking: physical (e.g., liver damage, delirium tremens, gastric ulcer), vocational (e.g., joblessness, absenteeism, poor performance, decreased productivity), personal (e.g., divorce, alienation of children), interpersonal (e.g., increased friction with friends, colleagues, employers) or legal (e.g., arrests).

In the ECA survey, the total lifetime prevalence for both alcohol abuse and dependence was 14%, and when broken down according to gender, 5% for women and 24% for men.[12] Among our eminent people, 26% (20% by strict criteria) experience alcohol-related problems during their lifetimes, 23% for women and 27% for men. However, a wide disparity exists in the percentages of those affected within the different professions (see Figure 7.1). Actors or directors, musical entertainers, sports figures, fiction writers, artists, and poets (29 to 60%) have higher rates of alcohol dependence or abuse than natural scientists, soldiers, social scientists, social activists, and social figures (3 to 10%).[52] A life table analysis reveals that

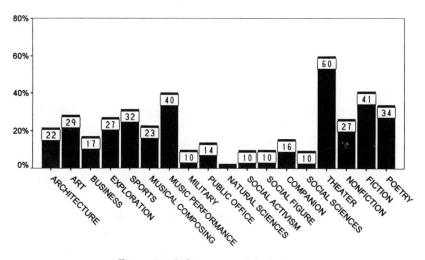

Figure 7.1. Lifetime rate of alcoholism.

progressively greater proportions of artistic types, compared to other types, succumb to alcoholism after age 20 and throughout much of the remainder of their lives.[S3a]

The finding that alcoholism should be so common among fiction writers, poets, and artists is hardly unexpected. Others have noted how alcoholism, especially among writers in the first half of this century, had almost reached epidemic proportions. It is well known that five of the seven Nobel laureates in literature in the United States were alcoholics: William Faulkner, Ernest Hemingway, Eugene O'Neill, Sinclair Lewis, and John Steinbeck.[13] It was the rare writer or artist who did not choose to meet with his or her compatriots in cafés, pubs or, settings in which alcohol flowed freely, either early in his or her career or later, as a result of growing fame or celebrity status. Under these circumstances, it is little wonder that vulnerable individuals incorporated alcohol more and more into their daily routines, until it inevitably began to interfere with their work. However, the fact that alcoholism does not seem to be as rampant among writers and artists in Europe suggests that the relationship between heavy alcohol use and creativity may be more an artifact of cultural expectations in the United States than a reflection of the biological predisposition in these people.

Drug-Related Problems

Besides signs of physical addiction, the criteria used to establish drug dependence or drug abuse included evidence of physical, vocational, personal, interpersonal, or legal problems related to compulsive, excessive, and sustained legal or illegal drug use. These criteria did not cover casual experimentation with certain psychoactive drugs, such as LSD, cocaine, stimulants, and barbiturates, or the infrequent use of marihuana.

With the ECA findings, about 31% of people—36% of men and 25% of women—used illicit drugs at some point in their lives. The lifetime prevalence of drug dependence or abuse, however, was about 6%, 8% for males and 5% for females.[14] Among our eminent persons, 12% experience drug-related problems sometime during their lives (9% with strict criteria), 10% in males and 17% in females. Musical entertainers, actors, and fiction writers have the highest lifetime rates of drug dependence or abuse (19 to 36%), and natural scientists, public officials, military officers, athletes, explorers, architects, and famous companions the lowest (0 to 5%)[S2] (see Figure 7.2). At a more general level, artistic types (18%) show rates of drug abuse three to ten times greater than those in other types. These differences

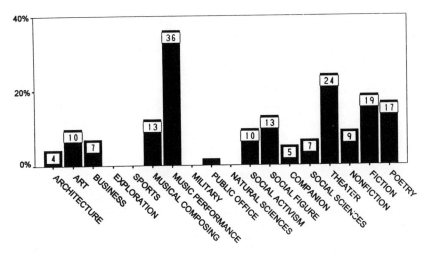

Figure 7.2. Lifetime rate of drug abuse.

begin to show up between the ages of 21 to 25 and become progressively more pronounced over the course of their lives.[S3b]

The exceptionally high rate of drug addiction among musical and popular entertainers has intriguing implications for the interaction between psychopathology and creative activity. First, however, we need to identify some of the people involved.

Judy Garland began her life-long struggle with drugs after her studio put her when she was 14 on diet pills and barbiturates to help her sleep. By her mid-30s, along with all the liquor she consumed, she was taking 40 Dexedrines a day and 10 to 12 Seconals to sleep at night. Both of the avant-garde jazz saxaphonists, John Coltrane and Charlie "Bird" Parker, were addicted to heroin. Marvin Gaye free-based cocaine and smoked huge amounts of marihuana. He nearly killed himself several times with overdoses, and was said to provoke people to the point of their trying to hurt him, both emotionally and physically. He allegedly pushed his wife to have sex with other men, and then became despondent. Some accounts of his death claim that he provoked his father, a Pentacostal minister, into killing him, in part because he bought the gun for him 4 months before he was shot. John Lennon relied on marihuana, LSD, amphetamines, methadone, and speedballs composed of cocaine and heroin to stay in a drugged haze for long stretches of time.

Perhaps because of their celebrity status, a portion of these entertainers were able to get their drugs legally. Elvis Presley, for instance, who found street drugs "despicable," got physicians to prescribe a limitless supply of legitimate drugs, including Seconals, Tuinals, Valiums, Nembutals, Placidyls, Quaaludes, amphetamines, and Percodans. The acerbic comedian Lenny Bruce traveled with what amounted to a portable drugstore, bringing along narcotics, sleeping pills, and assorted sedatives and stimulants to regulate his mood and consciousness. Remarkably, he even had a doctor's note saying that he was under professional care and had been taught how to inject Methedrine intravenously because he did not respond to the oral amphetamines prescribed for his "severe depression."

No discussion of musical entertainers with addictions can be complete without mention of the overdosing trio of Janis Joplin, Jim Morrison, and Jimi Hendrix. The recent addition of Kurt Cobain, the lead singer of the rock group Nirvana, indicates that the pattern still exists, although his own attempt at overdose was unsuccessful. All were famous rock stars who had become cult heroes by their early 20s. All drank heavily. Janis Joplin, for example, reached a point in her career where she would bring a bottle of Southern Comfort or tequila on stage and take sips between songs; Jim Morrison became known for his incredible binges. All abused and experimented with numerous drugs, including marihuana, barbituates, amphetamines, narcotics, cocaine, and psychedelics. Jim Morrison, lead singer of The Doors, who probably based the name of his group on Aldous Huxley's *Doors of Perception* (which gave an account of Huxley's personal experiences with mescaline), reportedly took LSD over 250 times, using it every other day for a long stretch of time. All were tormented, anguished, and unpredictable in behavior. But what beyond their artistic abilities will be remembered about them is that they all killed themselves at the age of 27, an act that in the case of Jim Morrison, who after the deaths of Janis Joplin and Jimi Hendrix used to tell his friends, "You're drinking with number three," did not seem completely coincidental. Kurt Cobain, who could not help but know when his predecessors died, shot himself at the same age, after attempting an overdose.

What does this fatal attraction to drugs say about many entertainers as people, about their lifestyles and their professions? All of the people mentioned were insecure, driven people who sought attention and adultation, but often rode on the fast track of success with mixed feelings about it and their places on it. Not only were drugs plentiful among their friends and within the circles they traveled, but they also began to rely on drugs to get their minds and bodies to do what they were not inclined to do. They became connoisseurs of a pharmacopeia of mind-altering chemicals. They used drugs to overcome their performance anxieties, to loosen their inhibitions, and to "wind down" so that they could sleep after being energized by their perform-ances. They began to rely on drugs as vital for their personal and professional existence. In time, usually when they had become increasingly exhausted by the pace of their careers and lifestyles, and the drugs no longer worked as they used to, a number also used drugs to end their lives.

Of course, these particular examples are extreme cases. Many of the other musical entertainers in my study used drugs moderately and did not experience so devastating an impact on their personal lives and careers. Some even used drugs at times to their creative advantage. And lest we fall in the trap of stereotyping all musical entertainers as drug addicts, we need to note that over half of them did not abuse drugs.

Depression/Melancholia

The criteria used to establish the existence of depression included at least one several-week episode of sustained depression, characterized by melan-choly mood, sleep disturbance, increased or decreased appetite, lack of energy, excessive tearfulness, sense of dread or futility, social withdrawal, and morbid thoughts or suicidal preoccupation. Unless evidence to the contrary existed, I interpreted the actual suicide attempts to be signs of depression. The "probable" indications of depression included continued moodiness, unhappiness, pessimism, gloominess, and general dysphoria. The designation of depression or melancholy was only reserved for those instances in which obvious precipitating causes, such as bereavement, imprisonment, ill health, or the loss of a job, did not seem to be responsible or when the response was out of proportion and lasted longer than expected. Common psychiatric conditions that qualified as depression included major depressive disorders, dysthymia or "neurotic" depressions, depressive episodes associated with bipolar disorders, and adjustment disorders with depression that lasted more than 6 months or resulted in severe consequences, such as a suicide attempt.

What needs emphasis is that depression can come in many varieties and forms. As with other kinds of psychopathology, depression, depending on its kind and severity, can have different kinds of effects on people's lives and works. Those who suffer from chronic, low-grade forms of depression may be affected differently by their disorder than those who have only one or two incapacitating episodes or those who experience depressions as preludes to highs or those who stay seriously depressed for many years.

The results of the ECA study revealed a combined lifetime prevalence of about 6% for major depression or dysthymia for the population at large,

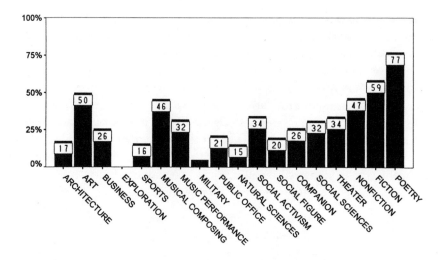

Figure 7.3. Lifetime rate of depression.

with the rate being over twice as high in females (9%) as for males (4%). Besides these formal diagnoses, the ECA study also reported that about 30% of the individuals experienced dysphoria, 28% experienced thoughts of death, and 24% had appetite changes lasting longer than 2 weeks—symptomatology generally associated with depression.[15] Even so, in our sample, the lifetime prevalence for severe depression was 38% (30% by strict criteria), 40% for females and 38% for males. About 15% of those who suffered from depression also had episodes of mania during the course of their lives.

Among the various professions, poets, fiction writers, artists, nonfiction writers, and musical composers have the highest lifetime rates of depression (46 to 77%), and explorers, military officers, natural scientists, athletes, and architects have the lowest (0 to 17%) (see Figure 7.3). Overall, the artistic types (50%) seem about twice as likely as social (27%), investigative (24%), and enterprising types (20%) to suffer from depression during their lifetimes.[S2] They also begin succumbing to depression at a greater rate than other types after the age of 25 and even more so after the age of 40.[S3c]

Mania

The criteria for mania or an emotional "high" included at least one sustained episode of several weeks' duration or longer of elation, grandiosity, excessive energy, unusually poor judgment, racing thoughts, social intrusiveness, prolonged insomnia, and excessive buying or juggling too many activities in comparison to the person's ordinary behavior. "Probable" indications of mania involved major mood swings with periods of heightened well-being, marked irritability, diminished sleep, lapses in judgment, and increased physical activity. Mania was not attributed to people if they simply felt "good" after a long period of depression, experienced a "flow state" or "creative high" while engaged in their work, or became "hyper" or energized during intense creative activity or the anticipation of a major performance or competition. In other words, mania or hypomania represented an "abnormal" level of arousal.

Mania usually has a chronic, relapsing course. Many people manage to endure these emotional peaks and valleys without irreversible damage to their personal relationships or work. For others, these recurrent episodes have devastating effects. In certain instances it is remarkable that certain people continued to be creative and productive, especially "rapid-cyclers" such as the noted art historian John Ruskin, who finally became incapacitated during the last 11 years of his life, and the poet Robert Lowell, who had annual breakdowns for 18 years before he pronounced himself "cured" by lithium.

In the ECA study, the lifetime prevalence of mania was 0.8%, with the range varying from 0.4 to 1.2% among the five research sites and with its rate in men (0.9%) and women (0.7%) being about the same.[16] In my sample, 7% (3% with strict criteria) of individuals, 7% in men and 7% in women, had at least one episode of mania during their lives. Actors (17%), poets (13%), architects (13%), and nonfiction writers (11%) have the highest rates of mania[S2] (see Figure 7.4). Overall, artistic types (10%) have much higher lifetime rates of mania than investigative types (0%). They also begin to succumb to mania at greater rates than other types after the age of 25.[S3d]

Schizophrenia-like Psychosis

Diagnostic criteria for schizophrenia have changed over the years, mostly with the tendency to shift many of those psychotic conditions with a major mood component to bipolar disorders. It is difficult to interpret earlier reports about the prevalence of schizophrenia in many eminent persons. Since individuals with mania or severe depression also can become psychotic and sometimes display symptomatology indistinguishable from schizophrenia, it no longer is feasible to assume that a schizophrenia-like

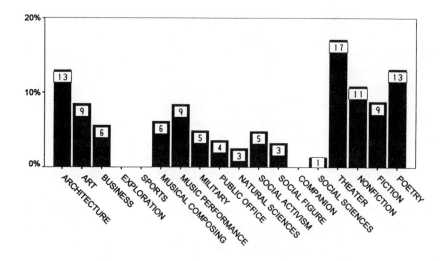

Figure 7.4. Lifetime rate of mania.

psychosis is necessarily equivalent to schizophrenia. Therefore, the more prudent course seems to be to identify "schizophrenia-like psychoses" rather than schizophrenia per se, bearing in mind that many of these psychoses may represent either schizoaffective disorders, atypical psychotic conditions, psychotic depressions, or, more likely, florid mania.

Part of the dilemma in interpreting the nature of these psychoses has to do with my choice of a syndromatic rather than diagnostic approach to the identification of psychopathology. A diagnostic approach requires that we try to establish a unitary diagnosis, when possible, on the basis of the entire pattern of emotional difficulties people show over their lifetimes. For example, if a man has what seems to be a schizophrenic episode in his early 20s and then in his 30s has a severe depression or manic episode, most clinicians will likely attribute all of these manifestations to a bipolar disorder. With a syndromatic approach, which as I discussed above has certain research advantages, no assumptions are made about a common link between different syndromes that occur at different points in peoples' lives. It is possible, at least in theory, for the man to have been schizophrenic, depressed, and manic at different times in his life without necessarily having a manic–depressive disorder. This observation has special relevance for roughly one-third of those in the sample who had a schizophrenia-like psychosis at one point and a clear-cut manic episode at another.

For the purposes of this study, the criteria for schizophrenia-like psychoses included at least one sustained psychotic episode, characterized by auditory or visual hallucinations, delusions of persecution, inappropriate affect, extreme suspiciousness, incoherent communications, bizarre behaviors, or impaired ability to care for oneself while clearly conscious. Lacking these symptoms, the diagnosis of schizophrenia or insanity by a qualified medical source also served to identify this condition. However, the legitimacy of these diagnoses at those particular times was perhaps debatable for people such as Robert Lowell, who earlier in his life was diagnosed as an "incurable schizophrenic" by no less an authority than Carl Jung, but who later clearly showed a manic–depressive disorder, or Ezra Pound, who was diagnosed by a panel of four noted psychiatrists as "suffering from a paranoid state that renders him unfit and mentally incapable" but who later, in retrospect, may have had an atypical mood disorder.

Despite these reservations, there are many other instances when the designation of a schizophrenia-like psychosis rather than an atypical mood disorder seemed the most judicious choice. For example, Zelda Fitzgerald, although she was sometimes credited with being the first American flapper, became famous especially because of her flamboyant lifestyle, her marriage to F. Scott Fitzgerald, and her long struggle with mental illness. Whatever promise she had as a short story writer, artist, or dancer was halted in her late 20s when she began having terrifying hallucinations. She heard extremely loud noises and felt the "vibrations" of everyone she met. People's bodies began to look distorted to her. She would write whole pages of text using only one word, and her communications in general became incoherent. She claimed to be in direct contact with Christ, William the Conquerer, Mary Stuart, and Apollo. Diagnosed as schizophrenic by Dr. Eugen Bleuler, the psychiatrist who coined the term "schizophrenia," she spent years in and out of mental hospitals, eventually dying in a fire after receiving a course of insulin coma therapy.

Bleuler also diagnosed Vaslav Najinsky, the great Russian ballet dancer and choreographer, as having schizophrenia. It was during his late 20s that Najinsky first began hallucinating, becoming increasingly withdrawn, having unpredictable bouts of rage, and behaving bizarrely. He was hospitalized for about 10 years in an asylum in Switzerland and, although he recovered somewhat, he spent most of the remainder of his life under treatment.

Antonin Artaud, the director, writer, and actor, abused drugs and suffered from depression as a young man, but in his early 40s became clearly psychotic and had to be hospitalized for years. Along with experiencing auditory hallucinations, he had delusions of communicating with Jesus or being tormented by the police. During this period, his behavior became very regressive. He reportedly played with and ate his own feces. He appeared to speak in tongues, often losing track of his ideas. He would telescope his syllables, make strange noises, go through a series of rituals, such as spitting, getting down on his hands and knees and singing psalms, drawing magic circles, talking with imaginary people, and belching in rhythmic patterns. His gestures were incomprehensible to others, and he was not able to complete the simplest of acts.

The ECA study estimated the lifetime prevalence of schizophrenia and schizophreniform disorders for the population as a whole to be 1.5%, and when broken down by gender, 1.2% in males and 1.7% in females. The remission rate for these disorders was 32%.[17] Among the eminent persons in my sample, 5% (3% by strict criteria) qualified as having had a schizophrenia-like psychosis, about 5% for men and 7% for women. Schizophrenia-like psychoses, which are probably not comparable to the designations of schizophrenia and schizophreniform disorders in the ECA study, have the highest representation among poets (17%), much higher than for any other professionals, and are not found at all among eminent military officers, natural scientists, politicians, and explorers[S2] (see Figure 7.5). Overall, the lifetime prevalence of these disorders is about two to seven

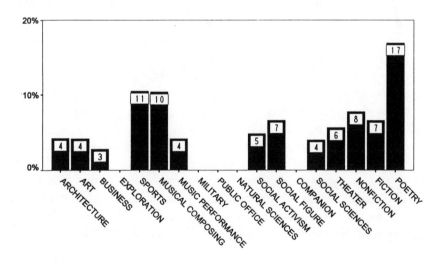

Figure 7.5. Lifetime rate of psychosis.

times higher for artistic types (8%) than other types. These differences between artistic and other types begin to become more marked after the age of 45.[S3e]

Pathological Anxiety

The criteria for pathological anxiety, usually resulting in some degree of incapacitation, included a prolonged period of fearfulness, apprehension, dread, agitation, restlessness, tension, and shakiness—all without any adequate physical or psychological basis. Besides representing a distinct syndrome in its own right, this symptom complex also covered obsessive-compulsive disorders, major phobias, post-traumatic stress responses, panic disorders, and cases of severe "nerves."

A couple of examples illustrate what is meant by pathological anxiety. The actress Joan Crawford was almost incapacitated by phobias, obsessions, and severe anxieties. Her claustrophobia, she believed, was due to having been locked in a closet by her older brother when she was 5. She dreaded elevators and never flew until she was middle-aged. Obsessed with cleanliness, she often scrubbed her floors herself, washed her hands over and over, and changed her clothes almost hourly. Even after becoming a star, she shook so much that her script had to be mounted on cardboard so it would not rattle, a bar had to be placed near her microphone so that she would have something to hold on to, and her physician had to be nearby.

William Dean Howells, considered by many to be the "Dean" of American letters at the turn of the century, was virtually immobilized for a period of time by his dread of being bitten by a rabid dog. Any mention of the word "hydrophobia," one of the symptoms of rabies, would nearly send him into a panic. While he was at his worst, a splash of water would leave him shaken and cause him to be seized by spasms. Even when writing about his fears many years later, he could not force himself to write or speak the word without experiencing a wave of anxiety.

The results of the ECA study revealed that about 9% of the general population experienced a generalized anxiety disorder, either as a separate syndrome or accompanied by another disorder. Instances when generalized anxiety was associated with another disorder varied from 58 to 65%, depending on the site.[18] Among the eminent people in my sample, the prevalence of generalized anxiety was 8% (4% by strict criteria), 12% for females and 7% for males. Nonfiction writers, actors, poets, and artists have the highest rates (13 to 16%), while explorers, athletes, politicians, businesspeople, musical composers, and entertainers have the lowest rates (0 to 4%)[S2] (see Figure 7.6). Overall, artistic types (11%) have the highest rate of anxiety, followed in turn by the investigative types (7%), social types (6%), and enterprising types (3%). The differences between artistic types and other types become accentuated between ages 25 and 30 and again after the age of 55.[S3f]

Somatic Dysfunction

The criteria for a "somatic" dysfunction included evidence of prolonged and excessive preoccupation with bodily functions or dysfunctions for which there was no physical basis or, conversely, for which there was a likely psychological cause. This category also included instances of emotionally caused paralyses, dramatic, attention- gaining, physical symptomatology, conversion hysteria, hypochondriasis, "psychosomatic" problems, and older diagnoses of "nervous exhaustion," nervous debilitation, or "neurasthenia."

A couple of examples of somatic dysfunctions should make the criteria for this syndrome clear. The world-renowned tenor, Enrico Caruso, had a chronic dread of infection. He would change shirts every 2 or 3 hours, have his room sprayed constantly with perfumed atomizers, and carry an assortment of syringes, medicines, and gargles with him on his travels.

The hypochondriasis of Glenn Gould, the concert pianist, was classical. He meticulously kept detailed lists of his symptoms, medicines, and tests. One typical entry read: "Palpitations . . . Heat in arm . . . Indigestive-style

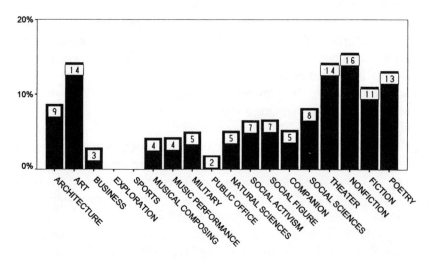

Figure 7.6. Lifetime rate of anxiety.

pains in chest . . . Wake-up pulse rate—dream episodes . . . Freezing sensations—shivers—top of nose . . . Recent month's lower abdomen problem—liquid consumption triggers pockets of 'ulcer-like' pains through to back—congestive sensations re bending over." He also recorded how many hours he slept, his pulse rate, sometimes at ½-hour intervals, when he woke up, and when he felt pressure on his bladder. There supposedly were times when he kept at least four doctors busy with his endless series of complaints.

The ECA study found the lifetime prevalence of somatization syndrome for the general population to be about 12%, 9% for males and 14% for females.[19] In my sample of eminent people, the lifetime prevalence of somatic dysfunctions was 11% (5% by the strict criteria), about 10% for males and 14% for females. Unlike other syndromes already discussed, the prevalence of somatic dysfunctions did not differ significantly among the 18 professions.[S2]

Adjustment (Stress) Reactions

The criteria for adjustment reactions included maladaptive but usually reversible responses to stress or trauma out of proportion to or lasting much longer than what is normally expected and usually associated with a decreased ability to cope, and accompanied by such symptoms as depression, agitation, fearfulness or work paralysis. In distinction to melancholia or generalized anxiety, there is always a triggering situation or legitimate precipitating cause.

Unfortunately, the ECA study did not establish the lifetime prevalence of such reactions for the population at large. For our sample, 36% (22% by strict criteria) experienced a difficulty of this sort at some point in their lives. The rate of these disorders was higher in women (46%) than in men (33%). Among the various groups, the prevalence was highest among sports figures, fiction writers and composers (44 to 58%) and lowest among architects, musical performers, and military officers (13 to 25%). Suitable information was not available for this syndrome to allow the construction of life tables.[S2]

Assorted Other Mental Problems

This category served as a catch-all for all mental disorders not included above that cause emotional, behavioral or social impairment and for which the available descriptions were imprecise or nonspecific. Examples included "nervous breakdown," "shell shock," and so on.

For the sample, the lifetime prevalence for these problems was 5% (3% by strict criteria), 9% for females and 4% for males. Since no significant differences existed among the 18 groups, there is no need to deal with this category further.

Suicide Attempts

Suicide attempts are common signs of depression. The criteria for a suicide attempt included any successful or unsuccessful effort or serious threat to end one's life, whether it was made for intentional, attention-gaining, manipulative, or other obscure purposes. The act itself, rather than motives for it or its degree of severity, qualified as a "suicide attempt."

Often, suicide attempts are impulsive, the result of a thwarted love affair or failure, and happen after prolonged drinking. Sometimes, during severe depressions, they become morbid obsessions that dominate every waking moment of the person's life. William Styron, who successfully overcame his own suicidal urges, vividly described this state of mind as that during which everything about him became a potential implement for his own death.[20] The attic rafters became a place to hang himself, the garage a place to inhale carbon monoxide. The bathtub became a receptacle for the blood from his slit arteries, the knives in the kitchen drawer were there for him to stab himself. His car became a means to have a fatal accident, and the nearby highway was a place for him to walk in front of a truck.

The lifetime prevalence of both unsuccessful and successful suicide attempts was about 11% for the entire sample (9% by strict criteria), 8% for men and 17% for women. Unfortunately, the ECA study did not provide rates for suicide attempts. In our sample, poets have the highest rates (26%), followed this time by actors (23%) and musical entertainers (17%). Overall, artistic types (14%) have at least twice the rate as all remaining types.[S2]

According to the mortality statistics, 1.0 to 1.4% of all deaths in the United States for people over 25 years of age were caused by suicide for seven sampling periods (1910, 1920, 1936, 1946, 1956, 1966, and 1988). The prevalence of suicide was 1.8% for males and 0.5% for females.[21] Among the eminent people in my sample, 4.4% succeeded in killing themselves. Table 7.1. lists their names and their means of death. The rate of suicide for poets (20%) is over twice that for musical entertainers (8%) and actors and directors (7%), the next highest groups[S4] (see Figure 7.7). Within the Holland classification of professions, investigative types (9%), surprisingly, have the highest suicide rates, followed next by artistic types

(5%). Survival analysis reveals that while artistic types are more likely than other types to commit suicide by the age of 30, greater proportions of investigative types begin taking their lives after the age of 60.[53g]

Any Psychiatric Disorder

Based on the above information, it is possible to determine the extent to which different groups of individuals experience any of the major disorders noted above over the course of their lifetimes. The ECA study found the lifetime prevalence for any psychiatric disorder to be 32%, 36% in women and 30% in men. My own results of 59% (45% for strict criteria) for lifetime

Table 7.1. Deaths by Suicide

Drug Overdose	Gunshot
Diane Arbus	Dora Carrington
Charles Bedaux	Harry Crosby
Lenny Bruce	Ernest Hemingway
Truman Capote	Vladimir Mayakovsky
Brian Epstein	Victor Tausk
Sigmund Freud (physician assisted)	Robert Ralph Young
Orlo Thomas Heggen	**Carbon Monoxide**
Janis Joplin	
Jimi Hendrix	Libby Holman
Alan Ladd	Ross Lockridge
Jack London	**Drowning**
Malcolm Lowry	
Aimee McPherson	Hart Crane
Marilyn Monroe	Donald Crowhurst
George Sanders	John Davidson
Jean Seberg	Virginia Woolf
Harry Stack Sullivan	**Poison**
Sara Teasdale	
	Alan Turing
Hanging	Charlotte Mew
	Erwin Rommel (forced)
W. J. Cash	
Sergei Esenin	**Other**
Maxim Gorky	John Berryman (jumped off a bridge)
Mitchell Kennerley	Sylvia Plath (oven)
Phil Ochs	Mark Rothko (slashed veins)
Alberto Santos-Dumont	
Marina Tsvetayeva	

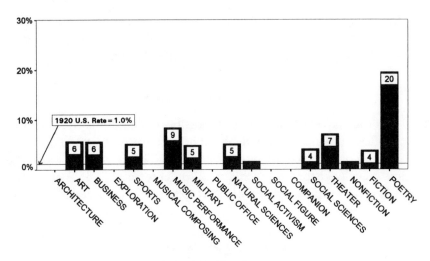

Figure 7.7. Suicide rate.

prevalence among those in my sample (excluding adjustment reactions), with a 59% rate for men and 61% for women, are higher, but are closer to the 57% prevalence found in the Stirling County study. From the results reported so far, it should come as no surprise to find that poets have the highest rates for *any* emotional disorder (87%), followed in descending order by fiction writers, actors, nonfiction writers, artists, musical composers, and musical entertainers (68 to 77%). Explorers, military officers, politicians, and natural scientists have the lowest rates (27 to 35%) (see Figure 7.8). Overall, 72% of artistic types, 49% of social types, 41% of investigative types, and 39% of enterprising types suffer from some form of mental illness over the course of their lives.[S2]

PSYCHIATRIC COMORBIDITY

With the establishment of the lifetime rates for different psychiatric disorders, we now need to find out whether certain disorders clump together or, put differently, whether people who have one kind of mental illness are likely to have another. A different picture of mental illness among members of a particular group emerges if the same people have the bulk of the disorders than if the different disorders are distributed uniformly over all members of a group.

According to the results of the National Comorbidity Survey, 52% of

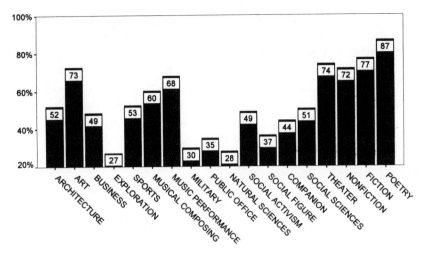

Figure 7.8. Lifetime rate of any mental disorder.

a national sample had no psychiatric disorders, 21% had one, 13% had two, and 14% had three or more disorders.[22] The finding that more than 60% of those with at least one lifetime disorder had two or more disorders suggested that most psychiatric disorders tended to be concentrated in a group of highly comorbid people.

Although the proportion of those in my sample with two or more psychiatric syndromes is higher than that in the National Comorbidity Survey (perhaps because I also included Adjustment Problems in my calculations), the findings are generally similar. About 28% of eminent people had one of the eight disorders I recorded, 20% had two, and 21% had three or more disorders. This meant that 59% of those with at least one lifetime disorder had two or more disorders. The rates of comorbidity were roughly similar for men and women.

Among the various professions, poets, fiction writers, actors, artists, and composers had the highest lifetime rates of psychiatric comorbidity (48 to 68%) and natural scientists, military officers, public officials, and explorers had the lowest (13 to 19%). Members of the artistic professions as a whole were about twice as likely to suffer from two or more psychiatric syndromes over the course of their lives than those in other professions.[55]

Not unexpectedly, certain combinations of psychiatric syndromes occur more frequently than others. All of these combinations are consistent with those commonly encountered in clinical psychiatric practice. People who have manic episodes almost always become depressed, but only

15% those who get depressed have episodes of mania. Almost three-quarters of those who suffer from severe anxiety suffer from depression, but only 15% of depressed people have distinct anxiety syndromes. Most of those who abuse drugs also abuse alcohol, but only 30% of those who abuse alcohol also abuse drugs. Interestingly, about one-half of those with severe anxiety or depression experience adjustment problems during their lifetimes as well, suggesting that they have a greater vulnerability to stress. Disappointments, job failures, or personal losses that others may handle without great distress seem more likely to become serious and prolonged emotional difficulties for these people.

MENTAL HEALTH CARE

Besides this information on the rates of psychiatric syndromes, documentation also was available on whether individuals received any treatment for their emotional problems. The different categories of therapy were as follows: *forced treatment* meant the person was pressured or forced to get help against his or her will; *voluntary hospitalization* represented total mental health care provided in a psychiatric hospital, sanitarium, or spa at the person's own initiative; *outpatient psychiatric care* referred to care outside the hospital, with or without medications; *psychotherapy* designated exposure to a course of therapy, ranging from psychoanalysis to counseling; *unorthodox therapy* referred to exposure to quasitherapeutic approaches, offbeat movements, fads, "cults," naturopathy, and so forth; and *other therapy* represented a catch-all for any approach designed to relieve emotional distress not included in the categories above (e.g., Christian Science, religious healings).

In the ECA study, the rates of any mental health care varied with the type of disorder, ranging from 10% for drug abuse or alcoholism to 47% for panic disorder and 67% for somatization syndrome. The average lifetime prevalence for *any* mental treatment for *any* psychiatric disorder was 13%, 10% for men and 16% for women.[23] In my study, the comparable rate is 26%, 23% for men and 35% for women. Among the various groups, poets, fiction writers, actors, musical composers, and musical entertainers have the highest rates (30 to 42%) and military officers, explorers, and politicians have the lowest rates (0 to 6%).[56]

These assorted results convincingly show that members of the artistic or creative arts professions have higher rates of various emotional disorders over the course of their lives than members of other professions. However, three important qualifications about these results must be made.

The first qualification is that no single pattern of psychopathology characterizes members of all the creative arts professions compared to those of other professions (see Figure 7.9).[24] Alcoholism is rife among creative artists, but not so among architects. Excessive drug use occurs mainly in musical entertainers and actors and to a lesser extent in fiction writers and poets but not in architects, artists, nonfiction writers, or musical composers. Depression is common to all the artistic groups, but not impressively so for architects or actors. Mania is not uncommon in poets and actors but is rare in other groups. Schizophrenia-like psychoses are prominent only in poets. Anxiety disorders occur mostly in artists, actors, and fiction writers, but do so largely before the age of 40. Adjustment reactions are just as likely to occur in certain artistic types as in other types, such as athletes. Poets, musical entertainers, fiction writers, and actors are more likely than other artistic types to attempt suicide.

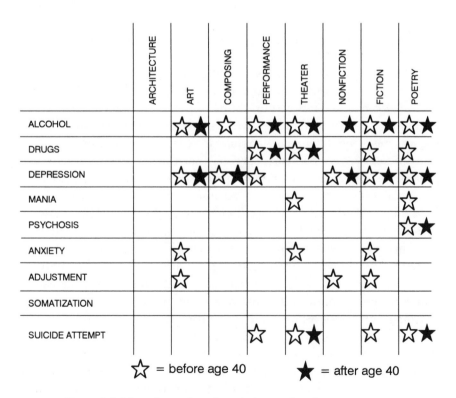

Figure 7.9. Major forms of psychopathology within the creative arts.

The second important qualification, which has not been emphasized in the discussion so far, is that no single form of mental illness occurs in more than half the members of any occupational group. Even with the mood disorders, which have received much attention of late, we find that 50% of artistic types give no evidence of having been clinically depressed and about 90% no evidence of mania. Of course, there are different ways to interpret this. It is possible that those who do not suffer from more severe forms of depression or mania actually have milder, subclinical forms that escape detection in this syndromatic approach. But it also is possible that they do not, and that mood disorders, while more likely to be found in artistic types, are not necessarily typical of individual members. However, because of the exceptionally high lifetime rates for *any* mental illness in these types, the presence of *some form of psychopathology* is definitely probable.[25]

The third qualification has to do with the relatively low rates of mental illness found in certain nonartistic professions, the investigative ones in particular. The fact that emotionally stable people in nonartistic professions, as we have noted, are likewise capable of exceptional creative achievement casts doubt on the existence of any absolute link between mental illness and creative achievement.

All told, these assorted results not only offer a different perspective on the linkage between psychopathology and exceptional achievement but on the functions of certain forms of psychopathology as well. The finding that members of the creative arts, even as youths, have significantly higher rates of mental illness than those in other professions, and that these rates increase over the years, suggests that certain of the creative arts professions either attract individuals predisposed to mental illness to them, aggravate their latent problems because of special stresses, particular life-styles, and professional status, or encourage them to cultivate certain psychopathology as a vehicle for fame and success. In addition, the finding that members of the different creative arts professions reveal different patterns of psychopathology suggests that certain forms of psychopathology may be advantageous and other forms disadvantageous for people pursuing different careers. Many musicians, for instance, may use alcohol and drugs not only because of a possible biological predisposition, the belief that drugs enhance performance, or the calming or stimulating properties of those substances but also because their immediate circles of friends pressure them to do so. Poets not only may be susceptible to depression, mania, psychoses, and suicide, and use their suffering as material for their work; they also may be influenced by the cultural expectation that they are supposed to struggle with their angst. In contrast, public officials and military officers who are accountable to the public or their superiors are less likely to be successful in their careers if they show obvious signs of mental instability or social deviance. While they may experience private distress, their public *persona* must be such that psychopathology could not be revealed. Otherwise, they would not gain the kind of public trust and approval essential for most leadership positions. Although some of these individuals suffer from mental illness, professions that operate in the public domain seem to be selective for people who are stable or who have the capacity to hide their psychopathology, perhaps even from themselves. This also applies to social scientists and natural scientists. Because of the demands for perseverance, rigor, impartiality, and often painstaking, laborious experimentation within the scientific and academic disciplines, people who experience certain psychiatric disturbances may be disadvantaged with respect to professional success.

MENTAL ILLNESS IN BIOLOGICAL RELATIVES

As a way of sorting out what role the professions themselves play in promoting mental illness, we need to know if certain people were predisposed to it before they entered their professions. Perhaps the best way to determine this is to learn whether certain professional types were more likely than other types to be exposed to emotionally disturbed parents or siblings while they were growing up. Unfortunately, hardly any systematic information exists on the prevalence of mental illness among the family members of eminent people. While there is evidence that the rates of mental illness are higher in the relatives of creative people than of others, most past reports, including my own, focus only on special populations, such as writers, and none settles whether the emotional disturbances found in eminent people are inherited or learned.[26]

The problems of establishing a genetic basis for the emotional difficulties of eminent individuals are formidable, mainly because there is no sure way to separate out the influences of nature and environment. The emotional trauma of being raised by mentally disturbed parents and the powerful role models provided by them are bound to confound any strict genetic explanation for mental illness in eminent persons, no matter how loaded with psychopathology their biological relatives may be. Ideally, to solve this problem, we should study the identical twins of eminent people, who preferably had been reared in different environments. But a sample of this sort is not available and is unlikely to be for the future. Nor do gene mapping studies seem options. Because of this, we must limit our search to the familial basis of mental disorders. The demonstration of a "familial" basis only means that the disorder runs in families, nothing more and nothing less.[27]

Here are examples of the kinds of emotional difficulties found in the parents and siblings of eminent people. Clara Bow's mother, Sarah Gordon Bow, who lapsed into long trances and experienced frequent depressions, eventually was committed to and died in a state mental hospital. During her manic episodes, Charlie Chaplin's mother would pray, swear, cry, shout, sing, and become indecent, hyperreligious and violently delusional. His father, who first worked as a mimic and later as a singer, became an alcoholic who developed cirrhosis of the liver. Jack London's mother, Flora Wellman, attempted suicide once with an overdose of laudanum and later shot herself in the head with a pistol. Indulged by her husband, Carrie Nation's mother had the fixed delusion that she was Queen Victoria and preferred to be called "Your Majesty." Earlier, she held the belief that she was a lady in waiting for the Queen. As befitting her station, she wore purple velvet gowns with a train and a crown of crystal and cut glass, and knighted several nearby farmers. She ended her days in an insane asylum.

Woody Guthrie's sister and both parents had mental problems. Clara, his sister, set fire to herself and died after an argument with her mother. His father was an alcoholic who lost all his money on risky ventures and ended up delivering groceries for a living. His mother experienced deep depressions, during which she would sit for hours crying and threatening to kill herself. One day she wrapped Guthrie's baby brother in a newspaper and put him in an oven. At another time she set fire to her husband and tried to stab the baby. Eventually she was committed to a mental hospital, where she was diagnosed as having Huntington's chorea.

Julia, one of Thomas Mann's sisters, abused drugs and hung herself, and Carla, another sister, was an unsuccessful actress and also committed suicide. Somerset Maugham's brother, Harry, who wrote unproduced plays and lyrical poetry, was phobic about trains and eventually committed suicide with a bottle of nitric acid; another brother, Charles, suffered from bouts of melancholy; and a third brother, Frederick, who later became Lord Chancellor, suffered from a general depression. Aldous Huxley's brother, Trevenen, who was a brilliant mathematician, became severely depressed and committed suicide; and Julian, another brother, who eventually was Knighted, experienced a series of "nervous breakdowns." Elinor Wylie's father, who served for a time as Solicitor-General under President Theodore Roosevelt, had a "nervous breakdown," which most likely was severe depression. One of her brothers, Henry, who was an artist, suffered from chronic depression and finally committed suicide by gassing himself. A sister, Constance, also killed herself. Morton, another brother, who had a fondness for alcohol, tried to commit suicide by jumping from a ship after his wife left him but was miraculously saved. William Butler Yeats' mother, father, and at least two sisters and one brother all suffered from periodic depressions over the years.

Orson Welles' father, who made his wealth by inventing a carbide bicycle lamp, was an alcoholic. Hank Williams' father, Elonzo, suffered from nerves after being "shell-shocked" during World War I and was committed voluntarily to a Veteran's hospital in Biloxi, Mississippi for 10 years. His sister, Irene, served several years in prison for possession of illegal drugs. Tennessee Williams' father had a reputation as a trouble-maker, fighter, card player, and heavy drinker, and his sister Rose lived in a psychotic dream world. In despair over the death of their child, the parents of Anna Akhmatova, the poet, made a suicide pact. Her father succeeded in killing himself, but her mother survived. Conrad Aiken's father, Dr. William Ford Aiken, was an ophthalmologist, inventor, photographer, amateur artist, and songwriter who began displaying manic–depressive mood swings, paranoid delusions, and more violent outbursts in his mid-thirties. Several years later, he attempted suicide by taking morphine and atropine. His wife awoke by accident, called a doctor, and he lived. Later, he took his wife's pleas that he should seek professional help as proof of her plotting against him and succeeded in killing her and then shooting himself. Fanny, the sister of Louis D. Brandeis, fell into a deep postpartum depression and killed herself shortly after giving birth to a child. Truman Capote's mother, whom Capote regarded as "the single worst person in my life," became an alcoholic and eventually succeeded in committing suicide with an overdose of Seconal. Peggy Guggenheim's mother repeated things three times and wore three watches, three wraps, and three sweaters. She was obsessed with hygiene and wiped everything repeatedly with Lysol. Peggy's sister, Hazel, flung her two sons off the roof of a hotel, killing them both, in order to teach her husband a lesson for deserting her. Mental illness ran in Ernest Hemingway's immediate family. Both his father, a physician, and a brother, Leicester, shot themselves, as did the novelist himself. His mother's father tried to shoot himself, but his son took the loaded gun from him. As another instance of particular problems being repeated in a family William Robert Wilde, the renowned father of Oscar Wilde, suffered from bouts of melancholy between periods of high activity, was also tried for a sexual offense, and also supposedly became a broken man afterwards.

Information of this sort was available on 965 mothers, 983 fathers, and 598 siblings. To simplify the interpretation of results, I comment only on comparisons between the immediate family members of persons in the creative arts and of those in other professions (see Table 7.2 below).[57] The results are consistent and clear. Mothers of persons in the creative arts reveal higher lifetime rates of alcohol abuse, drug use, depression, and psychoses. Fathers of those in the creative arts reveal higher lifetime rates of alcoholism. Siblings of those in the creative arts reveal higher lifetime rates of drug abuse and depression. The differences between the mothers, fathers, and siblings of members of the creative arts and those of other professions become amplified when the lifetime rates for *any* forms of mental disturbance are compared. All told, these results not only give dramatic evidence for a higher lifetime prevalence of mental illness among the biological, first-degree relatives of those in the creative arts but also suggest a familial basis for many later emotional problems in eminent people.[28]

Again, by using special analyses, it becomes possible to ascertain the extent to which mental disturbances in either parent predict mental

Table 7.2. Prevalence of Mental Problems in First Degree Relatives (by Percentage)

	Mother		Father		Any sibling	
	Creative arts (n = 537)	Other (n = 428)	Creative arts (n = 541)	Other (n = 442)	Creative arts (n = 330)	Other (n = 268)
Alcohol	2.4%	0.5%	12.2%	6.6%	10.6%	6.3%
Drugs	1.1%	0%	0.2%	0.2%	2.7%	0.4%
Depression	8.2%	4.7%	6.7%	4.8%	14.5%	9.3%
Highs	1.5%	0.5%	0.9%	0.7%	1.8%	1.9%
Psychosis	2.0%	0.5.%	0.6%	0.5%	3.9%	1.5%
Anxiety	1.5%	1.4%	0.6%	0.7%	1.2%	0.7%
Somatization	1.7%	1.9%	0%	0.2%	0.6%	1.1%
Unspecified	3.7%	2.8%	4.1%	2.0%	5.8%	3.0%
Suicide attempt	0.7%	0.2%	1.1%	1.6%	7.0%	4.1%
Any problem	15.5%	9.6%	21.4%	13.6%	31.2%	17.2%

Significant differences (*p* < .05) are underlined.

disturbances in their eminent offspring.[58] The results of these analyses, for the most part, reveal that certain kinds of mental disturbances tend to "run true," since the types of problems one or the other parent shows tend to surface later in their eminent offspring. As seems to be the case for the general public as well, alcohol abuse in mothers or fathers, for instance, predicts alcoholism in their eminent offspring. Somatic problems in mothers, along with psychoses, predict somatic problems, such as hypochondriasis or excessive health concerns, in their children. Suicide attempts by fathers and drug use by mothers predict suicide attempts by their eminent children. And "highs" in both parents and depression and unspecified emotional problems in mothers predict psychoses in their children. This heavy loading of depression and "highs" in the parents is of special interest, since it suggests that the schizophrenia-like psychoses that are observed sometimes in their eminent offspring may represent atypical manic–depressive episodes rather than schizophrenia per se.[29]

As a whole, the consistent pattern of these findings shows the strong familial contribution to the extent and nature of the emotional problems encountered by these eminent people. However, interpretation of these findings needs to be tempered by one important qualification. Although the predictive relationships are all statistically significant, *they are very weak*, generally accounting for less than 10% of the variation in the predicted variable. Simply put, this suggests that while the mental disturbances of eminent people are influenced by those of their biological parents, they are not inevitable consequences of them. Other factors obviously play an important role.

We have established that members of the various creative arts professions, as a whole, display higher rates of various emotional disorders than those in other professions; that certain kinds of mental illness are more likely to be associated with certain of these professions than others; that mental illness tends to run in families; and that mental illness does not seem necessary for exceptional achievement. The next logical step is to examine what relationship exists, if any, between the emotional disturbances of eminent people and their creative activities and accomplishments.

CHAPTER EIGHT

Mental Symptoms and Creative Activity

*L*ouis Wain, sometimes known as the "cat artist," illustrates some dilemmas about the link between creativity and madness.[1] Wain received so much fame for his illustration of cats in *Madame Tabby's Establishment* and many other books around the turn of the Century that H. G. Wells claimed, "He invented a cat style, a cat society, a whole cat world. English cats that do not look like Louis Wain cats are ashamed of themselves." To others, he was the Hogarth of cat life.

Born with a harelip and very shy, Louis was a strange, humorless and sickly child with a precocious mathematical faculty and interests in music, painting, writing, and chemistry. During his youth, he suffered from recurring nightmares. He claimed that he was haunted night and day by a vast globe with an endless surface that he saw himself climbing over in fright, and that he often saw thousands of pictures of extraordinary complexity.

Wain chose a career in art at the age of 20 and after a few years began illustrating books. Diffident and eccentric, he eventually met and married Emily Richardson, who was 10 years his senior. Not long afterward, his wife developed cancer, and he spent long hours with her during her decline. One of his main diversions and ways of amusing his wife during this time was to sketch a stray cat, called "Peter," while carrying on conversations with it. It was not too long after his wife's death that his obsession with cats began.

Cats soon began to find their way into most of his paintings and drawings, and continued to do so even when he was hospitalized for insanity. He became so adept at drawing cats that he could do so with lightning speed or draw two different cat pictures at once, one with each hand. More and more, a compulsive quality crept into his drawings and gave them a sense of urgency. Over the years, his behavior became more erratic and paranoid. He accused his sisters of robbing him and claimed that spirits were sending electric currents through him. A journalist wrote, in what is probably an apocryphal story, that Wain's insanity began when, for no apparent reason, he suddenly switched from drawing cats with his left hand to doing so with his right. The new cats appeared fiendish and bizarre. It supposedly was at the point that he struggled to start drawing with his left hand again that he began to go mad.

Even as he continued to draw reasonably coherent pictures, his thinking continued to deteriorate. For example, on the back of *The Perfect Cat*, painted about that time, his psychotic ramblings were obvious. "The solitary one more real Persian cat," he wrote, "is the one that is now going to be the one that is the real living animal left alone until the call is given to it at night time this evening at the same time as the rabbit can be again put to the test." In time, Wain became more violent, delusional, and unmanageable and eventually was certified as insane. While in the Bethlem Royal Hospital, he kept painting and drawing incessantly. He still drew cats, but now placed them in fantastic landscapes and complex geometrical patterns. As his delusional episodes increased in frequency, he became more incoherent and often made mistakes in identifying people. Sometimes he would do bizarre things, such as drinking liquid wax and pouring it on his hair. Although there were periods during his early hospitalization when he drew cats in his old style, the nature of his paintings gradually changed. The "wallpaper" series in which patterned fabric, carpets, curtains, and chaircovers dominated gave way to the "Persian carpet" design with elaborate rich blue–green patterning. Remarkably, he retained his skill in art until his eventual death in the mental asylum, even though he became increasingly psychotic.

Here are some issues. Would Louis Wain have achieved renown as a cat artist were it not for his obsessional preoccupation with cats? Once he was established in his profession, did the worsening of his psychosis lead to a deterioration in his artistic skills and creativity or did it free him up to be more creative? Can we construe the increasing fragmentation and patterning of his cats, which made them more unrecognizable and destroyed their commercial value, as adding to or detracting from their artistic value? Lastly, although we know that Wain's madness greatly affected his art, is it possible that his constant creative activity could have greatly affected his mind?

In this chapter, I address these issues as they apply to all creative artists by exploring the relationship between mental disturbances and creative activity. As I discuss below, many complexities are involved. People who are mentally disturbed are not necessarily incapable of being mentally lucid. A mental breakdown years before the initiation of a creative project may provide greater inspiration for that project than do emotional difficulties at the time. It may not be possible to say anything definite about the impact of mental disturbances on creativity without knowing the type and severity of the mental disturbance and the particular kind of creative activity. All inhibitions in creative activity may not be due to pathological processes, and all forms of creative activity are not necessarily meaningful. These are only some of the issues that we need to take into account.

WHAT PRECEDES WHAT

To clarify issues of this sort, we first must know if the mental problems of creative artists precede, follow, or occur during their creative activity. If people were struggling with mental illness during the time of their first professional success, for instance, we could not discount the influence of one on the other. If, instead, their emotional difficulties were resolved at least 1 year before their initial professional success, we could assume (perhaps arbitrarily) that these difficulties did not directly affect their creative work. And if the onset of their mental disturbances happened at least 1 year after their initial professional success, then we could assume that they played no role in their prior creative ability or productivity.

To get a sense of the extent to which mental illness preceded, overlapped, or followed a significant professional achievement, I examined whether people who had a mental illness at any point in their lives had a serious emotional disturbance around the time of their first career-launching success (e.g., publishing a story, designing a building, performing on stage, composing a song, winning elective office, presenting a scientific paper, having a gallery show, or obtaining a patent). The reason I selected this initial professional success as a marker of creative achievement was that it represented the only one uncontaminated by past professional successes and the later consequences of fame. It also was the easiest marker to identify.

Information of this nature was available on 632 persons. In about one-half of these persons, their first bout of mental illness happened at least 1 year after their initial professional success, and in about one-fourth, it happened and was resolved at least 1 year before. That meant that for about three-fourths of the sample, there was no obvious relationship or overlap between their first episode of mental disturbance and their initial professional achievement. In the remaining one-fourth, there was. Not surprisingly, artistic types (28%) were more likely than other types to show a linkage between a mental disorder and a career-launching event, suggesting that their mental symptoms played a greater role in their creative activity or that their professions had more tolerance for their display of psychopathology. However, it also was obvious that a linkage of this sort was not essential. Investigative types (3%), whose lifetime creative accomplishments rivaled those of artistic types, only rarely showed an overlap between a mental disorder and a career-launching event, suggesting a basic incompatibility between rigorous, scientific pursuits and mental instability and/or a greater intolerance of mental disturbances in their fields.[S1]

THE ARTS VERSUS THE SCIENCES

Finding a closer relationship between the mental symptoms and creative activities of artistic types than those of investigative types, despite similar degrees of creative achievement for both types, indicates that the arts and sciences use different criteria to judge the merits of creative activity. In the creative arts, what matters most is the individual's personal vision of the world, one that gives insight into human experience and offers new ways to appreciate it. With this as the goal, artists, writers, and composers can draw on their personal conflicts or the altered mental processes they artificially induce with alcohol and drugs to give people new ways of seeing nature and exploring the role of their minds in perception and experience. Even the insights gleaned from psychoses may help people to understand the irrationalities of their existence.[2]

To a large extent, creative artists focus on the personal and subjective, the world of meaning and significance rather than of knowledge and fact. With the exception of certain fields, individual expression is paramount. Creative artists can choose to turn inward for inspiration from their emotional turmoil, and to transform it into art.

What is advantageous for the creative artist is usually disadvantageous for the scientist or academician. Insights gained from psychotic, neurotic, or idiosyncratic experiences are not acceptable in the scientific community since they usually violate the fundamental assumptions of science, which are based on predictability, replicability, reliability, and testability. Objectivity and proof are more important in science than personal meaning or aesthetic appeal.

Social responses to the products of science and art also reveal certain differences between these forms of creative expression. Science seems to rely more on cumulative achievements. One discovery supplants another, and usually only the most recent theories command attention and value. Older discarded theories, while of historical interest, have little practical use. The situation is different in art, architecture, music, and certain forms of writing. There is a timeless quality to beauty and aesthetics. Classical works endure and are not necessarily displaced by new works or new schools of art.

What all this points to, as I mention above, is that the kinds of public and professional expectations about acceptable creative achievements influence whether or not mental illness may be advantageous or, at least, not detrimental to career success. What is especially intriguing is that these expectations not only are different between different major professional types but also seem to be operative for different fields within the creative arts. In general, fields that tolerate more ambiguity and less structure and proof in their permissible forms of expression and creative products appear to tolerate people with mental disturbances more and allow these people to capitalize on their highly personal visions. Art, for example, has a higher percentage of members with mental illness than architecture, a field that straddles art and engineering. Poets and fiction writers have higher rates of mental illness than nonfiction writers, including biographers, essayists, and literary critics. Improvisational jazz musicians and rock composers appear to have more emotional difficulties than more classical and traditional ones. And, interestingly enough, social scientists avail themselves of more mental health care than natural scientists. What this strongly suggests is that it is not appropriate to discuss whether mental illness is advantageous or not for creative achievement without taking into account the profession or the particular field.

CREATIVE BLOCKS

Before we examine the interplay between emotional disturbances and creative activity, we need to recognize that all inhibitions in creative expression are not necessarily due to mental illness. Prolonged disruptions in creative activity, commonly referred to as creative blocks, may arise for many reasons. The notion of creative blocks has become part of the conventional lore about the travails of writers, composers, and artists. During such dreaded times, these individuals supposedly become plagued with self-doubts and insecurities. Lacking in inspiration and new ideas, they believe their personal muse has left them, perhaps never to return again. Many weather these times by turning their energies elsewhere. Some become panicked at the prospect of enforced change and take desperate measures to break through their blocks, resorting to alcohol or drugs. Others become frustrated and confused, sometimes even suicidal, and believe that life is not worth living if they are no longer able to create.

Witness, for example, Joseph Conrad's desperation at a time when he was unable to write: "I sit down for eight hours every day—and the sitting down is all. In the course of the working day . . . I write 3 sentences which I erase before leaving the table in despair." Elsewhere he describes the extent of his disturbance: "Sometimes it takes all my resolution and power of self control to refrain from butting my head against the wall. I want to howl and foam at the mouth. . . . After such crises of despair I doze for hours till half conscious that there is that story I am unable to write. Then I wake up, try again—and at last go to bed completely done-up. So the days pass and nothing is done. In the morning I get up with the horror of that hopelessness I must face through a day of vain efforts."

That many should treasure their creativity and fear its loss is understandable. But when many believe it to be elusive and temperamental, something never to be taken for granted because it can disappear just as mysteriously as it comes, we may wonder whether there is any justification for this belief. It is not easy to find an answer, since much of what we know about creative blocks is hearsay and hardly any research has been done on them.

Although creative blocks are real phenomena, they apparently mean different things to different people. This was brought home to me by my study of 59 women writers, 36 of whom reported having extended periods of times when they were unable to write.[3] Of these people, 25% percent mentioned mental illness, such as depression, severe anxiety, or "mental chaos," as the reasons for their blocks; 28% mentioned negative personal attitudes, such as the lack of confidence, self-doubts, fear of failure, and worry about how others will view their work; 36% mentioned distracting external circumstances, such as family obligations, busy work schedules, lack of time, and being exhausted after they care for their families; 8% mentioned procrastination, problems getting started, difficulties meeting deadlines, or simply a lack of desire; and 3% gave other reasons.

The reasons for the creative blocks of eminent writers, although they may often be represented in more colorful and dramatic form, are not so different from those of noneminent women writers. Not surprisingly, the most common reason for prolonged periods of inactivity is mental illness. When depression, mania, anxiety, or alcoholism become intense enough, creative activity usually comes to a halt. "I have lapsed into a mere silence," Robert Lowell said about a poetry block that lasted throughout a period of depression of almost 2 years. During this difficult time, he turned to other less demanding activities, such as working on an adaptation of *Prometheus Bound* and translating a number of works. Albert Camus, when depressed, dealt with his inability to write by engaging in other pursuits, such as reading, writing letters, and getting involved in the theater.

At times, however, it is difficult to determine whether the person's mental disturbance caused the block or the block caused the disturbance. Sylvia Plath describes this conundrum well: "I just got into a vicious circle of the more I tried the less I could write, the less I could write, the more depressed I became about not being able to produce. . . . I just didn't think I was ever going to be able to write." Orlo Thomas Heggen, best known as the author of *Mr. Roberts*, also got caught up in a vicious circle of this sort. His depression and drug abuse made it hard for him to remain creative. Panicked over his worsening writing block, he sought therapy and later committed suicide.

Sometimes these writing blocks are precipitated by work difficulties, upsetting family events, or marital problems. After the death of a close friend and the breakup of his second marriage, John Steinbeck became frightened about losing his will to write. As his desire slowly returned, he commented on how strange it was that he could lose it so completely. After he lost his job at a newspaper and was forced to live with his parents, James Matthew Barrie, best known for his play *Peter Pan*, had a severe block during which his mind would go blank and he would be overcome with anxiety.

Agatha Christie had a long writing block after her husband told her he had fallen in love with another woman and wanted a divorce. In a state of shock, she ate little, slept little, and let her appearance deteriorate. During this time, she was unable to work on her next book. After about a month, she disappeared and her car was found abandoned. When she finally resurfaced in a hotel 10 days later, she had a complete loss of memory of who she was and apparently did not recognize her husband. She eventually was able to recover most her memory after undergoing a course of psychiatric therapy.

At other times creativity seems to be a finite source of energy that becomes depleted after a prolonged and especially difficult writing project. People describe the experience as feeling like their "wells have run dry" or their "creative juices have dried up," and they believe they have nothing original left to say. When this happens, all they can do is to wait anxiously until the elusive energy returns. Vladislav Khodasevich, the Russian poet, is a case in point. He attributed the inspirations for his prolific writings to "magic moments." Once these magic moments eventually left him, he was unable to write again.

Personal insecurities and idiosyncratic reactions also affect creative activity. Margaret Mitchell, author of *Gone With the Wind*, had a prolonged writer's block whenever she developed "the humbles." These were times when self-doubts arose after reading critical reviews of her work. Success also can have an inhibiting effect on inspiration. Gertrude Stein apparently had a long writing block after the phenomenal success of her book, *The Autobiography of Alice B. Toklas.*

Another obvious reason for writer's block is simply not wanting to write. Certain writers are terrible procrastinators and have trouble starting new projects. Dorothy Parker, noted for her mordant wit and cleverness, had constant difficulties meeting deadlines and commitments. Although some blamed her difficulties on her troubled marriage and her hectic social life, her editor at *Esquire* had a simpler answer. "She seemed sincerely to detest writing. She truly hated to write."

Of course, this list of the factors contributing to writer's block is not exhaustive. We have not considered debilitating physical illnesses, chronic pain, and other factors that lower energy and motivation. For present purposes, however, these anecdotal examples are sufficient to make an important point. There is some justification for the fear creative people feel about creative blocks. As prolific as they are, they cannot take their creativity for granted. Many circumstances can get in the way and interfere with their work. This is a frightening prospect for people who not only rely on creative expression for their livelihood but also often view it as their purpose for being. As Kafka wrote, "A non-writing writer is a monster courting insanity." However, what seems to be distinctive about those who become great writers is that they do not let these blocks get in their way. Most manage somehow to survive them. Later, many even write creatively about their blocks.

DIFFERENT POSSIBILITIES

It is not enough to establish an overlap between mental illness and creative activity at a critical juncture in people's lives. What we need to know is whether one has a harmful or beneficial effect on the other. Ample anecdotal information of this sort exists, not only about people's first professional success but also about other creative activities over the entirety of their lives.

As we examine the impact of mental disturbances on creative activity and productivity, certain matters have to be kept in mind. The effects of mental disturbances may depend on their severity. Mild depression or mania, for instance, may help creative activity or productivity, while more severe depression or mania may inhibit it. The same sorts of emotional disturbance may have different effects on creative activity at different periods in peoples' lives. A severe depression during a person's youth, for example, may have a far greater effect on his or her career than if it happens in later life. Different mental disturbances also may affect creative activity or productivity in different ways. Depression, for example, may slow thought processes, mania may speed them up, and schizophrenia may fragment them. Just as mental disturbances may influence creativity, creative activity may influence mental disturbances. What all this shows is that different kinds of relationships between mental disturbances and creative activity can occur in the same individuals over the courses of their lives and that one kind of relationship does not characterize them all.[4]

Mental Disturbance That Increases Creative Output

From examination of the various biographical materials, I found evidence that at least 16% of those persons who suffered from an emotional disorder showed an improvement in their creative activity at some point in their lives in response to a mental disturbance. This improvement involved greater productivity, overcoming writing blocks, the generation of new ideas, inspirations, or better performances. While examples of this improvement existed for most mental disturbances (with the exception of the psychoses), they were more plentiful in people with mania and alcoholism.

Among those with mood disorders, Theodore Roethke viewed his manic episodes as sources of creativity, and tried to preserve them and keep them under control. In his *Open Letter* he wrote that any history of the psyche is bound to be a succession of experiences, a "perpetual slipping-back, then a going forward but there is some progress made. . . . Dissociation often precedes a new state of clarity." Guillaume Apollinaire wrote that his sadness was not the impoverished kind that deadens everything: "Mine shines like a star, it illumines the path of art through the terrifying night of life." In 1876, after his parents' death the year before, Edvard Grieg wrote his longest and best composition for piano "with my life's blood in days of sorrow and despair." Periods of depression, rather than being disabling, inspired Joseph Pulitzer to greater activity and an increased flow of directives for the newspaper.

Others, such as Johan August Strindberg, exploited their inner chaos, sometimes deliberately stirring up turbulent emotions as inspiration for their work. Herman Hesse's creativity and productivity were intertwined with his tensions and conflicts. Frank O'Connor seemed to write better when he was tormented by adversity. Joseph Conrad claimed that he could not write unless he had the "nervous force"; writing was simply "the conversion of nervous force into phrases." Louise Bogan believed that she had achieved too much "normality," which had contributed to her spiritual death. After publication of *The Sleeping Fury*, when she proclaimed her neurosis cured, her productive days as a poet were essentially over.

Yet others relied on drugs to foster creativity and productivity. Andy Warhol used amphetamines to keep him going through 12-hour work days. Antonin Artaud used opium to aid him in the discovery of his identity and had a period of increased productivity while taking the drug. Jean-Paul Sartre used stimulants to heighten perception.

Instances also are plentiful of how people exploited alcohol in the service of their art.[5] The poet Robert Lowell who suffered from a debilitating manic–depressive disorder, wrote, "I seemed to connect almost unstopping composition with drinking. Nothing was written drunk, at least nothing was perfected and finished, but I have looked forward to whatever one gets from drinking, a stirring and a blurring." Delmore Schwartz, when manic, not only used alcohol to keep his writing from becoming more discursive and disorganized or, when depressed, to stimulate thought and creativity but, in time, for almost everything else as well: "I am an exaltation drinker, perhaps a sleep drinker or escape drinker too." Hart Crane gathered his raw material under the combined influence of alcohol and all forms of music, getting just drunk enough to link phrases easily. Then, after the phrases were assembled pell-mell, he would rework them for months until he came up with the exact words and structures for his poetry.

For many more people, alcohol appeared to exert a beneficial effect by removing roadblocks or impediments to creativity, such as relieving severe depression—as was the case for John Cheever early in his career—or by modulating the effects of other drugs, as was the case with Jean-Paul Sartre, who also relied heavily on stimulants and caffeine. William Faulkner once remarked, "The tools that I need for my trade are simply pen, paper, food, tobacco, and a little whiskey."[6] Others such as Jack Kerouac, who believed that drugs and alcohol helped him understand the human condition better, or Jackson Pollock, who claimed that alcohol made his paintings possible, although he seldom painted while he drank, apparently were referring to alcohol being helpful for the initiation of creativity rather than as fuel for the creative process itself. Kingsley Amis described this well: "And then, quaking, you sit down at the typewriter. And that's when a glass of Scotch can be very helpful as a sort of artistic icebreaker . . . artificial infusion of a little bit of confidence which is necessary in order to begin at all. . . . So alcohol in moderate amounts and at fairly leisurely speed is valuable to me—at least I think so. It could be that I could have written better without it . . . but it could also be true that I'd have written far less without it."[7] T. S. Eliot admitted to Elizabeth Bowen once that he needed alcohol to get him in the mood to write. With Tennessee Williams, however, the potential benefits of alcohol were not so clear. Describing his work routine, he wrote, "I go to my studio. I usually have some wine there. And then I carefully go over what I wrote the day before. You see, baby, after a glass or two of wine I'm inclined to extravagance, I'm inclined to excesses because I drink while I'm writing, so I'll blue pencil a lot the next day. Then I sit down, and I begin to write."[8]

Then there were those individuals physically dependent on alcohol who did not feel "normal" unless they could maintain a certain level of intoxication. Malcolm Lowry, who wrote his only novel, *Under the Volcano*, while intoxicated, was a case in point. His situation also demonstrated the dilemma of how to categorize the effects of alcohol: although alcohol made it possible for him to write, it was his addiction to alcohol that made it so vital for his functioning.

One possibility that needs to be considered is that the supposed beneficial effects of alcohol on the creative process are illusory, an artificial result of alcohol itself. Because of its pharmacologic properties, alcohol has the capacity to imbue perceptions, ideas, and experiences with a heightened sense of meaning, of making things seem "more utterly utter." Of course, the most objective way to test the validity of the claim that alcohol helps inspiration—or, at worst, does not impair creative performance—is to ascertain how well writers, artists, actors, and composers function when they are completely detoxified and no longer suffering from the unsettling effects of alcohol withdrawal. We do have available certain anecdotal observations that bear on this matter. John Cheever, who once claimed to get inspiration from alcohol, wrote his most acclaimed book, *Falconer*, after he stopped drinking. Eugene O'Neill had a very productive period in his life after he stopped drinking, as did John O'Hara. George Simenon claimed he could not write without drinking, but then later did. And during an extended sober period in the 1950s, Jackson Pollock, who previously had felt that alcohol made his paintings possible, had a burst of creativity, producing 32 paintings, including four of his greatest.

Mental Disturbance That Decreases Creative Output

Instances of mental disturbances that had harmful effects on creative output were far more frequent than those that had beneficial effects. From my examination of the biographical materials, I found evidence that at least 35% of those with emotional difficulties suffered from diminished productivity, impaired performances, or deterioration in the quality of their creative work because of a mental disturbance at some point in their lives. Although all major forms of psychopathology—alcoholism, drug abuse, depression, mania, anxiety, and psychoses—had potentially devastating effects on creativity, not surprisingly this was more likely to happen during psychotic episodes.

Examples of the detrimental effects of mental illness are plentiful. The experience of Delmore Schwartz illustrates the potentially detrimental effects of mood disorders. Although he never ceased to write, the quality of his writing changed drastically, depending upon whether he was depressed or manic. When depressed, he had trouble concentrating and thus writing, taking solace instead in recording his daily life with clinical exactitude. In his last years, when high his poems were diffuse, suffered from excessive spontaneity, and sometimes were inane ravings. After his emotional breakdown, Max Weber's productivity and creativity were impaired for years, and he was completely unable to carry on his academic duties. In 1892, while H. Rider Haggard was still in despair over his son's death, his father died. He stopped seeing friends, stopped writing, and made no public appearances for over 2 years. Warren G. Harding suffered from recurrent major depressions and was treated at Dr. J. P. Kellogg's sanitarium in Battle Creek, Michigan, on at least five occasions over a 12-year period. During severe depressions and manic episodes, John Ruskin was unable to write in any concerted and coherent way. This, however, did not keep him from treasuring his affliction. In his preface to *The Storm-Cloud of the Nineteenth Century*, he wrote, "I am indeed, every day of my yet spared life, more and more grateful that my mind is capable of imaginative vision, and liable to the noble dangers of delusion which separate the speculative intellect of humanity from the dreamless instinct of brutes." During a bout of depression at age 61, Anton Dvorák noted, "For more than 14 months I have done no work and been unable to make up my mind, and I don't know how long this state of affairs will continue." Andrè Gide experienced many depressions over the years, during which his creativity was stifled. He had a fallow period after completing *The Moralist* in 1901. "A mournful torpor of mind," he wrote, "has made me vegetate for three years. . . . The least sentence is effort: talking moreover is almost as much effort as writing." When depressed, Picabia stopped painting and shifted his attention to writing. Paul Gauguin's depression affected his work in a more dramatic way. In 1898, he went into the mountains, swallowed some arsenic and prepared to die. Because he had taken so much, however, he could not keep the poison down and began vomiting uncontrollably. After remaining on the mountain for hours, he struggled to make his way home when his strength returned. His life and artistic career changed dramatically after his failed suicide attempt. He was no longer interested in being a great artist. He began working as a yellow journalist, paid young girls for sex, produced pornographic art and displayed it around his house, and became involved in local politics.

Other forms of psychopathology also may take a toll. In the early years of her career, Judy Garland used "uppers" to help her perform, but as she came to rely on them more and more, she began to fall apart. She was late for performances, often could not hit her high notes, stuttered, and frequently stumbled and fell on the stage. Vaslav Nijinsky's insanity eventually made it impossible for him to continue to dance. Drugs dulled Clara Bow's exuberance in front of the camera, made her irritable and short-tempered, and at times made it impossible for her to perform. Glenn Gould's hypochondriacal concerns caused him to cancel many concerts. His airplane and travel phobias kept him from accepting invitations to perform and shifted his interests toward radio and television as the main media for displaying his musical talents. Arthur Conan Doyle experienced periods of anxiety when he was barely able to pursue his normal schedule of work.

One of the more bizarre situations involved John Jay Chapman, the post-Civil War poet, dramatist, and critic. As a law student, he held his hand over fire after beating the imagined suitor of his wife-to-be with a stick, and then calmly went to the hospital to have it amputated. Later in his life, he suffered a severe "nervous collapse," during which he remained bedridden for a year, was tormented by upsetting thoughts, crawled around on all fours, and labored under the delusion that he had lost use of his legs. It was almost 10 years before he recovered enough to resume his career.

Although many individuals who drank could consume large quantities of alcohol over many years without apparent detriment to their work, they were not able to do so indefinitely. Ernest Hemingway, for example, could spend his evenings carousing and drinking and then write without difficulty his customary 500 words the following morning when he was younger, but not when he became older. Alcohol ruined Buster Keaton's timing and eventually destroyed his career. As his alcoholism got worse, Jack London's stories became more conventional and repetitious, and his vocabulary and imagination deteriorated. Intoxication interfered with John Barrymore's ability to recall his lines. John Coltrane began taking heroin in 1953. By 1957 he realized that alcohol and heroin were adversely affecting his music. Inspired by his readings in religion and philosophy, he managed to beat his addictions by locking himself in a room and going cold turkey. When Phil Ochs sang under the influence of alcohol, he often forgot the songs or repeated certain lines. For Jack Kerouac, the quality of his writing diminished as his alcoholism progressed, and much of what he planned to write was never written. Bix Beiderbecke, the jazz cornetist, began having increasing trouble finding his "embouchure" with the mouthpiece and, later, began relying more on a derby and other devices to mute his tone in an attempt to disguise his deficiencies. Eugene O'Neill stated, "I will never, nor never have written anything good when I am drinking or even when the miasma of drink is left."[9] Elsewhere, he compared the consistency of the brain after exposure to too much alcohol to the raw white of an egg that becomes hardened when cooked.

But the detrimental effects of alcohol did not necessarily affect all forms of creative expression. Sometimes certain kinds of activity suffered and others did not. F. Scott Fitzgerald, for instance, claimed that the finest discernments of judgment and the perception or organization of a long book did not go with liquor, but writing a short story did.

What we observe anecdotally about the detrimental effects of alcohol receives support from the scant research in this area. My own earlier survey on 34 well-known, heavy-drinking writers, artists, composers, and musical performers showed that alcohol proved detrimental to productivity in over 75% of the sample, especially in the later phases of their drinking careers.[10]

Another older study on 17 established artists who drank showed that most avoided drinking alcohol while painting.[11] All but one of the artists regarded the short-term effects of alcohol as deleterious to their work, and none used alcohol to overcome technical difficulties. The general sentiment was that alcohol provided the freedom to paint but impaired the discipline. Interestingly enough, alcohol consumption also seemed to play a role in artistic style. All of the moderate drinkers, who were also the most well adjusted, were realistic painters. The steady social drinkers had a wide range of styles. And the excessive drinkers showed greater shifts in their style of painting.

Creative Activity That Increases Mental Disturbance

What has to be remembered about the relationships between creativity and mental disturbance is that they can go both ways. Just as mental disturbances can increase creative activity, creative activity can increase psychopathology. From available biographical sources, I could find evidence of such a reversal in about 6% of all persons with emotional disorders, especially those who suffered from alcoholism, depression, and anxiety. In interpreting some of these anecdotes, we also have to bear in mind that some of the post-creative depressions may represent the aftermaths of hypomanic episodes that often are indistinguishable from creative highs.[12]

Instances of creativity-induced psychopathology usually involved the arousal of severe emotional difficulties; the surfacing of dormant psychological conflicts; experiencing a profound and sustained emotional letdown; becoming agitated and frustrated; or increasing alcohol or drug use after a period of sustained, creative activity. Sometimes, when people delved into their pasts or wrestled with their emotions, they seemed unable to put the psychological lid back on their personal Pandora's Box.

Joseph Conrad was among those who became seriously depressed after completing a creative work. After writing *Under Western Eyes*, he had a 4-month "breakdown" during which he was unable to complete the revision. Shirley Jackson became depressed after she completed *The Bird's Nest* in 1954. As John Cheever worked on *The Wapshot Chronicle*, his mood grew darker and he became suicidally depressed; this "absurd melancholy" continued despite the novel's success. A similar mood overtook him several years later when he finished *Bullet Park*. In 1925 after publishing his latest book, Van Wyck Brooks became extremely depressed and began talking of suicide. Ivor Gurney experienced prolonged bouts of depression following periods of intensive creativity. John Steinbeck's mood swings coincided with periods of intensive creative activity and post-completion depression. Marc Blitzstein became despondent after composing *Cain*. After writing *Anna Karenina*, Leo Tolstoy suffered an emotional and spiritual collapse. Although Dora Carrington was happiest while she painted, her completed paintings frequently depressed her. Other creative artists showed anxiety, exhaustion, or an increase in alcohol use. On occasion, after periods of frantic, extended creative activity in preparation for an exhibit, Francis Picabia would suffer from "neurasthenia." William Dean Howells broke down and became overwhelmed with tremendous anxiety and depression during the writing of several books. Antonin Artaud was terrified of being creative, of exploring the depths of his unconscious, because he was afraid it would drive him insane. Truman Capote expressed a common reason for increased alcohol use after creative activity: for winding down and falling asleep. He said that once he began writing in earnest, his mind "zoomed all night every night, and I don't think I really slept for several years. Not until I discovered that whiskey could relax me."

What these anecdotes show is that creative activity is not without its dangers. Perhaps this partly explains why many approach it with some degree of apprehension. People often employ a variety of psychological defenses to keep emotional conflicts unconscious so that they can go about their daily business without constant anxiety or distractions. Creative activity often penetrates these defenses and brings to conscious awareness unresolved feelings and painful recollections, which after they are examined, may not be easily ignored.

Creative Activity That Reduces Mental Disturbance

Creative activity may not only aggravate mental problems, it may reduce them as well. For many people, creative activity seems to serve a therapeutic purpose, enabling them to organize their emotional chaos, to work out personal conflicts, or simply to distract themselves from worrisome concerns or their compulsion to drink. In certain instances, individuals feel compelled to engage in these creative pursuits to preserve their mental health. Whether the therapeutic benefits of the creative activity are due to problem solving, a pleasurable, neurophysiological "flow state," or the release of brain endorphins is hard to say. Whatever the reasons for these benefits, I could document their existence in about 13% of those persons with mental disturbances, although I suspect that the percentage in actuality is much higher. Instances of the therapeutic effects of creative activity were more common in those suffering from depression than from any other mental disturbance.

Clara Barton coped with depression mainly through activity and work, but when the work became excessive, it created incapacitating "nervous" symptoms. Pablo Picasso provides an excellent example of the salubrious effects of work. "Where do I get this power of creating and forming?" he said, "I don't know. I have only one thought: work. I paint just as I breathe. When I work I relax; doing nothing or entertaining visitors makes me tired." Eugene O'Neill claimed, "Writing is my vacation from living." During a tense and difficult time, Carson McCullers threw herself into her writing as a way of coping with her problems. Sherwood Anderson claimed that writing was "curative" because it helped him to face himself. He believed that when he was writing, he could not lie. If he hedged or was not honest, he could detect the misrepresentation immediately. When he wrote in a way that seemed to him right, he felt clean and pure, no longer a "smooth son of a bitch." When upset or depressed over some remark by her husband, Elinor Glyn typically turned to her diary or writing. Josephine Baker was "cured" of her severe depression after consulting a female doctor and taking on the task of editing a book on women. In 1915 the "Muse of Painting" rescued Winston Churchill from the "Black Dog," a term he used to describe his depressions. Puccini coped with his bouts of despair and troubled mood through work. William Faulkner used his writing as a form of exorcism and ventilation for various torments. When asked the name of his analyst, Ernest Hemingway replied, "Portable Corona No. 3." John O'Hara began writing his first novel as a way of coping with his divorce from his first wife. "In order to save myself from what is commonly referred to as 'nerves,'" Franz Kafka wrote, "I have lately begun to write a little. From about seven at night I sit at my desk, but it doesn't amount to much. It is like trying to dig a foxhole with one's fingernails in the midst of battle."

COMMENTS

Some general observations are in order. Despite our detailed examination of the ways mental disturbances and creativity actively affect the other, we should note that no evidence of this relationship exists for the vast majority of eminent persons, especially early in their careers when the prevalence rates of mental illness are lower. The career choices of individuals have an important bearing on this matter. Almost ten times as many artistic as investigative types, for example, display mental disturbances at the time of their initial professional success, suggesting that certain mental disturbances, such as excessive alcohol or drug use, far from being incompatible with creative accomplishment, may become part of the very fabric of their professional lives. While severe forms of emotional difficulties usually have devastating effects on their creativity, this does not necessarily hold for milder forms. Most individuals manage to function and work despite their mental problems, especially when they are not so severe, and a sizeable number even manage to use their psychopathology in the service of their art, much as artists use their palettes.

While creative activity can be therapeutic and self-reinforcing for many individuals, particularly for those who suffer from depression, it is not without inherent dangers, sometimes stirring up problems that cannot be readily contained. Those who delve inward and use emotional experiences as the raw material for their creative output are more likely to experience the double-edged sword of creative activity. While the creative process lets them master and channel their painful experiences through the power of their expression, they sometimes cannot contain the emotional forces unleashed through their probing.

Since psychopathology can be beneficial or harmful for creative activity and creative activity can be beneficial or harmful for mental health, a complex situation exists that cannot be accounted for easily by any simple, categorical claims about the healthy or unhealthy functions of creative activity. Any conclusions about the nature of this relationship, then, need to be tempered by a number of qualifications about the kind, severity, and timing of the mental disturbance and the type of creative activity involved.

So far my observations have been based entirely on anecdotes to illustrate the effects of mental disturbances and creative activity on one another at given points in time. While these anecdotes are instructive, they do not inform us about the impact of mental disturbances over the course of a lifetime on the lifetime accomplishments of people. Only this latter relationship matters, since greatness tends to be based on cumulative achievements. As it happens, statistical analyses designed for this purpose revealed that the various forms of psychopathology are only weak predictors of lifetime creative achievement.[13,S2] A definite relationship exists, but it is an unimpressive one, accounting for less than 10% of the variance in the achievement scores. This is an encouraging sign. If mental disturbances can weakly predict the extent of creative achievement in individuals, then perhaps they, in combination with other measures, can prove to be even more powerful predictors. This is what I explore in the next chapter.

CHAPTER NINE

Predicting "True" Greatness

Any plausible theory about the relationship between mental illness and creative activity must do two things. It must account for why certain people who do not suffer from mental illness are as capable of great creative achievements as other people who do. It also must be able to predict accurately which individuals will accomplish great deeds and which will not.

So far the results show that various mental health measures that establish different rates of mental illness for different professional types are not strong predictors of lifetime creative achievement. The question is why. Is it simply due to not using the right approach? Or is it because only a weak significant relationship exists? One likely reason for this situation was that the heterogeneity of the sample obscured any meaningful link between mental disturbances and creative achievement. Another reason was that my choice of predictors was too restricted. This prompted me to adopt a new approach, taking both possibilities into account.

Instead of trying to identify potential predictors of creative achievement within the entire sample, I decided to focus only on those who are truly great and those who are less so. The existence of these two groups should remind us that while most eminent people are remarkable, some are more outstanding than others. The most remarkable people—*the truly great*—are not simply celebrities, champions, gold medalists, highly successful professionals, or winners of important prizes. Thomas Carlyle and later William James noted that these are the people who, once accepted by their societies, modify them in original and particular ways, much like a new biological species changes the equilibrium of the vegetation and animal life in its region.[1] They are one-of-a-kinds, masters, the ultra-elite, virtuosos, the *crème de la crème*, the *ne plus ultra*, nonpareils, superstars within their fields, people whose lives and accomplishments have become legendary, and have come to represent the "gold standards" against which most forms of human achievement are measured. Thus if we wish to assess the relationship of mental illness to extraordinary achievement, we should concentrate our efforts on these individuals.

With a sample of over 1,000 eminent persons, the dilemma is where to draw the line that separates the ordinary eminent from the extrordinary eminent. Does the category of extrordinary achievement include the top 1%, 5%, 10%, 25% or 50% of eminent individuals? If we confine our study to the extreme 1% or 5% of these exceptional people, then we should be dealing with a greater concentration of genius. But this choice leaves so few individuals represented in the various specialties that the possibility of detecting any common characteristics among them becomes remote. On the other hand, if we compare the top half of the sample to the lower half, then the large number of people with overlapping, mid-range accomplishments will obscure the very qualities we are searching for. We need to find a compromise that will allow us to distinguish between those of greater and lesser eminence and yet provide sufficient numbers of people for the analyses.[2]

My strategy was to compare those individuals scoring in the upper quartile of creative achievement with those scoring in the lower quartile. Readers should remember that the creative achievement scores, which represented the basis for separating these two groups, were more than arbitrary numbers. Besides measuring the magnitude of the professional accomplishments of eminent individuals, they corresponded to the number of lines allotted to them in the *Encyclopaedia Britannica* and the *Encyclopedia Americana* and other external indicators of relative greatness. Those with higher scores commanded more page space than those with lower scores. This relationship of achievement scores to line space held not only for those in the arts and sciences but those in politics, exploration, business, social activism, and the military as well. In essence, these achievement scores served as a rough gauge of relative eminence or greatness.

For our purposes, the 250 people in the upper quartile of creative achievement represented the *truly great* or upper elite. In contrast, those 249 people in the lower quartile represented the *less great* or lower elite.[3] With rare exceptions, a listing of the people selected by this method should remove any doubts about how well this approach identified true greatness (See Appendix A).

GREATER VERSUS LESSER DEGREES OF EMINENCE

When we compare the upper and lower elite on certain general characteristics, several immediate differences emerge. While they share many similarities—life span, race, and birth order—they differ in the nature of their professional choice and their gender mix. Individuals at the upper level of eminence are largely in the creative arts professions, especially architecture, art, musical composition, musical entertainment, theater, fiction, and poetry, as well as the natural and social sciences. Those at the lower level are mostly in business, sports, exploration, the military, public office, or are social figures, companions, and nonfiction writers.[S1] Also, about three times the percentage of males as females are in the upper elite (59% versus 20%).[S2]

The family backgrounds of these individuals are revealing not only for their differences but for their similarities. Although parents of both the upper and lower elites have similar divorce rates and come from similar social classes and religious backgrounds, the parents of the upper elite earn less income and are more creative and aesthetically inclined. The mothers of those in the upper elite also have a greater likelihood of being emotionally disturbed.[S3]

As children and adolescents, the upper and lower elite show many important differences. Compared to members of the lower elite, those in the upper elite are about twice as likely to be sickly, physically handicapped, or have serious medical illnesses as youths.[S2] Besides the greater likelihood of others portraying them as moody, solitary, or "odd," four times as many members of the upper elite as lower elite have major emotional difficulties before age 13, and about twice as many have them between the ages of 13 and 20 years.[S2]

Not all the differences between these groups involve physical or emotional problems. At least four times as many ultra elite as lower elite show signs of precocity before the age of 13.[S2] About twice as many get superior grades in high school or college, read avidly, and win academic awards. Greater percentages have personal mentors, and about four times as many enjoy a major professional success before they are 21. They also are less likely than the lower elite to enter professions similar to those of their fathers.[S2]

As we found in the comparison of professional types, those who differ as youths usually differ as adults. With both groups of elites, this turns out to be the case. Members of the upper elite are more likely to be solitary, moody, nonaffiliative, and aesthetically inclined.[S2] They also are about twice as likely to be atheists or agnostics, or to hold idiosyncratic beliefs about God.

While those at the upper and lower levels of eminence do not differ in their rates of marriage and divorce or their sexual orientations, those who achieve true greatness within the creative arts are disproportionately heterosexual compared to those in the other professions. Why this is so is a matter for speculation. My suspicion is that the moral climate of the times was largely responsible. Many of these individuals grew up during the tail end of the Victorian era, which affected moral attitudes in Western society well into this century. The fact of homosexuality was a taboo topic, which must have been especially constraining for those in the creative arts where people often reveal so much of themselves. When people have to be more discreet and circumspect in what they paint, sculpt, or do, they surely must be at a competitive disadvantage in terms of the content and scope of their art or even in developing a supreme confidence in themselves. This may not have prevented them from becoming eminent, but it may have hampered many from becoming "truly great," a designation that requires their work to have broad influence over others and some degree of universal appeal.

Members of the upper elite also differ from those of the lower elite in their physical and mental well-being. Those in the upper elite are more likely to suffer from chronic medical illnesses both before and after the age of 50. They also suffer more from mental disturbances throughout their adult lives—especially depression, alcoholism, adjustment difficulties, and somatic problems—and are more likely to receive treatment for them.[52] This is an especially important finding for our purposes, since it documents for the first time a significant, positive relationship between mental illness and the extent of creative achievement in eminent persons, across a variety of vocations. It also offers justification for using certain mental health measures as predictors of professional achievement.

These assorted results clearly establish that members of the upper elite differ from those of the lower elite in many ways. The sheer number of the significant differences between them is impressive. With all their differences, those in the upper elite and lower elite appear to be fundamentally different types. The challenge is how to capitalize on this for predictive purposes.

A PREDICTION MODEL

In one anecdotal survey of the early lives of gifted men and women, the authors concluded that it was impossible to forecast achievement or to identify the best home and scholastic background for enabling a child to develop to his or her full potential. They write:

We cannot possibly say whether the men . . . achieved their fame in spite of their homes and their schools or because of them—even when the homes were thoroughly deplorable, and the education was as unsatisfactory as it could be. Boys who had unhappy childhoods because of their homes, or who were bullied and derided at school, or were beaten unmercifully by their teachers, might never have achieved what they did if they had been brought up differently. *Life is so complex that no man can say.*[4]

If true, this is a discouraging conclusion, but it happens to be premature.

The very fact that many personal characteristics and circumstances successfully distinguish the upper elite from the lower elite raises the question of whether some combination of them can be used to predict the relative greatness of people, if not in advance then at least retrospectively.[5] Since these subjects were equally divided between the upper and lower quartiles of creative achievement, the laws of chance, like the tossing of a coin, dictate that we should be able to guess correctly if they are in the lower or upper quartile, even without knowing anything about them, in about 50% of the cases. But any useful prediction model should be much more accurate than chance. With human behavior, a predictive accuracy of 75% to 85% is good, and anything above that is excellent. The closer the odds are to 100% of correctly classifying all individuals, the greater the likelihood that a causal relationship exists between the predictors and what is predicted if the predictors precede the event of interest. This, of course, represents a theoretical ideal, seldom realized in the behavioral sciences. Still, it is one to which we can aspire.

My approach was to use a logistic regression model to determine which combination of variables best predicted whether individuals belonged to the upper or lower quartiles of achievement.[6] At first, I simply used the extensive mental health information about individuals to learn how well this predicted the extent of their professional achievement. This information correctly classified 63% of all persons, significantly better than chance but not impressively so. Next I broadened the list of potential predictors to 30 promising variables (including some of the mental health items), mainly those that distinguished the lower from the upper elite.The results revealed that this model fit the data almost exactly, correctly classifying 92% of all cases on whom complete information was available, with a smaller subset of these predictors correctly classifying almost as much. This was far better than could have been expected by chance, and given the nature of the measures, as close to a perfect prediction as I could hope for. [S4]

A TEMPLATE FOR TRUE GREATNESS

These results, in their entirety, help to identify the essential elements of exceptional achievement. Not only can we distinguish individuals at the upper level of eminence from those at the lower level based on many personal attributes and developmental events, but even more important, we can predict with great accuracy their relative eminence from certain of these same attributes and events, including their mental health. Rather than any single attribute being identified with greatness, the findings reveal that a special combination of elements distinguishes the truly great from those at the lower rung of eminence. From a theoretical standpoint, this special combination of elements, along with the significant findings from the many comparative analyses, seems to comprise a "template" for exceptional achievement and public recognition. This combination of elements includes a special talent or ability, the right kind of parents, contrariness, being a loner, physical vulnerability, a "personal seal," a drive for supremacy, and psychological "unease." Under proper social conditions, fortune favors those who possess this template over those who do not, and adversity does not deter them as much. Because this template seems so essential for exceptional achievement, a discussion of each of its elements follows.

Special Ability

Being "gifted" represents an important element of this template. Individuals with extraordinary talents, abilities, or gifts as youths, such as perfect pitch, photographic memory, great mathematical skills, physical agility, superior draftsmanship, an ear for languages, or a keen intelligence that allows them to grasp complex concepts in certain areas easily, appear to have a decided edge over those who do not. But being gifted is not, however, sufficient for greatness. Only a very small percentage of gifted children become eminent and far fewer ever reach the heights of greatness. Experts now agree that most accomplishments of any social value require that the gifted be thoroughly trained and grounded in their particular fields.[7] The time necessary to do this varies among the different professions. Classical composers, for instance, require about a 10-year period of intense musical training before completing their first enduring work. For artists, writers, and actors, the amount of time is usually less. The greater the genius of individuals, naturally, the less preparatory time they require to realize their full creative potentials.[8]

With a need to hone their skills, high percentages of those at the upper level of eminence get college degrees and doctorates or attend special schools, such as music conservatories or art academies. People on the path toward greatness exploit every possible opportunity to exercise and perfect their special talents or intellectual gifts. As youths, they are self-learners, and do more than their formal training requires them to. They read widely, practice incessantly, study under the top tutors, win important awards, give special recitals and become increasingly adept in their preferred media of expression. At some time during their training, many deliberately seek out or manage to attract influential mentors who recognize their unique abilities, help them to refine their talents, and aid them in their careers. It is no accident that future Nobel laureates tend to study under other Nobel laureates, that the future top academicians attend the best schools, that great composers and artists choose to study under masters, or that many young artists, writers, and musicians with great promise tend to congregate together. Excellence attracts excellence. What this suggests is that those destined for greatness have become servants to their own talent. They constantly seek ways to perfect and express it and construct much of their world around it as well.

The "Right" Kind of Parents

In general, parents of the truly great seem to recognize the exceptional qualities of their offspring and provide them with the necessary tutors, educational opportunities, and other resources to pursue their professional goals. Although those in both the upper and lower elite mostly come from solid, middle-class, professional backgrounds with lawyers, physicians, teachers, ministers, professors, scientists, artists, writers, and small businessmen as fathers, the parents of those in the upper elite, while comfortable financially, are not apt to be as wealthy. It seems that families that provide "optimal" material resources—not too many or too few—are not as likely to dull their children's need to achieve or discourage them from trying to achieve.

There is good reason why too many or too few material resources should hinder great achievement. When children are born into families with high social status and ample wealth, they already have much of what eminent people are striving for. If they come from aristocratic or wealthy families, they have a certain degree of name recognition, people already defer to them and treat them as special, and they can essentially do as they please. There is no need for them to work incessantly or take risks that may jeopardize what they already have. Most important, they have not been inculcated with the work ethic, nor need they be.

Among the truly great in my sample, less than 8% have landed gentry, aristocrats, tycoons, or wealthy socialites as parents, and of those who do, most seem to have encountered special events during childhood that set them apart. Guillaume Apollinaire's father, supposedly a nobleman, deserted his wife before Apollinaire was born. Both of Bertrand Russell's parents died when he was a child. Henri Toulouse-Lautrec, whose father and mother belonged to the nobility, had to cope with his small stature and deformity. Winston Churchill, whose father was Lord Randolph Spencer Churchill, a brilliant speaker in Parliament, stuttered as a child. Count Leo Tolstoy lost his parents and other close relatives at an early age. Vladimir Nabokov and his aristocratic parents fled Russia during the Revolution. Later, he had to endure the assassination of his brilliant and beloved father.

If having upper-class, wealthy parents can be disadvantageous for eminence, having very poor parents may be more so, but in a different way. The problems associated with poverty can be enormous. Not only do children with unemployed or unskilled parents often have to work to contribute to the family finances, but they also lack many cultural advantages. Even more important, without accomplished parents, they are not exposed to professionally successful role models and, because of the family's struggle for survival, are not as likely to embrace a broader vision. Due to these factors, people from very poor backgrounds who manage to reach the pinnacle of success are more likely to do so in fields such as business, art, social activism, or the entertainment industry, which do not require costly training.

But other ingredients also go into making the proper parental mix. Having creative or aesthetically inclined parents also benefits children. Growing up in these family environments, children are exposed to many culturally enriching influences and imbued with the value of creative expression.

But parents engaged in creative activities are not always the most stable or well-adjusted. The mothers of the truly great, in particular, often tend to be emotionally disturbed, perhaps understandably so, given the temper of the times and the limited opportunities for intelligent and talented women to realize their personal potentials. Their fathers, too, also seem to have their share of emotional difficulties. Children raised in these households are bound to sense that all is not well in their immediate worlds.

Simone de Beauvoir's parents, for example, fought constantly over money. Her mother, who encouraged her daughter to write, was the eldest child of a banker who went bankrupt. Her father, who had banked on his wife becoming wealthier, was an amateur actor and avid reader. He instilled in de Beauvoir a love of reading, often claiming that nothing in the world was finer than an author. Meaning to compliment his daughter, he once claimed, "Simone has a man's brain; she thinks like a man; she is a man."

Georgia O'Keeffe's father was an inventive farmer, the first in his area to own a telephone and harvest tobacco. Her mother, who played the piano and sang, held strong views about the values of education. She supported her daughter's aspirations and encouraged her to be self-reliant. Although her parents had been reasonably prosperous, they had financial troubles while Georgia was growing up.

The mother of Rudyard Kipling was a witty, attractive, and brilliant woman who alternated between periods of gaiety and serious depression. Immensely talented, she played musical instruments, sang, composed songs, and wrote poetry and stories. Before his parents married, they remained engaged for 4 years because his father, also a writer of stories, did not have enough money to support a family. Eventually he secured a teaching position at an art school in India and made an adequate living.

Frank Lloyd Wright's mother was a teacher who idolized her son and stimulated his interest in architecture. Wright's father was a preacher and later a lawyer who was subject to depression, moved around a lot, and never made much money. Some thought him to be a musical genius because he played at least six instruments. Growing up in this household must have been difficult for Wright. His mother would have spells when she supposedly had "mad hysterics," "raved like a maniac," and occasionally attacked her husband. This continued until his parents divorced.

Contrariness

Talented, well-trained, and highly motivated individuals may either choose to work within the framework of existing paradigms or radically depart from them to pursue novel, unacceptable views. When they work within the framework of existing paradigms, individuals may achieve respectability and success but will not be likely to leave a distinctive mark on their societies. To create new schools of thought, blaze new trails, make major discoveries, propose radical solutions, or promote new products, they must show irreverence toward established authority and a readiness to discard prevalent views. For the upper elite, antagonism toward their parents, unwillingness to follow "in their fathers' footsteps," and the greater likelihood of rejecting formal religion and embracing atheistic, agnostic, or idiosyncratic religious views all point toward an early eagerness to reject the status quo.

These individuals often have an attitude set that is oppositional in nature.[9] It is almost as though this response style is part of their very natures. Given their tendencies toward iconoclasm, these individuals are often at odds with others. Their style may seem confrontational, sarcastic, and challenging, prompting other people to feel attacked. They also may be outwardly modest and unassuming, while not backing down from their unpopular views. Sometimes their mental perversity may even put them in mortal danger. A good example of this is when the Gestapo made Sigmund Freud sign a statement saying that he had been treated well by them as a condition for his being able to leave Germany. Freud responded by writing that he recommended the Gestapo highly. None of the Gestapo, fortunately, detected his sardonic wit.

This antagonism to traditional beliefs and practices and established forms of authority assumes many forms. George Bernard Shaw, for instance, displayed it in his satirical comedies and essays, in which he attacked such sacrosanct social institutions of the times as medicine, the legal profession, religion, marriage, and the status of women. C. Wright Mills was a loner and rebel, whom few liked personally. He reacted strongly against his domineering father and was contemptuous of the political system. Fascinated with authorities and leaders, he offered an indictment of the social power structure in The Power Elite, his best known work. Henrik Ibsen, the Norwegian playwright, was rebellious during his youth and had a hatred toward all authority figures. Although outwardly conforming, he decided that Christianity was the enemy of society and espoused many other controversial views about other cherished beliefs. Some, such as Francis Picabia, displayed this contrariness almost in caricature. Picabia, known for his mechanomorphic style and his dadaist paintings and writings, was antieverything: antiestablishment, antiauthority, and antitradition. He lambasted various social institutions and schools of thought. In one of his attacks against religion, he offered the following theorem to prove that God was a fantasy: (a) God = a creation of man in man's image; (b) Machine = a creation of man in man's image; (c) God = Machine. Perhaps the best display of his natural contrariness was that he eventually became an anti-Dada Dadaist.

Where this automatic contrariness or almost reflexive antagonism to established beliefs comes from is hard to say. Those who adopt a psychological approach are likely to seek answers in the relationships children have with their parents. In some cases this may be relevant. But we also cannot discount the possibility that it may be biological in origin. We know that in the animal world certain animals are born mavericks or, like the rogue elephants, prefer to travel alone. As Ivan Pavlov noted with his dogs, certain ones naturally resist classical conditioning and even show contrary responses. A streak of wildness never leaves them, and they are difficult to train.

In a related manner, it may be the case that many of those who achieve true greatness have a feral outlook in their work, which resists attempts at domestication and social programming. While this wild streak may have irrational roots, it is not necessarily misguided. What distinguishes these individuals from others is that they do not simply rebel. These are not people who just see that the emperor has no clothes; they offer their own brand of attire for him to wear. Also, when dominant ideologies challenge reason, morality, or "truth," they feel obliged to speak out, do what they believe is right, or pursue their own goals, even when they may be punished for doing so.

Loners

Others have commented on the importance of solitude in the life of creative persons.[10] With a relative lack of outside distractions, they have a chance to turn inward and reflect, focusing all their energies on the task at hand. This capacity for aloneness or solitude seems important for the truly great.

As children, members of the upper elite are more likely to be loners and regarded by others as a bit strange. As adults, they engage in solitary pursuits and don't seek out social affiliations. Reluctant to collaborate, they do not work well in groups. When they do participate in groups or organizations, they take over, function only in a symbolic capacity, or accept only honorary positions. They are disinterested in interacting socially with others on an equal basis. Less reliant on other people, organizations, and social activities, they view their work as an extension of themselves and resist outside demands that detract from it. Many have stormy relationships with friends, neglect their families and have conflicts with fellow professionals. While others may interpret this behavior as self-centered, these individuals have practical reasons for their self-sufficiency, independence, and solitariness. If they kept up active social lives, spent lots of time with their families, became actively involved in professional organizations, and participated in community activities, they simply would not have time and energy left for their work.

Being a loner can take different forms. George Orwell, best known for his novels *1984* and *Animal Farm*, wandered about Paris and London on his own, looking to experience the underbelly of society. Paul Gauguin, who alienated his friends and peers, retreated to Tahiti to paint. While there, except for the many women who served as his models and sex partners, he led a relatively solitary existence. Arnold J. Toynbee, the historian, had few friends while in school and only pursued solitary sports such as cross-country running or walking. At Oxford, he rebelled against his parents' and tutors' instruction in religion and social values. As a father, he withdrew from family responsibilities. He preferred to work only with a research assistant because he had difficulty collaborating with others. He also showed little active involvement in any social or professional organizations.

Physical Vulnerability

As children, members of the upper elite are more likely than those less eminent to be sickly and frail, to experience a life-threatening illness, or to have a physical disability. They are thus likely to have disruptions in their schooling and spend more time at home in the company of often solicitous and attentive parents. Separated from their peers, they tend to develop solitary interests, like reading, and perhaps begin to feel different from others. Along with these shaping influences on their psyches, physical problems during childhood may screen out those who possess especially effective coping skills from those who don't. As we discussed in an earlier chapter, the ability of people to cope with adversity as children may immunize them to many of the stresses they will encounter later in their lives.

For some, the influence of a childhood affliction on their later careers seems obvious; for others its impact is more obscure. In James Thurber's case, his affliction had an indirect effect. When he was 7 years old, his older brother accidentally shot an arrow in his left eye. With a 2-week delay in removing the blinded eye, Thurber developed a "sympathetic ophthalmia" in his good eye, which plagued him in his later life and eventually caused his total blindness. Although he was able to see for 40 years well enough to read, write, and draw, his visual difficulties seemed to have contributed to the distinctive nature of his cartoons.

While the physical disorders of childhood may pursue some of our eminent people all their lives, many other members of the truly great only begin to develop some form of chronic medical illness as an adult. Although others may find these illnesses to be daunting and professionally detrimental, these individuals do not seem to let them get in their way. On the contrary, they learn to work around them or find ways to turn them to their advantage. Because of their pain, discomfort or physical fragility, they may experience a greater sense of urgency, which spurs them on to increased productivity. It is almost as though they were in a race against time, a race against their failing health and the imminence of death. They realize that they have much to say and much to do but not enough time in which to do it. Their chronic illnesses, which heighten their sense of mortality, perhaps stimulate them to perpetuate their identities through their works. For these individuals, creation becomes a defense against physical deterioration.

This pressure to be creative as a way of dealing with failing health may have been operating in Friedrich Nietzsche. Knowing that the syphilis he had contracted in his 20s would cause later agonies and shorten his life, he went on to produce an enormous body of work. Subject to strange fits of paralysis, which left him unconscious, and other signs of poor health, he resigned from the university in his late 30s and increasingly withdrew from professional and social life. Even as he became more incapacitated, he somehow managed to channel his remaining energies into his writings, when his mental and physical condition allowed him to do so.

In his novel *Straight Is The Gate*, André Gide described how his convalescence from tuberculosis gave him a fresh vision of the physical world and heightened joy in his senses. When Edgar Degas was 37, he developed a recurrent infection of his right eye, which left him with the continuing fear that his artistic career would be ruined by blindness. At age 29, Isak Dinesen contacted syphilis from her husband, Bror Blixin. The crippling abdominal pains and physical consequences of this disease took a large toll on her life and, undoubtedly, affected her writing career. During the last 15 years of her life, Margaret Bourke-White shifted more of her energies from photography to writing after she was diagnosed as having Parkinson's disease. James Joyce's recurring eye difficulties had a major impact on his writing. At age 35, he was operated on for glaucoma. When he was 36, he had an attack of iritis in both eyes that left him almost incapacitated. Over the years, he had numerous operations, each time recommencing writing after the pain subsided. By the age of 44, he could write only in large, exaggerated letters. After the age of 21, H. G. Wells became a semi-invalid for 12 years because of his many physical ailments, which may have been caused by diabetes or tuberculosis. It was after this long seige of illness that Wells showed a great spurt of productivity.

What these examples suggest is not that chronic physical illnesses are beneficial to creative achievement but rather that certain individuals can take advantage of them. For most people, chronic physical ailments are usually wearying and debilitating. Certain exceptional people, in contrast, find ways to become creatively energized and even motivated by them.

A Personal Seal

The influence that eminent people can exert on their disciplines, their societies, and their times is enormous. Famous leaders such as Winston Churchill, Cecil Rhodes, Franklin Delano Roosevelt, or Golda Meier can define an era. The names of discoverers, inventors, and thinkers such as Alexander Graham Bell, Thomas Edison, William James, and others, have become linked with their scientific discoveries and philosophical contributions. Artists, composers, and performers such as Paul Cézanne, Pablo Picasso, Sergei Rachmaninoff, Fred Astaire, George Gershwin, Jackson Pollock, Auguste Rodin, and Vaslav Nijinsky have left their distinctive seals on their art. Revolutionaries, social activists, or religious leaders such as Martin Luther King, Jr., Mary Baker Eddy, or Margaret Sanger have transformed their societies or founded new movements. The identities of certain people have merged with their creations or characterizations: Charlie Chaplin with The Little Tramp, Walt Disney with his cartoon characters, Alfred Hitchcock with movie thrillers, Harry Houdini with grand illusions, H. G. Wells with science fiction. Other eminent people have become immortalized in their works, their names defining new branches of science (e.g., Freudian and Jungian psychology, Einsteinian physics), philosophical, literary, or psychological outlooks (e.g., the adjectives Kafkaesque, Nietzschean, Schweitzerian) and many major discoveries (e.g., Bohr's atom, the Stanislavsky method of acting, Turing's universal machine, the Tesla coil).

What this indicates is that individuals are not likely to assume the mantle of true greatness unless their works and achievements bear their personal seals or distinctive signatures. Whatever they do, their accomplishments have to become specifically identified with them. History does not usually accord greatness to people who are good at working in groups, participating in joint projects, carrying out others' instructions, or sacrificing personal glory for the sake of their organizations. Like tombstones, the works, products, deeds, and creations of people need to serve as ways of personally identifying them. Perhaps that is why membership in the arts and sciences represents an important predictor of greatness. Successes in these fields, far more than in other professions, involve advances, break-throughs, inventions, and discoveries that are credited to the originators. While people may also become great by providing inspiring leadership at critical times, exploring uncharted lands, developing new business prod-ucts or strategies, offering new political alternatives, or showing great bravery under duress, they only can do so when their exploits are consid-ered distinctive and specifically identified with them.

Drive for Supremacy

While those who become great live and breathe their work and their work becomes extensions of them, it is not their persistence *per se*, as some have proposed, that is unique to extraordinary persons but the special way that it is expressed. These persons have a drive for dominance, supremacy, preeminence, or power, which goes beyond professional ambition and influences the scope and nature of their goals. They behave as if they felt compelled to be the leader, champion, prophet, pioneer, master, founder, discoverer, originator, hero, or god-like creator. When they encounter social resistance, they try to shape and bend their environments to suit them, rather than adapting to their environments. Although they attract many followers and make many converts, they antagonize and alienate many people as well.

Naturally, a drive of this nature is not likely to be found in people who doubt their abilities, have modest goals, or are unsure of their values. This drive for dominance or supremacy tends to be found mostly in people with supreme self-confidence or with expansive aspirations. Many of those in the upper ranks of the eminent fit this description.

Sometimes it is difficult to distinguish the confidence that people express in themselves from arrogance or hubris. Take, for example, Charles de Gaulle's claim that he *was* France ("Je suis la France") and that he was destined to save the French nation during and after World War II. Later, after liberating Paris, he proclaimed, "I felt I was fulfilling a function beyond myself. . . . I was an instrument of destiny." In his assessment of De Gaulle, Jean-Paul Sartre wryly said, "I do not believe in God. But if I had to choose between God and De Gaulle, I would vote for God. He is more modest."

There are some who believe that General Douglas MacArthur, the one-time Supreme Commander of Allied Powers who ruled Japan after World War II and wrote its constitution, could hold his own with De Gaulle. Exposed to stories of military daring from an early age, MacArthur believed that when he grew up he would accomplish great feats. Following in the footsteps of his revered father, who was a lieutenant-general and former military governor of Manila, he tried to get into West Point but flunked his preliminary physical because of curvature of the spine. This did not deter him. He worked with a doctor to correct it and to develop the erect bearing for which he was later famous. With his remarkable memory and determination, he went on to graduate first in his class at West Point. Seemingly born to lead, he advanced rapidly in his career and was promoted to general at the age of 38. A remote and authoritarian man, whose character was marked by personal boldness, magnetism, and flair, he insisted on utter loyalty from others while reserving the right to disagree strongly with his own superiors. By middle age, he seemed so taken with himself that he began speaking of himself in the third person. He also installed a 15-foot mirror behind his office chair in Washington to amplify his image.

Cecil Rhodes also exuded this kind of self-confidence. Caught up with the British imperialist fervor as a youth, he had a keen sense of destiny, forsaking intimate sexual relationships with anyone, male or female, and pursuing his almost "divine" mission to extend the influence of the English-speaking people in Africa. After gaining control of 90% of the world's diamonds and various gold mines, he founded Rhodesia and, as an international statesman, helped to transform Southern Africa and much of the British Empire. Because Rhodesia was later renamed Zimbabwe, Rhodes is probably best known today for the scholarships bearing his name.

Other examples of great self-confidence are plentiful. Paul Gauguin claimed, that "I am a great artist, and I know it," and that he personally was the future of modern art. T. E. Lawrence believed that he was ordained to free a people from bondage. Leo Tolstoy longed to be persecuted and jailed for his extreme views, announcing to Maxim Gorky, "Were I to suffer for my ideas, they would have a greater influence." Jean-Paul Sartre said, "I could not detach myself from the symbol I had become." Ezra Pound resolved in his early teens to know more about poetry by the age of 30 than any other living person. William Saroyan proclaimed himself at age 20 to be the world's greatest writer. Frank Lloyd Wright claimed that he was the world's greatest living architect and that if he had to choose between honest arrogance and hypocritical humility, honesty dictated that he choose the former.

With truly great people, this self-confidence, while immodest, seems deserved. They accomplish what they set out to. Often, however, even when these people do not boast of their intentions, their very deeds bespeak of an underlying expansiveness in their attitudes. How else should we interpret the activities of Einstein, who strove to develop a unified field theory of the universe; Freud, who worked out a system of psychology that embraced all humanity; Arnold Schoenberg, whose 12-note scale changed the structure of music; Arnold Toynbee, who set out to write a history of mankind; or Margaret Mead, whose anthropological theories applied to all cultures?

The reason, I suspect, for the proportionately greater predominance of men than women within the upper elite is an indirect reflection of this drive for professional dominance and the greater availability of professional outlets that allow this drive to be expressed. Women can be as competitive and aggressive as men, and as capable of great achievements, but historically they could not express their personal ambitions in the same ways as men, either in their overt behavior or in more respected kinds of professional work. In addition, valued "female" qualities like humbleness, humility, self-sacrifice, tactfulness, compassion, sensitivity, and empathy may be admirable, but they are not conducive to the grand visions, large-scale projects, ambitious and risky undertakings, and monumental achievements associated with this drive for mastery and supremacy.

Psychological "Unease"

Extraordinary achievements do not arise from emotional contentment, nor do they necessarily confer peace of mind. Members of the upper elite are inclined to be restless, discontent, impatient, and driven people whose success does not necessarily satisfy them for long. No sooner do they complete one project than they are ready to tackle another. This holds for those who struggle with mental illness and those who do not.

This tendency toward being driven helps to explain why mental disturbances may contribute to exceptional achievement. Mental disturbances seem to have an indirect, rather than direct, effect on creative expression and productivity. By keeping individuals on edge or in a state of psychological "unease," they can serve as a source of creative tension. This creative tension tends to be relieved when these individuals are busily at work and in the midst of problem solving.

The notion of psychological unease forms a conceptual bridge between those in the upper elite who suffer from mental disturbances and those who do not. Those with mental disturbances that are not too severe or incapacitating experience a constant source of inner tension. Those who are not emotionally troubled seem to have the natural capacity to generate their own psychological "unease."

Aside from its many important functions, the human brain is a problem-solving organ. When it does not have problems to solve, it generates them. When it cannot generate them, it begins to seek them out. People with great curiosity and intelligence need to keep their brains active solving problems.[11] Those who suffer from mental disturbances often have an abundance of psychological problems to solve, or if they are not trying to solve them through their writing or art, may gain relief from their own problems by solving problems not particularly related to their personal histories. Those who are not bothered by psychological conflicts or troubled pasts seek out other challenging problems to solve, usually the bigger the better.[12] Once they seize on these problems, the problems take possession of them and begin to dominate most aspects of their lives. When no solution is forthcoming or the task is not going well, they may not eat, sleep, or relax well, and become irritable and short-tempered, much like those who are mentally disturbed.

What is especially impressive about all these individuals is their ability to "turn the power on" in their brains when they are involved in important tasks. Those who experience mood swings may capitalize on the inexhaustible energy, heightened confidence, and abundance of ideas that arise spontaneously during mild forms of mania or the need to distract themselves from the negativity and pessimism that comes with depression. Those who do not suffer from mood swings may have comparable experiences during creative "highs" or "flow states" that bear many resemblances to hypomania.[13] They are able to work steadily on projects without tiring for extended periods of time. These creative highs can be highly pleasurable or they can become dysphoric, especially when people have trouble winding down or turning them off. Sometimes the intensity with which these people become immersed in their work suggests that they have become addicted to their own thought processes.

What all this points to is that while mental disturbances may be important for providing individuals with an underlying sense of unease that seems necessary for sustained creative activity, these disturbances are not the only source for inner tension. People who are reasonably stable are also able to generate this kind of creative tension when they tackle challenging problems. What leads to great achievement, however, is not the existence of this unease but the ability of these people to use it to their advantage, either as a spur to productivity or in the service of their art, social ventures, or scientific pursuits.

These appear to be the essential elements for exceptional creative achievement. All represent integral parts of a whole. *No single element in this template takes on special significance without reference to the others.* Few individuals possess all the elements of this template; most have several. This fact presents no problem if key elements of the basic template remain, and elements that ordinarily do not comprise this template substitute for absent ones that do. Much depends upon the way individuals interpret a particular event: losing a parent at an early age, for example, may instill a similar sense of vulnerability or fragility in them as sickliness or physical disabilities during childhood. Legal difficulties due to political or social actions could replace contrariness and irreverence toward parental, religious, or professional authorities. And being a member of a minority or socially marginal group—feeling like a social "outsider"—may substitute for being a loner.

This set of attributes, predictive of exceptional creative achievement, suggests a definite relationship between mental illness and genius, but not in the usual sense. What becomes clear is that the presence of a psychological "unease," potentially but not necessarily produced by any mental disturbance that is not too incapacitating, contributes to the realization of true greatness—but only in the presence of other elements of the template. When most of these elements are not present, people may not be able to exploit their inner tensions, which may make all the difference between phenomenal success and abysmal failure.

Inevitably, the question arises about whether the potential price of greatness—all the hard work, confrontations with authorities, conflicts with colleagues, time away from the family, constant pressures and tensions, and living in the limelight—is worth it. There is no way to answer the question definitively because the inevitable companion question, "Worth it in reference to what?" is itself unanswerable. No persons, including the eminent individuals themselves, can ever know what would have happened if they had taken a different course. Whatever the personal toll of their quest, they cannot tell if it would have been greater if, instead of achieving phenomenal success, they had fallen short of realizing their dreams or even more important, had never dreamed at all.

Notes

CHAPTER 1

1. See Aristotle's *Metaphysics*, trans. H. G. Apostle (Grinnell, IA: Peripatetic Press, 1979) and Plato's *Phaedrus*, trans. R. Hackworth (Indianapolis: Bobbs-Merrill, 1952). An excellent discussion of these different views may be found in C. R. Hausman's *A Discourse on Novelty and Creation* (The Hague: Martin Nijhoff, 1975). Also see E. R. Dodds, *The Greeks and the Irrational* (Berkeley: University of California Press, 1968).

2. It is important to point out that certain authors, such as A. Rothenberg (*The Emerging Goddess: The Creative Process in Art, Science, and Other Fields* [Chicago: The University of Chicago Press, 1979]), emphasize that creative achievement is based on healthy mental processes. D. W. MacKinnon ("The Nature and Nurture of Creative Talent," *American Psychologist*, 17 [1962]: 484–495) believed that emotional stability was necessary for success in architecture. Positions such as these receive some support from the long-term follow-up Stanford studies on child geniuses: L. M. Terman, *Genetic Studies of Genius*, Vols. 1–6, (Stanford: Stanford University Press, 1925–1959); M. Oden ("A 40-year Follow-up of Giftedness: Fulfillment and Unfulfillment," in *Genius and Eminence: The Social Psychology of Creativity and Exceptional Achievement*, 2nd ed., R. S. Albert, ed. [London: Pergamon Press, 1992]); and D. Goleman ("1,528 Little Geniuses and How They Grew," *Psychology Today*, February 1980, pp. 28–43). Certain well-known but methodologically flawed studies likewise report exceptionally low rates of mental illness among eminent persons. H. Ellis, in *A Study of British Genius*, (Boston: Houghton-Mifflin, 1926) reported a 4% prevalence of mental illness. In a little-known survey of American "geniuses," modeled after Ellis', W. G. Bowerman (*Studies in Genius* [New York: Philosophical Library, 1947]) reported only a 2% prevalence of mental illness. V. Goertzel and M. G. Goertzel (*Cradles of Eminence* [Boston: Little, Brown, 1962]) reported about a 2% rate of mental illness, and M. G. Goertzel, V. Goertzel, and T. G. Goertzel (*Three Hundred Eminent Personalities* [San Francisco: Jossey-Bass, 1978]) reported about a 10% rate of mental illness in their respective samples. Although the study by E. Raskin ("Comparison of Scientific and Literary Ability: A Biographical Study of Eminent Scientists and Men of Letters of the Nineteenth Century," *Journal of*

Abnormal and Social Psychology, 31 [1936]: 20–35) did not support a close association between genius and mental instability, 46% of the literary group as compared to 17% of the scientific group showed evidence of "neurotic breakdown."

These views and findings stand in stark contrast to clinicians who find a close link between mental illness and creativity. Older views on the potential role of schizophrenia or psychosis on creativity may be found in C. Lombroso, *The Man of Genius* (New York: Charles Scribners' Sons, 1910); W. Lange-Eichbaum, *The Problem of Genius* (New York: Macmillan, 1932); J. L. Karlsson, *Inheritance of Creative Intelligence* (Chicago: Nelson-Hall, 1978); and A. Juda, "The Relationship Between Highest Mental Capacity and Psychic Abnormalities," *American Journal of Psychiatry*, 106 (1949): 296–307. Most recently, H. J. Eysenck ("Creativity and Personality: Suggestions for a Theory," *Psychological Inquiry*, 4 [1993]: 147–148) has argued that "psychoticism," characterizing a mode of thought, underlies most forms of creativity.

More recent studies, which emphasize the importance of mood disorders, include N. C. Andreasen, "Creativity and Mental Illness: Prevalence Rates in Writers and Their First-Degree Relatives," *American Journal of Psychiatry*, 144 (1987): 1288–1292; K. R. Jamison, "Mood Disorders and Patterns of Creativity in British Writers and Artists," *Psychiatry*, 52 (1989): 125–134; and R. Richards, D.K. Kinney, I. Lunde, M. Benet, and A. P. C. Merzel, "Creativity in Manic-Depressives, Cyclothymes, Their Normal Relatives, and Control Subjects," *Journal of Abnormal Psychology*, 97 (1988): 281–288.

For excellent overviews of the relationship of psychiatric disorders to creativity, see R. Richards, "Relationship Between Creativity and Psychopathology: An Evaluation and Interpretation of the Evidence," *Genetic Psychology Monographs*, 103 (1981): 261–324; K. R. Jamison's chapter, "Manic–Depressive Illness, Creativity and Leadership," in *Manic-Depressive Illness*, F. K. Goodwin and K. R. Jamison, eds. (New York: Oxford University Press, 1990) and recent book, *Touched by Fire* (New York: Free Press, 1993); and R. A. Prentky, *Creativity and Psychopathology: A Neurocognitive Perspective* (New York: Praeger, 1980).

3. N. C. Andreasen, "Creativity and Mental Illness: Prevalence Rates in Writers and Their First-Degree Relatives," *American Journal of Psychiatry*, 144 (1987): 1288–1292.

4. A. M. Ludwig, "Creative Activity and Mental Illness in Female Writers," *American Journal of Psychiatry*, 151 (1994): 1650–1656.

5. M. Atwood, *Cat's Eye* (London: Virago, 1988), p.90.

6. H. Carpenter, *Geniuses Together: American Writers in Paris in the 1920's* (Boston: Houghton Mifflin Company, 1988).

7. See R. Richards, D.K. Kinney, I. Lunde, M. Benet, and A. P. C. Merzel, ("Creativity in Manic–Depressives, Cyclothymes, Their Normal Relatives, and Control Subjects") for a discussion of the "inverted-U" function of psychopathology in bipolar disorders. Also, Kay R. Jamison, "Manic-Depressive Illness, Creativity and Leadership" provides an excellent discussion of the relationship between mood disorders and creativity.

8. Cited in P. Sandblom, *Creativity and Disease: How Illness Affects Literature, Art and Music* (Philadelphia: George F. Stickley Co., 1982).

9. A. M. Ludwig, "Culture and Creativity," *American Journal of Psychotherapy*, 46 (1992): 454–469.

CHAPTER 2

1. A. L. Kroeber in his study of great civilizations (*Anthropology: Culture Patterns and Processes* [New York: Harcourt, Brace and World, 1963]), claims that while genius was inherited, cultural factors kept 75–90% of potential genius from being realized.

2. S. J. Gould, "Losing the Edge," in *The Flamingo's Smile: Reflections in Natural History* (New York: W. W. Norton & Co., 1985).

3. As a cousin of Charles Darwin and a grandson of Erasmus Darwin, Francis Galton was a firm believer in the hereditary basis of genius. With an I.Q. estimated to be 200, he had a far-ranging and probing intelligence that sometimes ventured into controversial areas, such as developing a "rational" basis for eugenics and evaluating the "statistical efficacy of prayer." Despite some of his debatable views, his statistical studies on eminence, presented in *Hereditary Genius: An Inquiry Into Its Laws and Consequences* (New York: D. Appleton & Company, 1870) and *English Men of Science: Their Nature and Nurture* (New York: D. Appleton & Company, 1875) represent landmarks in the field. See K. Pearson, *The Life, Letters and Labours of Francis Galton*, 3 vols. (New York: Cambridge University Press, 1914–1930) for an overview of his life and works.

4. R. S. Albert ("Toward a Behavioral Definition of Genius," *American Psychologist*, 30 [1975]: 140–151) offers a convincing argument for this view. Also see D. K. Simonton's *Genius, Creativity, and Leadership: Historiometric Inquiries* (Cambridge, MA: Harvard University Press, 1984) and *Scientific Genius* (Cambridge, England: Cambridge University Press, 1988).

5. Harriet Zuckerman, *Scientific Elite: Nobel Laureates in the United States* (New York: The Free Press, 1977).

6. F. Galton, *English Men of Science*.

7. F. Galton, *Hereditary Genius*.

8. J. McKeen Cattell, "A Statistical Study of Eminent Men," *The Popular Science Monthly*, 62 (1903): 359–377. Also see D. J. De Solla Price's discussion of these findings in *Little Science, Big Science* (New York: Columbia University Press, 1963) and those reported by S. S. Visher, "Scientists Starred: 1903–1943," in *American Men of Science* (Baltimore: Johns Hopkins Press, 1947).

9. See M. N. Marger's *Elites and Masses: An Introduction to Political Sociology* (New York: D. Van Nostrand Company, 1981) for a fuller explication of the sociology of elitism.

10. Jonathan R. Cole and Stephen Cole, *Social Stratification in Science* (Chicago: The University of Chicago Press, 1973).

11. The Ortega hypothesis is discussed by Jonathan R. Cole and Stephen Cole in *Social Stratification in Science*, p. 228.

12. Jonathan R. Cole and Stephen Cole, *Social Stratification in Science*.

13. These figures are based entirely on the work of A. Moles, *Information Theory and Aesthetic Perception*, trans. J. E. Cohen (Urbana: University of Illinois Press, 1966).

Percentages of Works Played by Different Composers

No.	Composer	Percent	No.	Composer	Percent
1	Mozart	6.1	26	Purcell	1.0
2	Beethoven	5.9	27	Puccini	1.0
3	Bach	5.9	28	Grieg	0.95
4	Wagner	4.2	29	Weber	0.95
5	Brahms > 25%	4.1	30	Prokofiev	0.95
6	Schubert	3.6	31	Berlioz	0.95
7	Handel	2.8	32	Rossini	0.95
8	Tchaikovsky	2.8	33	Ravel	0.95
9	Verdi	2.5	34	Rimski-Korsakov	0.85
10	Haydn 40%	2.3	35	D. Scarlatti	0.85
11	Schumann	2.1	36	Franck	0.7
12	Chopin	2.1	37	Gounod	0.7
13	Liszt	1.75	38	Vaughan Williams	0.7
14	Mendelssohn	1.75	39	Bizet	0.65
15	Debussy	1.7	40	Couperin > 75%	0.65
16	Wolf > 50%	1.65	41	Mahler	0.6
17	Sibelius	1.6	42	Rameau	0.6
18	R. Strauss	1.4	43	St. Saens	0.6
19	Moussorgsky	1.3	44	Massenet	0.6
20	Dvorák	1.3	45	Donizetti	0.55
21	Stravinsky	1.3	46	De Falla	0.45
22	Fauré	1.2	47	Scriabin	0.45
23	J. Strauss	1.2	48	Meyerbeer	0.45
24	Smetana	1.1	49	Gluck	0.45
25	Rachmaninoff	1.0	50	Paganini	0.45

14. Robert K. Merton introduced the notion of the 41st chair in his widely quoted article, "The Matthew Effect in Science" (*Science, 159* [1968]: 56–63). The "Matthew effect" referred to the finding that only a very small number of people have a disproportionately large influence in their fields or society at large and was aptly named after the *Gospel According to St. Matthew*, which states, "For unto every one that hath shall be given, and he shall have abundance: but from him that hath not shall be taken away even that which he hath." For further discussions of the importance of the Matthew effect in science, see H. Zuckerman, *Scientific Elite* and D. K. Simonton, *Scientific Genius*.

15. Of course, there are many exceptions to this notion. In her article on "The Proliferation of Prizes: Nobel Complements and Nobel Surrogates in the Reward System of Science" (*Theoretical Medicine, 13* [1992]: 217–231), Harriet

Zuckerman describes the proliferation of rich prizes and large honoraria in science over the last 2 decades. This proliferation was the result of the marked limitations on the numbers and types of scientists eligible for Nobel prizes and consequent increases in the number of uncrowned laureate equivalents. Although these rich prizes extend the reward system of science to new fields and add new members to the scientific ultra elite, Zuckerman concludes that no fundamental change in the nature or structure of science has occurred.

16. In an eloquent discussion of the use of biographical evidence, M. J. A. Howe ("Biographical Evidence and the Development of Outstanding Individuals," *American Psychologist*, 37 [1981]: 1071–1081) lists seven advantages of biographical evidence. Among these advantages are being able to draw on a collection of relatively detailed accounts of the growth of knowledge and abilities in the early years of distinguished individuals, being able to answer questions about the relationship of early precocity to later mature achievements, having available information about childhood and family circumstances, gaining information on special events during the lives of individuals, and potentially having access to information about the phenomenon of specialization, career interest, and commitment at an early stage of life. Further discussion on the use of biographical materials can be found in A. M. Ludwig, "Who Is Someone?" *American Journal of Psychotherapy*, 44 (1990): 516–524; W. M. Runyan, *Life Histories and Psychobiography: Explorations in Theory and Method* (New York: Oxford University Press, 1984); and I. B. Nadel, *Biography: Fiction, Fact and Form* (New York: St. Martin's Press, 1984).

17. From this point forward references to the Method and Statistics section of this book are called out in text by a number preceded by "S."

18. Selected descriptive characteristics

Time Period of Birth

Years	Number	Percent
1800–1824	15	1.5
1825–1849	86	8.6
1850–1874	261	26.0
1875–1899	416	41.4
1900–1924	183	18.2
1925–1949	43	4.3

Average Birth Year = 1882 (SD = 24)
Average Life Span = 68.0 (SD = 16.3)

Nationalities Represented
Australia (.6%); Austria (1.3%); Belgium (.3%); Canada (.7%); Czechoslovakia (.5%); England (17.6%); France (6.0%); Germany (3.3%); Greece (.2%); Hungary (.5%); Ireland (2.4%); Italy (1.3%); Mexico (.2%); Poland (1.0%); Russia (4.4%); South and Central America (.4%); Scandinavia (i.e.,, Denmark,, Sweden,, Finland,, or Norway) (1.3%); Scotland (.7%); South Africa (.4%); Spain (.6%); United States (54%); Wales (.7%); Yugoslavia (.2%); Assorted other (1.1%); Unknown or missing (.2%).

19. Because of space and fiscal considerations, the long list of bibliographic sources could not be published here. Readers who wish to learn which references provided the material for the anecdotes scattered throughout the book as well as for much of the information used in the various analyses may obtain copies of the selected bibliographic references on floppy disk or hard copy for a nominal fee by writing Mark Runco, Ph.D., Editor, *Creativity Research Journal*, c/o Erlbaum Associates, 365 Broadway, Hillsdale, NJ 07642.

20. *Book Review Digest (BRD)* (New York: H. W. Wilson Co., 1964, 1969, 1974, 1979, 1984, 1989); V. Goertzel and M. G. Goertzel, *Cradles of Eminence*, M. G. Goertzel, V. Goertzel, and T. G. Goertzel, *Three Hundred Eminent Person-alities*; *Biographies of Creative Artists: An Annotated Bibliography*, S. M. Stievater, ed. (New York: Garland Publishing, 1991); and *St. James Guide to Biography*, P. E. Shellinger, ed. (Chicago: St. James Press, 1991).

21. The oppressive influence of professions reached its height in Italy in the late 13th and early 14th centuries, when the artistic guilds proscribed religious obligations, guided the education of apprentices, supervised contracts, regulated relationships with patrons, and assumed authority over the physical and moral well-being of their members. See R. Wittkower and M. Wittkower, *Born under Saturn: The Character and Conduct of Artists* (New York: W. W. Norton, 1963).

22. See L. S. Gottfredson, "Circumscription & Compromise: A Developmental Theory of Occupational Aspirations," *Journal of Counseling Psychology Monograph*, 28 (1981): 545–579; D. E. Super and M. J. Bohn, Jr., *Occupational Psychology* (Belmont, CA: Wadsworth Publishing Co., 1970); and A. Roe, *The Psychology of Occupations* (New York: John Wiley and Sons, 1956).

23. Because of suggestive evidence in the literature that expository writers, poets, and fiction writers differed with respect to psychopathology, they were assigned to separate groups. See K. R. Jamison, "Mood Disorders and Patterns of Creativity in British Writers and Artists," *Psychiatry*, 52 (1989): 125–202 and K. R. Jamison, "Manic–Depressive Illness, Creativity and Leadership," in *Manic–Depressive Illness*.

The designation of "Companion" includes persons, such as Eleanor Roosevelt, Cosima Wagner, Grace Coolidge, Clara Ford, Alma Schindler Mahler, or Edith Wilson, who often were remarkable in their own right even though their main avenue to fame and opportunity came through their relationships with famous people.

24. PRIMARY PROFESSIONS OF SAMPLE: ARCHITECTURE (Architect, Commercial Artist, Designer); ART (Painter, Photographer, Sculptor); BUSINESS (Advertiser, Publicist, Banker, Entrepreneur, Manager, Agent, Producer, Publisher); EXPLORATION (Adventurer, Explorer); SPORTS (Athlete, Manager/Coach, Other); MUSICAL COMPOSITION (Choreographer, Composer, Conductor); MUSICAL PERFORMANCE (Dancer, Musician, Singer); MILITARY (Soldier, Spy); PUBLIC OFFICE (Policy Advisor, Elected Official, Judge, Lawyer, Appointed Public Official, Religious Official, Royalty); NATURAL SCIENCES (Inventor, Physicist, Mathematician, Naturalist, Scientist); SOCIAL ACTIVISM (Human Rights Advocate, Labor Leader, Persuader, Revolutionary); SOCIAL FIGURE (Collector/Aesthete, Host(ess), Curator, Patron, Philanthropist); COMPANION (Spouse, Lover); SOCIAL SCIENCES (Anthropologist, Economist, Educator, Historian, Philosopher, Political Theorist,

Psychologist, Sociologist, Theologian); THEATER (Actor, Broadcaster, Director); NONFICTION (Biographer, Critic, Editor); FICTION (Novelist, Short-Story Writer, Lyricist, Multimedia Writer, Playwright, Screen Writer); POETRY (Poets).

25. John L. Holland, *Making Vocational Choices: A Theory of Vocational Personalities and Work Environments* (Englewood Cliffs, NJ: Prentice-Hall, 1985). See Appendix B.

26. See *Dictionary of Occupational Titles*, 4th ed. (Washington, D.C.: U.S. Printing Office, 1977) for the most extensive classification of occupations.

CHAPTER 3

1. See R. S. Albert, "A Developmental Theory of Eminence," in *Genius and Eminence*, 2nd ed., R. S. Albert, ed. (New York: Pergamon Press, 1992), and R.S. Albert and M.A. Runco, "The Achievement of Eminence: A Model of Exceptionally Gifted Boys and Their Families," in *Conceptions of Giftedness*, R. J. Sternberg and J. E. Davidson, eds. (New York: Cambridge University Press, 1980).

2. Despite the extensive writings about geniuses, we hardly know anything with certainty about their early lives. Of all the scholarly investigations on this topic, only the reports by the Goertzels on two separate samples of eminent persons, the first on about 400 and the second on 300, offers a fairly comprehensive picture of their childhoods. See V. Goertzel and M. G. Goertzel, *Cradles of Eminence*; and M. G. Goertzel, V. Goertzel, and T. G. Goertzel, *Three Hundred Eminent Personalities*. Unfortunately, since their classifications and methods differed substantially from mine, direct comparisons of results are not always possible even when terminology is the same. Still, the Goertzels deserve credit for their early probes into this important area.

3. The measures and criteria below were used to determine social status: See S1 in the Method and Statistics section for correlations among these measures.

1. *Occupational Status (Social Level) of Major Wage-Earning Parent*: Royalty/Upper Class/Aristocrat/Power Broker (e.g., landed gentry, "gentleman farmer," financier, tycoon, mogul, independently wealthy, entrepreneur). Certified/Licensed/Degreed Professional (e.g., doctor, lawyer, minister, architect, teacher, scholar). Noncertified/Non-licenced Professional (e.g., artist, entertainer, writer, musician, soldier, adventurer, businessman, merchant, professional athlete, journalist). Skilled Laborer (e.g., carpenter, plumber, mechanic, clerk, bookkeeper). Unskilled Laborer (e.g., factory worker, farmer, manual laborer, peddler). Dependent/Unemployed (persons who did not work for their livelihood but were dependent on noninherited income [e.g., homemakers or individuals who were supported by friends, relatives, etc.]). Other.

2. *Occupational Success of Father*: Unsuccessful (the inability to keep a job or develop a successful business [e.g. being disabled, enslaved, bankrupt, or unable to work for whatever reason, such as prolonged hospitalization, prison, etc.]). Steady Employment (borderline business success or steady work with no advancement or promotions beyond the norm [e.g. government clerks, blue collar workers, craftsmen, salesmen, and businessmen with only meager success, usually

illustrated by lower-class status]). Successful Professional or Businessman (e.g., doctors, lawyers, businessmen, politicians, social leaders, military officers, and missionaries). Limited Social Fame (social recognition limited to local communities or to a select group [e.g., small town mayors, civic leaders, etc.]). Eminence/National Reputation (individuals who are likely to have encyclopedia entries written about them [e.g., a mayor of a major city, writers or artists of national reputation, etc.]). Unknown (those who never knew their father, or information was not available in the biography or offered conflicting evidence).

3. *Vocational Activities of Mother*: Homemaker. Unskilled Worker. Skilled or Technical Worker. Business or Managerial Work. Service, Academic, or Applied Profession. Creative Profession. Other.

4. *Family Income*: Upper Income (the parents are landed, wealthy, and can afford leisure and exhibit a life-style beyond mere comfort [e.g., own a yacht, expensive art collection, estate, etc.]; as such, the subject of the biography has no economic restrictions with regard to pursuit of his or her career). Middle Income (the parents are dependent on their profession or employment; their economic circumstances allow them to own a home or live in the neighborhood of their choice; the parents are employed in relatively secure careers regardless of their skills as long as the general economy is sound [e.g., a well-paid factory worker]; the subject of the biography is not denied adequate medical care or a higher education, though he or she may or may not attend an elite school). Lower Income (the parents have various restrictions put on them based solely on income [i.e., not race or religion]; income is marginal and, at times, inadequate; as a result, there are restrictions on where they can live, the consistency of employment, the success of their economic endeavors; the subject of the biography may live in an inner city or rural environment and be denied the opportunity to attend college or receive adequate health care).

4. L. Iremonger, *The Fiery Chariot: A Study of British Prime Ministers and the Search for Love* (London: Warburg, 1970).

5. For figures on orphanhood, see J. Marvin Eisenstadt, "Parental Loss and Genius," *American Psychologist, 33* (1978): 211–223.

6. For information about early parental loss, see V. Goertzel and M. G. Goertzel, *Cradles of Eminence*; M. G. Goertzel, V. Goertzel, and T. G. Goertzel, *Three Hundred Eminent Personalities*; F. Brown, "Depression and Childhood Bereavement," *Journal of Mental Science, 107* (1961): 754–777; F. Brown, "Childhood Bereavement and Subsequent Psychiatric Disorder," *British Journal of Psychiatry, 112* (1966): 1035–1041; C. Martindale, "Father Absence, Psychopathology, and Poetic Eminence," *Psychological Reports, 31* (1972): 843–847; H. J. Walberg, S. P. Rasher, and J. Parkerson, "Childhood and Eminence," *Journal of Creative Behavior, 13* (1980): 225–231; R. S. Albert, "Cognitive Development and Parental Loss Among the Gifted, the Exceptionally Gifted and the Creative, *Psychological Reports, 29* (1971): 19–26; and A. Roe, *The Making of a Scientist* (New York: Dodd Mead, 1953).

7. Although the figures are not strictly comparable, the Metropolitan Life Insurance Company (*Family Responsibilities Increasing* [New York: Metropolitan Life, 1959], cited by J. Marvin Eisenstadt, "Parental Loss and Genius,") estimated that by the age of 20, 32.1% and 21.7% of persons experienced the deaths of their

fathers or mothers, respectively, if these parents were middle-aged (45 to 50) at the time of their births, and 12.1% and 9.7% if their parents were 20 to 25 years old during 1900 to 1902. This is an ideal time period for comparison since it conforms to a time when the average age of the subjects in my sample was also about 20. For the sample, the cumulative death rate of 28% for fathers and 23% for mothers for individuals under 21 years of age was comparable to the Metropolitan estimates for those whose parents were middle-aged at the time of their birth and substantially higher than those whose parents were younger at the time of their birth. Unfortunately, the nature of my data does not allow more specific comparisons. (For further discussion, see J. M. Eisenstadt, "Parental Loss and Genius," in M. Eisenstadt, A. Hayal, P. Rentchnick, and P. De Senarclens, *Parental Loss and Achievement* [Madison, CT: International Universities Press, 1989].)

8. A recent study (M. A. Fristad, R. Jedel, R. A. Weller, and E. B. Weller, "Psychosocial functioning in children after the death of a parent," *American Journal of Psychiatry*, 150 [1993]: 511–513) shows that 8 weeks after the death of a parent, children from stable families did better than depressed inpatients and normal children on their school behavior, interest in school, peer involvement, and self-esteem.

9. A. Cahen, *Statistical Analysis of American Divorce* (New York: AMS Press, 1968), revealed a divorce rate of 18% for the general U. S. population in 1928.

10. See Kevin Leman, *Growing Up First Born, The Pressure and Privilege of Being Number One* (New York: Delacorte, 1989); M. Hennig and A. Jardim, *The Managerial Woman* (Garden City, NY: Anchor Books, 1981); D. Coleman, "The Link Between Birth Order and Innovation," *New York Times*, 8 May 1990, sec. B, p. 1; D. S. P. Schubert, M. E. Wagner, and H. J. P. Schubert, "Family Constellation and Creativity: First-Born Predominance Among Classical Music Composers," *Journal of Psychology*, 95 (1977): 147–149; R. Eisenman, "Birth Order, Development and Personality," *Acta Paedopsychiatrica*, 55 (1992): 25–27, 1992; W. R. Altus, "Birth Order and Its Sequelae," *Science*, 151 (1966): 44–48; L. Belmont and F. A. Marolla, "Birth Order, Family Size, and Intelligence," *Science*, 182 (1973): 1096–1101; and H. M. Breland, "Birth Order, Family Configuration, and Verbal Achievement," *Child Development*, 45 (1974): 1011–1019.

Besides the potential influence of birth order on professional achievement and innovation, others have linked it to schizophrenia, alcoholism, delinquency, and suicide as well. Some authors found, for example, that early-born males and later-born females were more likely to be schizophrenic, maladjusted, delinquent, or troublemakers; later-born males were more often schizophrenic; later-born females were overrepresented among alcoholics; and first and last borns were more likely than middle children to commit suicide. While intriguing, these results lack confirmation. (See C. Ernst and J. Angst, *Birth Order: Its Influence on Personality* [New York: Springer-Verlag, 1983] and B. N. Adams, "Birth Order: A Critical Review," *Sociometry*, 35 [1972]: 411–439). One monumental review of all the available studies on birth order concluded that there was little evidence to support the effect of birth order on any attribute, including creativity. (See C. Ernst and J. Angst, *Birth Order: Its Influence on Personality*.) A variety of methodological problems, such as the lack of adequate control groups or the failure to control for family size, child spacing within families, social class, and rural versus urban background, could account for the differences attributed to birth order. One researcher, who controlled for these problems in her study of over 100,000 people, found that birth order made no difference in how intelligent they were or how far they went in school or their conformity, sociability, anxiety, or assertiveness. (See J. Blake, *Family Size and Achievement* [Berkeley: University of California Press, 1989]).

11. Frank J. Sulloway, *"Orthodoxy and Innovation in Science: The Influence of Birth Order in a Multi-Variate Context"* (paper presented at the meeting of the American Association for the Advancement of Science, New Orleans, February, 1990).

12. A. S. Phillips, A. G. Bedeian, K. W. Mossholder, and J. Touliatos ("Birth Order and Selected Work-Related Personality Variables," *Individual Psychology*, 44 [1988]: 492–499) offer indirect support for these claims, finding that first borns scored higher than later borns on tests of leadership and dominance, achievement through conformity, and the desire to make a good impression.

13. See C. Ernst and J. Angst, *Birth Order: Its Influence on Personality* (New York: Springer-Verlag, 1983) and B. N. Adams, "Birth Order: A Critical Review," *Sociometry, 35* (1972): 411–439.

14. R. B. Zajonc ("The Decline and Rise of Scholastic Aptitude Scores," *American Psychologist* [August 1986]: 862–867) explains this difference in intelligence on the basis of a "confluence model," while R. D. Retherford and W. H. Sewell offer evidence against it ("Birth Order and Intelligence: Further Tests of the Confluence Model," *American Sociological Review, 56* [1991]: 141–158.

15. See J. Blake (*Family Size and Achievement* [Berkeley: University of California Press, 1989]) for an excellent review of the methodological problems involved in evaluating the relationship of birth order to achievement.

16. M. G. Goertzel, V. Goertzel, and T. G. Goertzel (*Three Hundred Eminent Personalities*), F. Galton (*Hereditary Genius: An Inquiry into its Laws and Consequences* [New York: D. Appleton & Co., 1877]), and H. Ellis (*A Study of British Genius* [London: Hurst and Blackett, 1904]) reported an overrepresentation of first borns in their samples, but their methods for establishing this overrepresentation were not well spelled out.

17. As a prelude to the presentation of results, the guidelines used for establishing birth order need to be explained. Birth order only applied to the children mutually produced by the individual's natural parents. Stillborns and infants who did not survive the first year were not counted as siblings. Step-siblings and half-siblings were eliminated from these analyses, as were cases for which information was insufficient for classification purposes.

18. For our purposes, the actual birth order of persons within their families (i.e., first, second, third, fourth, fifth, etc.) is less important than whether they are only children, first borns or later borns. With these three groups, we can judge the relative contributions of congenital and developmental factors to whatever differences these groups display. If only children differ from first and later borns, these differences should be due to developmental or psychological factors associated with being an only child. This is because similar uterine conditions and difficulties in labor should exist in the mothers

both for only children and for first borns. If only children and first borns do not differ, but both groups differ from later borns, these differences presumably should be due to differences in uterine physiology or special psychological and developmental factors associated with first-born status. And if only children and later borns do not differ, but both groups differ from first borns, these differences should be due to the special role and responsibilities assumed by first borns within families. By comparing these three groups, we also reduce the need to control for family size—the big bugaboo of many birth order studies—since the influence of family size, with only children, represents the very factor we will be evaluating.

19. With greater proportions of only children (particularly males) drawn to the creative arts, we should not be surprised to find that they are likewise more susceptible to various mental disturbances. Only children are at far greater risk for alcoholism, drug use, mania, anxiety, and psychoses than first borns or later borns. They also are more likely to experience severe psychopathology over a longer period in their lives and to be treated voluntarily or forcibly for their problems. See S17 in the Methods and Statistics section.

Why being an only child should be associated with higher rates of mental illness requires comment. While it is possible to blame this on the psychological burdens of being an only child, other factors are more likely. The most obvious one has to do with the finding that the single children in this study had more emotionally troubled mothers. The mental illness of these mothers likely contributed to their having only one child and also to their increased tendency to divorce.

Harry Stack Sullivan's mother had a mental breakdown and tried to kill herself. Alexander Blok's mother, Alexandra Beketov, a poet, translator, and musician, suffered from "fits of morbid melancholy and suicidal mania" and tried to take her life three times. Judy Holliday's mother, who experienced serious depressions, was hospitalized and received electric shock therapy after putting her head in an oven. Robert Lowell's mother, Charlotte, suffered from irritability and nervousness and was in and out of psychiatric treatment over many years. Marilyn Monroe's mother, Gladys, was hospitalized during her daughter's childhood with a diagnosis of paranoid schizophrenia. Clara Bow's mother had fainting spells and trances that lasted for hours and eventually was committed to a state mental hospital. Hart Crane's mother had many bouts of melancholia for which she was hospitalized. The mothers of Katherine Cornell, John Paul Vann, Peter Sellers, and Elvis Presley were alcoholics. Cary Grant's mother, Elsie, was a manic-depressive who spent 20 years in an insane asylum. Alan Ladd's mother, Inia, was an alcoholic who eventually killed herself by ingesting arsenic and ant paste. A spiritualist who presided at seances, Jack London's mother Flora attempted suicide with laudanum and, another time, shot herself in the forehead. Robert Peary's mother suffered from an inconsolable melancholy. Evelyn Scott's mother displayed fits of hysteria and a "paranoiac cast of mind." Allene, mother of Howard Hughes, had an intense fear of cats and was phobic about exposure to germs. Hettie Green's mother, Abby, took to her bed after the death of her infant son and never fully recovered. H. P. Lovecraft's mother, Sarah, who had vague artistic leanings, was eventually confined to a mental institution. And Dorothy

Sayers' mother, Helen, suffered from "acute nervous attacks" that made it difficult for her to speak or move.

20. See W. Lange-Eichbaum, *The Problem of Genius*, E. Paul and C. Paul, trans. (New York: Macmillan, 1932); G. Pickering, *Creative Malady* (New York: Dell Publishing Co., 1974); P. Sandblom, *Creativity and Disease: How Illness Affects Literature, Art and Music* (Philadelphia: George F. Stickley Co., 1982).

21. M. G. Goertzel, V. Goertzel and T. G. Goertzel, *Three Hundred Eminent Personalities*.

22. According to the *International Classification of Impairments, Disabilities, and Handicaps* (Geneva: World Health Organization, 1990) a handicap represents a disadvantage for a given individual, resulting from an impairment or disability, which limits or prevents the fulfillment of a role that is normal (depending on age, sex, and social and cultural factors) for that individual.

23. See Chapter 9 for the discussion about how illness contributes to the template of greatness.

24. The Goertzels (*Three Hundred Eminent Personalities*) estimated that 34% of their subjects were precocious; Havelock Ellis (*A Study of British Genius*) reported that 28%, mostly musicians and artists, were gifted; and W. C. Bowerman (*Studies in Genius*) reported that 5% were precocious.

25. See D. H. Feldman, *Nature's Gambit: Child Prodigies and the Development of Human Potential* (New York: Basic Books, 1986), and D. H. Feldman, "A Developmental Framework for Research with Gifted Children," in *Developmental Approaches to Giftedness and Creativity*, ed. D. H. Feldman (San Francisco: Jossey-Bass, 1982). Also see M. Csikszentmihalyi and R. E. Robinson, "Culture, Time and the Development of Talent," and A. J. Tannenbaum, "Giftedness: A Psychological Approach," both in *Conceptions of Giftedness*, R. J. Sternberg and J. E. Davidson, eds.

26. Not all researchers agree about the relationship of formal education to professional achievement. Distinguishing between those who are leaders and those who are creators, D. K. Simonton (*Genius, Creativity and Leadership: Historiometric Inquiries*), for instance, concluded that progressively fewer leaders were likely to be found among those with higher levels of education and that fewer creators were likely to be found at the lower and upper educational levels than at the middle level. My own findings suggest other interpretations.

27. Harriet Zuckerman, *Scientific Elite*.

28. D. K. Simonton *Genius, Creativity and Leadership*.

29. J. Walters and H. Gardner, "The Crystallizing Experience: Discovering an Intellectual Gift," in *Conceptions of Giftedness*, R. J. Sternberg and J. E. Davidson, eds.

30. See the classic studies by H. C. Lehman, *Age and Achievement* (Princeton, NJ: Princeton University Press, 1953). Wayne Dennis ("Variations in Productivity Among Creative Workers," *Scientific Monthly*, 80 [1955]: 277–278 and "Age and Productivity Among Scientists," *Science*, 123 [1956]: 724–725) has shown that differing life spans may bias the achievements reported at the different ages. See D. K. Simonton, *Genius, Creativity and Leadership*, for a fascinating statistical assessment of this relationship.

CHAPTER 4

1. H. Gardner, *Creating Minds* (New York: Basic Books, 1993).

2. See B. T. Eiduson, "Early Influences on Research Scientists," in *Genius and Eminence*, R. S. Albert, ed. (New York: Pergamon Press, 1983) pp. 182–202; R. J. Shapiro, *Creative Research Scientist* (Johannesburg: National Institute for Personnel Research, 1968); A. Roe, *The Making of a Scientist* (New York: Dodd, Mead, 1952); D. K. Simonton, *Genius, Creativity and Leadership*; M. G. Goertzel, V. Goertzel, and T. G. Goertzel, *Three Hundred Eminent Personalities*; R. B. Cattell and H. J. Butcher, *The Prediction of Achievement and Creativity* (Indianapolis: Bobbs-Merrill, 1968); and J. A. Chambers, "Relating Personality and Biographical Factors to Scientific Creativity," *Psychological Monographs: General and Applied*, 78 (1964): 1–19.

3. See D. W. MacKinnon, "The Nature and Nurture of Creative Talent," *American Psychologist*, 17 (1962): 484–495, and D. W. MacKinnon, "The Highly Effective Individual," in *Genius and Eminence*, ed. R. S. Albert.

4. See F. Barron, "Creative Writers," in *Genius and Eminence*, ed. R. S. Albert; and R. B. Cattell and H. J. Butchers, *The Prediction of Achievement and Creativity*.

5. F. Barron, "Creative Writers."

6. Catherine M. Cox, *Genetic Studies of Genius: Volume II, The Early Mental Traits of Three Hundred Geniuses* (Stanford: Stanford University Press, 1959).

7. V. Goertzel and M. G. Goertzel, *Cradles of Eminence*; M. G. Goertzel, V. Goertzel, and T. G. Goertzel, *Three Hundred Eminent Personalities*; and D. K. Simonton, *Genius, Creativity and Leadership*.

8. See L. M. Terman, "Psychological Approaches to the Biography of Genius," *Science*, 92 (1940): 293–301, and R. S. Illingsworth, and C. M. Illingsworth, *Lessons from Childhood: Some Aspects of the Early Life of Unusual Men and Women* (Baltimore: William and Wilkins Company, 1966).

9. See J. A. Chambers, "Relating Personality and Biographical Factors to Scientific Creativity"; B. T. Eiduson, "Early Influences on Research Scientists"; and R. B. Cattell and H. J. Butcher, *The Prediction of Achievement and Creativity*.

10. D. J. Weeks, *Eccentrics: The Scientific Investigation* (London: Sterling University Press, 1988).

11. J. A. Chambers ("Relating Personality and Biographical Factors to Scientific Creativity"), B. T. Eiduson ("Early Influences on Research Scientists"), and A. Roe (*The Making of a Scientist*) have commented on the lack of religious involvement of scientists.

12. B. A. Kosmin and S. P. Lachman, *One Nation Under God* (New York: Harmony Books, 1993).

13. See A. Kinsey, W. B. Pomeroy, and C. E. Martin, *Sexual Behavior in the Human Male* (Philadelphia: W. B. Saunders and Co., 1948). Also see J. O. G. Billy, K. Tanfer, W. A. Grady, and D. H. Klepinger, "The Sexual Behavior of Men in the United States," *Family Planning Perspectives*, 25 (1993): 52–60, "Landmark French and British Studies Examine Sexual Behavior, Including Multiple Partners, Homosexuality," *Family Planning Perspectives*, 25 (1993):

91–92, and J. H. Gagnon, R. T. Michael, E. O. Laumann, and G. Kolata, *Sex in America: A Definitive Survey* (New York: Little, Brown, 1994).

14. H. Ellis (*A Study of British Genius*) reported that 26% of his subjects were unmarried; W. G. Bowerman (*Studies in Genius*) reported 9% unmarried; and M. G. Goertzel, V. Goertzel, T. G. Goertzel (*Three Hundred Eminent Personalities*) reported 18%. Except for the Goertzel report, whose findings approximate my own, the other reports cover entirely different time frames.

15. A. Cahen (*Statistical Analysis of American Divorce* [New York: AMS Press, 1932, 1968]) reported an 18% divorce rate in the United States for 1928.

16. W. G. Bowerman's subjects had an average of 5.5 children and came from families with an average of 7.5 children. Because his study covers a 300-year period, it is difficult to place these averages in a suitable context.

17. H. Ellis (*A Study of British Genius*) reported that 10% and the Goertzels (*Three Hundred Eminent Personalities*) reported that 25% of their entire sample suffered from chronic physical illness, with no difference in the rates among professions.

CHAPTER 5

1. See R. E. Park, *On Social Control and Collective Behavior: Selected Papers* (Chicago: University of Chicago Press, 1967); R. E. Park, *Race and Culture* (Glencoe, IL: The Free Press, 1950). D. K. Simonton offers a brief discussion of this topic in *Scientific Genius, Creativity and Leadership*.

2. See J. Abra and S. Valentine-French ("Gender Differences in Creative Achievement: A Survey of Explanations," *Genetic, Social, and General Psychology Monographs, 117* [1991]: 235–284) for an excellent overview and critique of these theories.

3. See L. M. Terman, "Psychological Approaches to the Biography of Genius," *Science, 92* (1940): 293–301, as well as discussion in L. S. Gottfredson, "Circumscription and Compromise: A Developmental Theory of Occupational Aspirations," *Journal of Counseling Psychology Monograph, 28* (1981): 545–579. Also see L. F. Fitzgerald and N. E. Betz, "Issues in the Vocational Psychology of Women," in *Handbook of Vocational Psychology*, Vol. 1, W. B. Walsh and S. H. Osipow, eds. (Hillsdale, NJ: Laurence Erlbaum Associates, Publishers, 1983), pp. 83–159.

4. See S. L. Bem and D. J. Bem, "Case Study of a Nonconscious Ideology: Training the Woman to Know Her Place," in *Beliefs, Attitudes, and Human Affairs*, D. J. Bem, ed. (Monterey, CA: Brooks/Cole, 1970). In a series of studies, R. Helson ("Which of Those Young Women with Creative Potential Became Productive? Personality in College and Characteristics of Parents," in *Genius and Eminence*) examined the characteristics of 31 women in their early 40s who were nominated earlier by faculty members in a women's college from a sample of 141 women for their creative potential. In brief, she found that creative achievers were characterized in adolescence and adulthood by confidence, dominance, and originality. They tended to identify with their fathers and were alienated from their mothers.

5. G. Greer, *The Obstacle Race* (New York: Farrar Straus Giroux, 1979).

6. See L. Nochlin, "Why Are There No Great Women Artists?" in *Women in Sexist Society: Studies in Power and Powerlessness*, V. Gornick and B. K. Moran, eds. (New York: New American Library, 1972).

7. According to the *Statistical Abstract of the United States* (Bureau of the Census, U.S. Department of Commerce), the percentage of blacks varied from 10% to 12% over these years. All but a couple of blacks in the study were born in the United States.

8. See H. Zuckerman, *Scientific Elite*. Also see supporting views by Colin Berry, "The Nobel Scientists and the Origins of Scientific Achievement," *British Journal of Sociology*, 32 (1981): 381–391, and N. Weyl, *The Creative Elite in America* (Washington, D.C.: Public Affairs Press, 1966).

9. See S. M. Lipset and E. C. Ladd, Jr., "Jewish Academics in the United States: Their Achievements, Culture and Politics," *American Jewish Yearbook* (1971): 89–128.

10. These findings generally support those previously reported by H. Zuckerman (*Scientific Elite*) for Nobel laureates.

11. A. C. Kinsey, W. B. Pomeroy and C. E. Martin, *Sexual Behavior in the Human Male* (Philadelphia: W. B. Saunders Co., 1948).

12. J. O. E. Billy, K. Tanfer, W. R. Grady, and D. H. Klepinger, "The Sexual Behavior of Men in the United States"; and K. Tanfer, "National Survey of Men: Design and Execution," *Family Planning Perspectives*, 25 (1993): 83–86.

13. J. R. Cole and S. Cole, *Social Stratification in Science* (Chicago: University of Chicago, 1973).

14. J. R. Cole, *Fair Science: Women in the Scientific Community* (New York: Free Press, 1979).

15. F. E. Crossland, "Graduate Education and Black Americans" (New York: Ford Foundation, 1968).

16. See S. M. Lipsett and E. C. Ladd, Jr., "Jewish Academics in the United States."

CHAPTER 6

1. The *Creative Achievement Scale* (CAS) consists of three groups of items, as suggested by C. E. Gray ("The Measurement of Creativity in Western Civilization," *American Anthropologist*, 68 [1966]: 1384–1417), each with different weightings depending upon its presumed relative importance. Each item can be rated on a continuum from "none," to "minimal," "moderate" or "maximal" with proportional scores assigned to each level.

The first grouping of items, regarded as "major" criteria, received a weighting of "3." Item 1 pertained to degree of posthumous recognition; Item 2, the universality of the contribution; Item 3, the anticipation of social or future needs; Item 4, the influence on contemporary and subsequent professionals; Item 5, the originality embodied in the person's main work, product, or accomplishment; and Item 6, the extent of innovative accomplishments over the person's adult lifetime.

The second grouping of items, regarded as "intermediate" criteria, received a weighting of "2." Item 7 pertained to the degree of the person's versatility and many-sidedness; Item 8, productivity; and Item 9, fame, admiration, and acceptance.

The third grouping of items, regarded as "minor" criteria, received a weighting of "1." Item 10 pertained to the degree of technical competence and skill, and Item 11, creative involvement in nonvocational pursuits.

The cumulative scores from all 11 Items constitute a "Total Score." Total Scores potentially can range from 0 to 78.

Detailed instructions and examples for the rating of each item may be found in Appendix G.

In any assessment of general creativity, at least four dimensions need to be accounted for: creativity as a reflection of the person; creativity as a process; creativity as manifested in actual products, performances, or works; and creativity as determined by social and cultural judgments. See R. Richards, ("Relationship Between Creativity and Psychopathology"), and R. Richards, D. K. Kinney, M. Benet, and A. P. C. Merzel ("Assessing Everyday Creativity: Characteristics of the Lifetime Creativity Scales and Validation With Three Large Samples," *Journal of Personality and Social Psychology*, 54 [1988]: 476–485). With regard to these different dimensions of creativity, Items 5, 7, 8, 10, and 11 may be presumed to apply mostly to personal variables (i.e., originality, versatility, productivity, skill and aesthetic interests); Items 2, 3, 5, 6, and 8, to the nature of the product, work or performance (i.e., general applicability, trend-setting, novelty, and extent and number of original contributions); and Items 1, 4 and 9, to contemporary and historical factors (i.e., posthumous recognition, influence, and general acceptance). Some overlap exists among these groupings. From the various analyses performed, the CAS appears to be a reliable and valid instrument. Internal consistency among scale items was high. Scale validity was initially demonstrated by correlating CAS Total Scores for two separate samples ($n = 12$ and $n = 50$) with the number of lines allotted to each subject in the *Encyclopaedia Britannica* (*Micropaedia*) ($r = .64, p < .05$ and $r = .40, p < .01$, respectively) and the *Encyclopedia Americana* ($r = .65, p < .05$ and $r = .29, p < .05$, respectively). A comparable analyses performed later with 150 individuals who were selected at random from the sample revealed remarkably high correlations of .59 ($p < .000$) for the *Encyclopedia Britannica* (*Micropaedia*) and .42 ($p < .000$) for the *Encyclopedia Americana*. In addition, the four trained raters' scores were correlated with the average ratings of a panel of 10 expert judges from different professions for 12 designated subjects (Pearson r values ranged from .86 to .92, $p < .05$ for all values).

The CAS scores for the 1,004 subjects in the current study appear to be normally distributed, ranging from 1 to 71. The actual quartile scores assigned to each individual can be found in Appendix A. The above description largely comes from my article on "The Creative Achievement Scale" (*Creativity Research Journal*, 5 [1992]: 109–124), which contains further conceptual, methodological, and statistical details about the CAS.

2. D. K. Simonton ("Latent-variable Models of Posthumous Reputation: A Quest for Galton's G," *Journal of Personality and Social Psychology*, 60 [1991]:

607–619) offers a statistical demonstration of the relative stability of posthumous fame. Also see R. Over, "The Durability of Scientific Reputation," *Journal of the History of the Behavioral Sciences*, 18 (1982): 53–61.

3. T. Kuhn, *The Nature of Scientific Revolutions* (Chicago: The University of Chicago Press, 1962).

4. T. Amabile, *The Social Psychology of Creativity* (New York: Springer-Verlag, 1983).

5. R. K. White, "The Versatility of Genius," *Journal of Social Psychology*, 2 (1931): 460–489.

6. R. S. Root-Bernstein, *Discovering* (Cambridge, MA: Harvard University Press, 1989).

7. R. S. Root-Bernstein, M. Bernstein, and H. Garnier, "Correlations Between Avocations, Scientific Style, Work Habits, and Professional Impact of Scientists," *Creativity Research Journal* (in press).

8. R. S. Root-Bernstein et al. believe that their findings confirm the usefulness of H. Gruber's concept of "networks of enterprise." See H. Gruber, "The Evolving Systems Approach to Creative Work," in *Creative People at Work*, D. B. Wallace and H. E. Gruber, eds. (Oxford: Oxford University Press, 1989), and H. Gruber, "Networks of Enterprise in Creative Scientific Work," in *Psychology of Science and Metascience*, B. Gholson, A. Houts, R. A. Neimayer, and W. Shadish, eds. (Cambridge, England: Cambridge University Press, 1988).

9. See R. S. Albert ("Toward a Behavioral Definition of Genius" and D. K. Simonton (*Creativity, Leadership & Genius*) for an excellent discussion of this issue.

10. R. S. Root-Bernstein, M. Bernstein, and H. Garnier, "Identification of Scientists Making Long-Term, High Impact Contributions, with Notes on Their Methods of Working," *Creativity Research Journal*, 6 (1993): 329–343.

11. W. Lange-Eichbaum, *The Problem of Genius*, E. Paul and C. Paul, trans.

CHAPTER 7

1. See Edmund Wilson, "Philoctetes: The Wound and the Bow," in *Art and Psychoanalysis*, ed. W. Phillips (New York: Criterion, 1957), p. 532, and L. S. Zegans, "Beyond the 'Wound and the Bow': An Interdisciplinary Survey of Theories Related to the Nature of Creativity," *Psychiatric Quarterly*, 38 (1964): 717–732.

2. R. Richards, "When Illness Yields Creativity" (paper presented at the 101st Annual Convention of the American Psychological Association, Toronto, Canada, 24 August 1993).

3. World Health Organization, *Mental Disorders: Glossary and Guide to Their Classification in Accordance with the Ninth Revision of the International Classification of Disease* (Geneva, 1978).

4. J. B. Persons, "The Advantages of Studying Psychological Phenomena Rather Than Psychiatric Diagnoses," *American Psychologist*, 41 (1986): 1252–1260.

5. R. E. Kendall, "What is a Case?: Food for Thought for Epidemiologists," *Archives of General Psychiatry*, 45 (1988): 374–376.
6. L. N. Robins and D. A. Regier, eds., *Psychiatric Disorders in America: The Epidemiological Catchment Area Study* (New York: The Free Press, 1991).
7. The results of the ECA study show substantial differences from those of an Icelandic study that used the Diagnostic Interview Schedule and DSM-III criteria to establish the lifetime prevalence of various psychiatric disorders (J.G. Stefánsson, E. Líndal, J. K. Björnsson, A. Guomundsdóttir, "Lifetime Prevalence of Specific Disorders Among People Born in Iceland in 1931," *Acta Psychiatrica Scandinavica*, 84 [1991]: 142–149.) These results are summarized below.

Disorder	% men (n = 441)	% women (n = 421)	% total (n = 862)
Any Disorder (except tobacco use)	59.2	54.9	57.1
Alcohol Abuse/Dependence	45.6	8.5	27.5
Substance Abuse	0.5	1.0	0.7
Schizophrenia/Schizophreniform	0.9	0.9	0.9
Bipolar (includes manic)	0.9	0.9	0.9
Depression (includes dysthymia)	8.0	25.5	16.5
Generalized Anxiety	11.8	32.2	21.7
Somatization Disorder	0.0	0.5	0.2

The most recent U.S. mental health survey of 8,098 people ages 15 to 54 (R. C. Kessler et al., "Lifetime and 12-Month Prevalences of *DSM-III-R* Psychiatric Disorders in the United States," *Archives of General Psychiatry*, 51 [1994]: 8–19) revealed the following lifetime prevalences for various mental disorders: Any Mental Disorder = 48%; Major Depressive Episode = 17.1%; Dysthymia = 6.4%; Manic Episode = 1.6%; Alcohol Dependence = 14.1%; Other Alcohol Abuse = 9.4%; Drug Dependence = 7.5%; Other Drug Abuse = 4.4%; Any Anxiety Disorder = 24.9%; and Psychosis (including Schizophrenia) = 0.7%.

8. See D. C. Leighton, J. S. Harding, D. B. Macklin, A. M. MacMillan, and A. H. Leighton, *The Character of Danger: Psychiatric Symptoms in Selected Communities* (New York: Basic Books, 1963). It should be noted that the lifetime prevalence for any psychiatric disorder was identical to that obtained in the Icelandic Study. (See reference 7 above.)
9. L. Srole, T. S. Langer, S. T. Michael, M. Opler, and T. Rennie, *Mental Health in the Metropolis: The Midtown Manhattan Study* (New York: McGraw-Hill, 1962).
10. Inter-rater reliability was high for the identification of specific forms of psychopathology. The percentage of agreement between pairs of raters averaged almost 92%. Kappa values between pairs of raters ranged from .51 to .76 (mean = .65).
11. For excellent descriptions of the advantages and limitations of survival analyses, see R. Peto et al., "Design and Analysis of Randomized Clinical Trials Requiring Prolonged Observation of Each Patient: Introduction and Design," *British Journal of Cancer*, 34 (1976): 585–612; R. Peto et al., "Design and Analysis

of Randomized Clinical Trials Requiring Prolonged Observation of Each Patient: Analysis and Examples," *British Journal of Cancer*, 35 (1977): 1–39; and D. G. Altman, *Practical Statistics for Medical Research* (London: Chapman and Hall, 1991).

12. J. E. Helzer, A. Burnam, and L. T. McEvoy, "Alcohol Abuse and Dependence," in *Psychiatric Disorders in America*, L. N. Robins and D. A. Regier, eds.

13. See D. Goodwin (*Alcohol and the Writer* [Kansas City: Andrews and McMeel, 1988) for an excellent discussion of the use of alcohol by writers.

14. J. C. Anthony and J. E. Helzer, "Syndromes of Drug Abuse and Dependence," in *Psychiatric Disorders in America*.

15. M. M. Weissman, M. Livingston Bruce, P. J. Leaf, L. P. Florio, and C. Holzer, III, "Affective Disorders," in *Psychiatric Disorders in America*.

16. M. M. Weissman, M. Livingston Bruce, P. J. Leaf, L. P. Florio, and C. Holzer, III. "Affective Disorders," in *Psychiatric Disorders in America*.

17. S. J. Keith, D. A. Regier, and D. S. Roe, "Schizophrenic Disorders," in *Psychiatric Disorders in America*.

18. D. G. Blazer, D. Hughes, L. K. George, M. Swartz, and R. Boyer, "Generalized Anxiety Disorder," in *Psychiatric Disorders in America*.

19. M. Swartz, R. Landerman, L. K. George, D. G. Blazer, and J. Escobar, "Somatization Disorder," in *Psychiatric Disorders in America*.

20. Although William Styron ("Darkness Visible," *Vanity Fair* 52 [December, 1989]) was not in the study, his observations seemed most apt.

21. For suicide rates, see *Mortality Statistics* for the years 1910, 1920, and 1921 (Bureau of the Census, United States Department of Commerce); *Vital Statistics of the United States* for the years 1946, 1956, and 1966 (U. S. Department of Health, Education and Welfare); and the *Statistical Abstract of the United States 1991* (Bureau of the Census, U. S. Department of Commerce), which also contains the suicide statistics for men and women.

22. R. C. Kessler et al., "Lifetime and 12-month Prevalence of DSM-III-R Psychiatric Disorders in the United States," *Archives of General Psychiatry*, 51 (1994): 8–19.

23. L. N. Robins, B. Z. Locke, and D. A. Regier, "An Overview of Psychiatric Disorders in America," in *Psychiatric Disorders in America*.

24. These findings are explained in more detail in my article on "Creative Achievement and Psychopathology: Comparison Among Professions," *American Journal of Psychotherapy*, 46 (1992): 330–356.

25. These results, while confined to eminent persons, conform closely to those obtained in my study on women writers (A. M. Ludwig, "Mental Illness and Creative Activity in Female Writers," *American Journal of Psychiatry*, 151 (1994): 1650–1656.

26. See K. R. Jamison, "Manic-Depressive Illness, Creativity and Leadership"; J. L. Karlsson, "Creative Intelligence in Relatives of Mental Patients," *Hereditas*, 100 (1984): 83–86; N. C. Andreasen, "Creativity and Mental Illness: Prevalence Rates in Writers and Their First-Degree Relatives," *American Journal of Psychiatry*, 144 (1987): 1288–1292; A. M. Ludwig, "Creativity and Mental Illness in Women Writers", and R. Richards, D. K. Kinney, I. Lunde, M. Benet,

and A. P. C. Mercel, "Creativity and Manic-Depressives, Cyclothymes, Their Normal Relatives and Control Subjects."

27. Some mention needs to be made of the increasing difficulty in obtaining detailed, reliable information about the mental symptomatology of relatives of eminent persons the farther removed they were in consanguinity, especially if they were deceased and not famous in their own right. Because information about the emotional status of relatives was seldom as rich, detailed, or extensive as that for their eminent kin, the more permissive criteria for the identification of psychopathology often had to be used. But even with these constraints, the clear and consistent nature of the results appears to override whatever "static" might be inherent in data of this kind.

28. Although an attempt was made to secure comparable information on the children of the subjects, the quality of this information was not as complete or consistent as that for other first-degree biological relatives, probably because many of these children were still alive or only recently deceased.

29. Before the introduction and general use of lithium for the prevention and treatment of manic–depressive disorder, clinicians were more inclined to diagnose various psychotic conditions as schizophrenia. In more recent times, with changing diagnostic criteria and a greater emphasis on the importance of affective symptoms as indications of mood disorders, clinicians would probably diagnose many of these same conditions as variants or atypical manifestations of mania. The finding that depressive and manic symptomatology in the parents significantly predicted the presence of schizophrenic-like psychoses in their eminent offspring lends support to the legitimacy of these changing diagnostic practices.

CHAPTER 8

1. None of Louis Wain's biographies were reviewed in the New York Times Book Review, so he is not included in the sample. Nevertheless, that does not preclude using material about his life and work to highlight important issues that apply equally well to our eminent people. For information about this intriguing person, see R. Dale, Louis Wain: The Man Who Drew Cats (London: William Kimber, 1968); R. Dale, Catland (London: Duckworth, 1977); and H. Latimer, Louis Wain: King of the Cat Artists (New York: Papyrus, 1992). Because controversy exists about certain details of Wain's life and works, I cannot vouchsafe for the reliability of reported material.

2. I am indebted to Robert Root-Bernstein for his comments on this matter.

3. Unpublished data.

4. For an excellent conceptual analysis of the potential interactions between creativity and psychopathology, see R. Richards, "Relationship Between Creativity and Psychopathology." In an earlier anecdotal report (A. M. Ludwig, "Alcohol Input and Creative Output," British Journal of Addiction, 85 [1990]: 953–963), I attempted an analysis of the relationships between creativity and alcoholism that was based largely on her schema. For present purposes, a

simpler categorization of potential interactions seemed appropriate. Also see Kay R. Jamison (*Touched by Fire*) for an excellent discussion of the relationship between mood disorders and creativity.

5. See my article, "Alcohol Input and Creative Output," for a detailed discussion of this matter.

6. Quoted in T. J. Schlereth, *Cultural History and Material Culture* (Ann Arbor: U.M.I. Research Press, 1990), p. 422.

7. See G. Plimpton, ed., *Writers at Work, Fifth Series* (New York: The Viking Press, 1981), pp. 191–192. This quote was included because of its aptness, even though Kingsley Amis was not one of the subjects.

8. G. Plimpton, ed., *Writers at Work: The Paris Interviews, Sixth Series* (New York: Viking Press, 1984), p. 99.

9. L. Schaeffer, *O'Neill: Son and Playwright* (Boston: Little, Brown and Co., 1968), p. 424.

10. A. M. Ludwig, "Alcohol Input and Creative Output."

11. A. Roe, "Alcohol and Creative Work," *Quarterly Journal of Studies in Alcohol,* 6 (1946): 415–467.

12. K. R. Jamison, R. H. Gerner, C. Hammen, and C. Padesky, "Clouds and Silver Linings: Positive Experiences Associated with Primary Affective Disorders," *American Journal of Psychiatry, 137* (1980): 198–202.

13. In an earlier report (A. M. Ludwig, "Creative Achievement and Psychopathology: Comparison among Professions," *American Journal of Psychotherapy, 46* [1992]: 330–356), a multiple regression analysis with a somewhat different set of independent variables showed that lifetime anxiety and lifetime depression scores were significant predictors of creative achievement, but the magnitude of the relationship also was fairly low (total R^2 = .04).

CHAPTER 9

1. See William James' two essays on this topic, "Great Men and Their Environments" and "The Importance of Individuals," in *The Will to Believe and Other Essays in Popular Philosophy* (Cambridge, MA: Harvard University Press, 1979) and T. Carlyle, *On Heroes, Hero Worship, and the Heroic in History,* C. Niemeyer, ed. (Lincoln: University of Nebraska Press, 1966).

2. L. M. Terman ("Psychological Approaches to the Biography of Genius," in *Creativity: Selected Readings,* P. E. Vernon, ed. [Baltimore: Penguin, 1970]) reported a similar strategy in comparing the attributes of the upper and lower quartiles of 600 men who were rated on the basis of "life success." D. W. MacKinnon ("The Personality Correlates of Creativity: A Study of American Architects, *Proceedings of the 14th International Congress on Applied Psychology* [Munksgaard, 1962]) adopted a somewhat different approach in his study of architects. The attributes of a highly distinguished group were compared to two groups of less well-known architects.

3. The uneven numbers of persons in the upper and lower quartiles was generated by the computer program that excluded cases with overlapping scores.

4. R. S. Illingsworth and C. M. Illingsworth, *Lessons From Childhood: Some*

Aspects of the Early Life of Unusual Men and Women (Baltimore: William and Wilkins Company, 1966), p. 350.

5. D. K. Simonton ("Emergence and Realization of Genius: The Lives and Works of 120 Classical Composers," *Journal of Personality and Social Psychology*, 61 [1991]: 829–840) adopted an intriguing approach to the prediction of genius. According to his longitudinal model of genius, individuals differ on their initial "creative potential," defined as the total amount of contributions they theoretically can produce during an unrestricted life span. Once their careers begin, a two-step process of ideation and elaboration converts their initial creative potential into actual products. The expected rates of ideation and elaboration depend upon the fields in which creativity occurs. Fields such as mathematics and poetry have fast information-processing rates, and fields such as philosophy and history have slower ones. These differences in information-processing speed have repercussions for the optimal age at which individuals are likely to achieve maximum professional productivity, complete their best works, and realize their creative potentials.

This approach seems sound enough. But I have taken an entirely different approach to the prediction of greatness. That is mainly because certain of the measures Simonton used to predict genius—namely, productivity and "best work"—are already incorporated in my measure of creative achievement. I also am less interested in the relationship of productivity and creative potential to the recognition of genius than in the relationship of certain personal attributes and life circumstances to the productivity and creative potential of individuals.

6. In seeking a causal model for greatness, I initially explored the use of certain artificial intelligence programs that might provide the best explanation for the data. Dr. Peter Spirtes, in the Department of Philosophy at Carnegie Mellon University, was kind enough to test out TETRAD II, a computer software package that exploits artificial-intelligence techniques to run a heuristic search for optimal reformulations of the initial model. Once TETRAD II narrowed the range of possible models, the EQS program was used to estimate the structural coefficients. For excellent discussions of this approach to model-building, readers should secure the following sources: C. Glymour, R. Scheines, P. Spirtes, and K. Kelly, *Discovering Causal Structure: Artificial Intelligence, Philosophy of Science, and Statistical Modeling* (Orlando, FL: Academic Press, 1987); P. Spirtes, R. Scheines, and C. Glymour, "Simulation Studies of the Reliability of Computer Aided Specifications Using TETRAD II, EQS, and LISREL Programs," *Sociological Methods and Research*, 19 (1990): 3–66; and K. Bollen, *Structural Equations with Latent Variables* (New York: Wiley, 1989). In addition to this approach, I also had an opportunity to explore the use of the LISREL 7.2 software program, developed by K. Jöreskog and D. Sörbom (*LISREL 7: A Guide to the Program and Application*, 2nd ed., [Chicago: SPSS Inc. 1989]). Dr. Joanne Ries and Dr. John V. Haley of the Department of Behavioral Science, University of Kentucky College of Medicine, should be credited with running this analysis. The LISREL program, comparable to ESQ, tested how well the available data fit a predetermined model. However, because of the nature of the data and the large number of explicit and latent variables to be accounted for, these models did not prove suitable for theory building or testing.

Fortunately, a logistic regression model, which estimates the probability of a particular event occurring (i.e., membership in the upper or lower quartile) in relation to various categorical variables, avoided many of the difficulties encountered with these other approaches.

The following sources discuss different approaches to model building and testing: P. M. Bentler, "Multivariate Analyses With Latent Variables: Causal Modeling," *Annual Review of Psychology, 31* (1980): 419–446; E. J. Pedhazur, *Multiple Regression in Behavioral Research: Explanation and Prediction*, 2nd ed. (New York: Holt, Rinehart and Winston, 1982); H. M. Blalock, Jr., ed., *Causal Models in the Social Sciences* (Chicago: Aldine Publishing Company, 1971); and J. M. McPherson, "Theory Trimming," *Social Science Research, 5* (1976): 95–105.

7. See M. A. Wallach, "Creativity Testing and Giftedness," in *The Gifted and Talented*, F. D. Horowitz and M. O'Brien, eds. (Washington, DC: American Psychological Association, 1985).

8. D. K. Simonton, "Emergence and Realization of Genius: The Lives and Works of 120 Classical Composers," *Journal of Personality and Social Psychology*, 61 (1991): 829–840, 1991.

9. A. Rothenberg, "Psychopathology and Creative Cognition: A Comparison of Hospitalized Patients, Nobel Laureates, and Controls," *Archives of General Psychiatry, 40* (1983): 937–942.

10. A. Storr, *Solitude: A Return to the Self* (New York: The Free Press, 1988).

11. See M. Runco, "Creativity and Its Discontents," in *Creativity and Affect*, M. Shaw and M. A. Runco, eds. (Noorwood, NJ: Ablex, 1994) for an excellent discussion of the relationship of discontentment to creativity.

12. See M. Csikszentmihalyi (*Flow: The Psychology of Optimal Experience* [New York: Harper & Row, 1990]) for a discussion of problem seeking and the kinds of mental states that problem solving produces.

13. See K. Jamison, R. H. Gerner, C. Hammen, and C. Padesky, "Clouds and Silver Linings.

APPENDIX A

Creative Achievement Scale Quartile* (1 = Lowest and 4 = Highest)

Name	Quartile	Profession
Ackerley, J. R	1	Multimedia writer
Adams, Ansel	4	Photographer
Adams, Charles Francis, Jr.	1	Public official
Addams, Jane	4	Reformer
Agee, James Rufus	3	Multimedia writer
Aiken, Conrad	4	Poet
Aitken, William Maxwell	3	Businessman
Akhmatova, Anna	2	Poet
Alexandra, Queen	1	Royalty
Algren, Nelson	2	Fiction writer
Alinsky, Saul	3	Reformer
Allen, Fred	2	Actor
Allen, Frederick Lewis	2	Editor
Anderson, Elizabeth Garrett	1	Reformer
Anderson, James Maxwell	3	Playwright
Anderson, Sherwood	3	Fiction writer
Andreas-Salome, Lou	3	Multimedia writer
Antheil, George	4	Composer
Anthony, Susan B.	3	Reformer
Apollinaire, Guillaume	4	Poet
Arbus, Diane Nemerov	4	Photographer
Arden, Elizabeth	1	Businesswoman
Arendt, Hannah	2	Political theorist
Armstrong, Louis	4	Performer
Artaud, Antonin	4	Multimedia writer
Ashton-Warner, Sylvia	3	Multimedia writer
Asquith, Herbert Henry	1	Elected official
Astaire, Fred	4	Dancer
Astor, Nancy (Lady)	1	Elected official
Attlee, Clement	1	Elected official
Auden, W. H.	4	Poet
Baker, Hobart A. H.	1	Athlete
Baker, Josephine	3	Dancer
Baker, Newton D.	1	Public official
Bakhtin, Mikhail	3	Philosopher

Name	Quartile	Profession
Balanchine, George	4	Choreographer
Baldwin, James	3	Fiction writer
Bankhead, Tallulah	2	Actor
Barbirolli, John	3	Conductor
Barnes, Albert C.	1	Aesthete
Barnes, Djuna Chappell	3	Multimedia writer
Barney, Natalie Clifford	1	Hostess
Barr, Alfred H., Jr.	1	Curator
Barrie, James Matthew	3	Playwright
Barrymore, John	2	Actor
Bartok, Bela	4	Composer
Barton, Clara	3	Reformer
Baruch, Bernard	1	Businessman
Bateson, Gregory	3	Anthropologist
Bazin, Andre	3	Critic
Beaton, Cecil	3	Photographer
Beauduin, Lambert	1	Theologian
Beauvoir, Simone De	4	Multimedia writer
Bechet, Sidney	4	Performer
Bedaux, Charles Eugene	3	Manager
Beecham, Thomas	3	Conductor
Beerbohm, Max	4	Caricaturist
Behan, Brendan	3	Multimedia writer
Beiderbecke, Bix	2	Performer
Bell, Alexander Graham	4	Inventor
Bell, Vanessa	2	Painter
Belloc, Hilaire	3	Multimedia writer
Bellows, George	3	Painter
Belushi, John	2	Actor
Ben-Gurion, David	4	Elected official
Benedict, Ruth	4	Anthropologist
Bennett, Arnold	3	Fiction writer
Bennett, James Gordon, Jr.	1	Publisher
Benny, Jack	4	Actor
Berenson, Bernard	3	Critic
Berg, Alban	4	Composer
Berle, Adolf A.	3	Policy advisor
Bernhardt, Sarah	3	Actor
Bernstein, Aline	2	Designer

*See Chapter 9 for explanation.

Name	Quartile	Profession
Berryman, John	3	Poet
Besant, Annie	2	Reformer
Bethune, Mary Mcleod	2	Reformer
Bevan, Aneurin	1	Elected Official
Bevin, Ernest	1	Elected Official
Bierce, Ambrose	3	Multimedia writer
Birkett, Norman	1	Judge/Lawyer
Black, Hugo Lafayette	3	Judge
Blackmur, R. P.	2	Multimedia writer
Blackwell, Elizabeth	3	Reformer
Blitzstein, Mark	3	Composer
Blixin, Bror	1	Adventurer
Bloch, Mark	2	Historian
Blok, Alexander	3	Poet
Blum, Leon	3	Elected official
Blunt, Anthony	1	Historian
Blunt, Wilfrid	2	Poet
Bogan, Louise	2	Poet
Bogart, Humphrey	3	Actor
Bohr, Neils	4	Physicist
Bonaparte, Marie	2	Psychoanalyst
Bonhoeffer, Dietrich	3	Theologian
Booth, Maud Ballington	4	Reformer
Borodin, Mikhail	1	Activist
Boulanger, Nadia	1	Conductor
Bourke-White, Margaret	4	Photographer
Bourne, Randolph	2	Nonfiction writer
Bow, Clara	2	Actor
Bowen, Elizabeth	3	Fiction writer
Bowles, Jane	1	Fiction writer
Bradden, Mary Elizabeth	2	Fiction writer
Brandeis, Louis D.	3	Judge
Brecht, Berthold	4	Playwright
Breton, Andre	4	Multimedia writer
Brett, Dorothy	1	Painter
Breuil, Abbe Henri	4	Anthropologist
Bronfman, Sam	1	Businessman
Brooke, Rupert	2	Poet
Brooks, Louise	2	Actor
Brooks, Romaine	1	Painter
Brooks, Van Wyck	2	Critic
Broun, Heywood	3	Journalist
Bruce, Lenny	2	Actor
Brundage, Avery	1	Sportsman
Bryan, William Jennings	1	Elected official
Bryant, Louise	2	Journalist
Buber, Martin	3	Theologian

Name	Quartile	Profession
Buchan, John	2	Fiction writer
Buckner, Emory	1	Lawyer
Bulgakov, Mikhail	3	Fiction writer
Burbank, Luther	4	Biological scientist
Burdett-Couts, Angela	2	Philanthropist
Burnham, Daniel H.	3	Architect
Burroughs, Edgar Rice	3	Fiction writer
Burt, Cyril	4	Psychologist
Burton, Richard	3	Actor
Butler, Josephine	2	Reformer
Cabot, Godfrey Lowell	3	Businessman
Cagney, James	3	Actor
Cain, James M.	3	Fiction writer
Callas, Maria	3	Singer
Campbell, Beatrice Stella	2	Actor
Camus, Albert	4	Fiction writer
Canary, Martha Jane	1	Adventurer
Capa, Robert	3	Photographer
Capote, Truman	4	Fiction Writer
Carnegie, Andrew	4	Businessman
Carr, Emily	3	Painter
Carrington, Dora	1	Painter
Carson, Rachel	3	Naturalist
Caruso, Enrico	4	Singer
Carver, George Washington	4	Scientist
Casals, Pablo	4	Performer
Casement, Roger	1	Reformer
Cash, W. J.	2	Journalist
Cassatt, Mary	4	Painter
Cather, Willa	3	Fiction writer
Catt, Carrie Chapman	2	Reformer
Cavafy, Constantine	2	Poet
Celine, Louis-Ferdinand	3	Fiction writer
Cézanne, Paul	4	Painter
Chaliapin, Fedor	3	Singer
Chamberlain, Joshua L.	1	Soldier
Chamberlain, Neville	1	Elected official
Chandler, Raymond	2	Fiction writer
Chanel, Gabrielle	4	Designer
Chaplin, Charlie	4	Actor
Chapman, John Jay	2	Nonfiction writer
Cheever, John	3	Fiction writer
Chekhov, Anton	4	Playwright
Chennault, Clairelee	2	Policy advisor
Chesterton, G. K.	3	Nonfiction writer
Chopin, Kate	1	Fiction writer
Christie, Agatha	4	Fiction writer
Churchill, Jennie Jerome	1	Hostess

Name	Quartile	Profession
Churchill, Winston	4	Elected official
Clark, Kenneth	3	Historian
Clark, Mark	1	Soldier
Clayton, Geoffrey Hare	1	Religious official
Clift, Montgomery	3	Actor
Cobb, Ty	2	Athlete
Cockerell, Sydney Carlyle	2	Aesthete
Cocteau, Jean	4	Multimedia writer
Cody, William F.	2	Adventurer
Coffin, Henry Sloane	2	Theologian
Cohn, Harry	1	Producer
Cohn, Roy	1	Lawyer
Colette, Sidonie	4	Fiction writer
Coltrane, John	4	Performer
Compton-Burnett, Ivy	2	Fiction writer
Conrad, Joseph	4	Fiction writer
Coolidge, Calvin	2	Elected official
Coolidge, Grace Anna	1	Companion
Cooper, Gary	4	Actor
Cornell, Katherine	3	Actor
Coward, Noel	4	Playwright
Cozzens, James Gould	2	Fiction writer
Crabtree, Lotta	2	Actor
Crane, Cora	1	Companion
Crane, Hart	3	Poet
Crane, Stephen	4	Fiction writer
Cranko, John	3	Choreographer
Crawford, Joan	3	Actor
Croly, Herbert	3	Political theorist
Crosby, Harry	1	Poet
Crosby, Percy	4	Cartoonist
Crouse, Russell	3	Playwright
Crowhurst, D.	1	Inventor
Cummings, E. E.	4	Poet
Cunard, Nancy	1	Patron
Curie, Marie	4	Scientist
Curzon, George	1	Public official
Curzon, Mary	1	Companion
Cushing, Harvey	4	Medical scientist
D Annunzio, Gabrielle	4	Multimedia writer
Daley, Richard J.	1	Elected official
Dalton, Hugh	2	Elected official
Daniels, Josephus	1	Editor
Darrow, Clarence	3	Lawyer
David-Neel, Alexandra	3	Nonfiction writer
Davidson, John	2	Poet
Davies, Marion	1	Actor

Name	Quartile	Profession
Davis, Elmer	2	Journalist
Davis, John W.	1	Judge/Lawyer
Davis, Richard Harding	2	Journalist
Day, Dorothy	2	Journalist
Day, F. Holland	2	Photographer
De Wolfe, Elsie	4	Designer
Dean, James	2	Actor
Debs, Eugene	1	Labor leader
Debussy, Claude	4	Composer
Degas, Edgar	4	Painter
DeGaulle, Charles	4	Elected official
Delius, Frederick	3	Composer
Demille, Cecil B.	3	Director
Demuth, Charles	2	Painter
Deutsch, Helene	3	Psychoanalyst
Devoto, Bernard	2	Multimedia writer
Dewey, John	4	Philosopher
Dewey, Thomas	1	Elected official
Diaghilev, Sergei	4	Producer
Dilke, Sir Charles	1	Elected official
Dinesen, Isak	4	Nonfiction writer
Disney, Walt	4	Producer
Dodge, Horace	4	Businessman
Dodge, John	2	Businessman
Donovan, William J.	1	Public official
Doolittle, Hilda	3	Poet
Dos Passos, John	4	Fiction writer
Douglas, Lewis W.	1	Public official
Douglas, Lord Alfred	1	Poet
Douglas, William O.	3	Judge
Doyle, Arthur Conan	4	Fiction writer
Dreiser, Theodore	4	Fiction writer
Duchamp, Marcel	4	Painter
Duff Gordon, Lady	2	Designer
Dulles, Allen	1	Lawyer
Dulles, John Foster	2	Public official
Duncan, Isadora	4	Dancer
Dupont, Alfred I.	2	Businessman
Durkheim, Emile	4	Sociologist
Duse, Eleanora	3	Actor
Duveen, Joseph	1	Businessman
Dvorák, Antonín	4	Composer
Eady, Dorothy Louise	1	Anthropologist
Eakins, Thomas	2	Painter
Earhart, Amelia	1	Explorer
Eastman, Max	2	Journalist
Eberhardt, Isabelle	1	Multimedia writer
Eddy, Mary Baker	4	Persuader
Eden, Anthony	1	Elected official
Edison, Thomas Alva	4	Inventor
Edward VII	1	Royalty

Name	Quartile	Profession
Edward VIII	1	Royalty
Ehrenburg, Ilya	3	Multimedia writer
Einstein, Albert	4	Physicist
Eisenhower, Dwight D.	2	Elected official
Elgar, Edward	4	Composer
Eliot, T. S.	4	Poet
Ellington, Duke	4	Composer
Ellis, Henry Havelock	3	Psychiatrist
Ellis, Perry	2	Designer
Emerson, P. H.	3	Photographer
Epstein, Brian	1	Manager
Esenin, Sergei	3	Poet
Eugenie, Empress Of France	1	Companion
Evans, Edward	2	Soldier
Evans, Sir Arthur	4	Anthropologist
Fanon, Franz	3	Activist
Farmer, Frances	2	Actor
Fassbinder, Rainer Werner	4	Director
Faulkner, William	4	Fiction writer
Faust, Frederick	3	Fiction writer
Feneon, Felix	1	Critic
Feodorov, Leonid	1	Theologian
Ferber, Edna	3	Fiction writer
Ferdinand, Franz	1	Royalty
Finch Hatton, Denys	1	Adventurer
Firbank, Ronald	1	Fiction writer
Fitzgerald, F. Scott	3	Fiction writer
Fitzgerald, Zelda	1	Fiction writer
Flagler, Henry	1	Businessman
Flagstad, Kirsten	3	Singer
Flaherty, Robert Joseph	4	Director
Fleming, Alexander	4	Biologist
Fleming, Ian	3	Fiction writer
Fletcher, Alice	2	Anthropologist
Flynn, Errol	3	Actor
Fontanne, Lynn	3	Actor
Ford, Clara	1	Companion
Ford, Edsel	1	Businessman
Ford, Ford Madox	3	Fiction writer
Ford, Henry	4	Inventor
Ford, John	4	Director
Forester, E. M.	4	Fiction writer
Fortas, Abe	2	Judge/Lawyer
Fortuny, Mariano	4	Designer
Fosse, Bob	4	Choreographer
Fossey, Dian	2	Anthropologist
Fowler, Gene	3	Journalist
France, Anatole	4	Multimedia writer
Frankfurter, Felix	2	Judge/Lawyer
Frazer, James George	4	Anthropologist

Name	Quartile	Profession
Frazier, Brenda Diana Duff	1	Hostess
Freeman, Richard Austin	2	Fiction writer
Freud, Anna	3	Psychoanalyst
Freud, Sigmund	4	Psychoanalyst
Frewen, Moreton	1	Businessman
Friedman, William F.	3	Physicist
Frost, Robert	4	Poet
Fry, Roger Elliot	3	Critic
Gable, Clark	3	Actor
Gaitskell, Hugh	1	Elected official
Gallimard, Gaston	1	Publisher
Galsworthy, John	3	Fiction writer
Garcia Lorca, Federico	4	Poet
Gardner, Isabella Stewart	1	Aesthete
Garland, Judy	3	Actor
Garvey, Marcus	2	Activist
Gauguin, Paul	4	Painter
Gautier, Judith	2	Critic
Gaye, Marvin	2	Singer
Gershwin, George	4	Composer
Getty, Jean Paul	1	Businessman
Giacometti, Alberto	4	Sculptor
Gibson, Josh	1	Athlete
Gide, Andre	4	Fiction writer
Gilbert, W. S.	4	Lyricist
Gill, Eric	3	Sculptor
Girandoux, Jean	3	Fiction writer
Gissing, George	2	Fiction writer
Glyn, Elinor	2	Fiction writer
Goddard, Robert	4	Inventor
Goldberg, Rube	4	Cartoonist
Goldman, Emma	1	Activist
Goldwyn, Samuel	1	Producer
Gollancz, Victor	2	Publisher
Gompers, Samuel	2	Labor leader
Gonne, Maud	1	Activist
Goodhue, Bertram Grosvenor	2	Architect
Goodman, Benjamin D.	3	Performer
Gordon, Caroline	1	Fiction writer
Gorky, Arshille	3	Painter
Gorky, Maxim	4	Fiction writer
Gosse, Edmund	3	Critic
Gould, Glenn	4	Performer
Grant, Cary	3	Actor
Gray, Eileen	3	Architect
Green, E. H. R.	1	Businessman
Green, Hettie	1	Businessman
Gregory, Lady	1	Patron
Grenfell, Julian	2	Poet
Grieg, Edvard	4	Composer

Name	Quartile	Profession
Griffith, Arthur	1	Activist
Griffith, D. W.	4	Director
Groesbeck, Alex J.	1	Elected official
Grosz, George	3	Painter
Guevara, Ernesto	3	Activist
Guggenheim, Peggy	1	Patron
Guilbert, Yvette	2	Singer
Guitry, Sacha	3	Playwright
Gurdjieff, George	3	Persuader
Gurney, Ivor	3	Composer
Guthrie, Woody	3	Composer
Hagar, Connie	1	Scientist
Haggard, Rider	3	Fiction writer
Haldane, J. B. S.	4	Scientist
Halifax, Lord	1	Public official
Hall, Radclyffe	3	Fiction writer
Hammarskjold, Dag	2	Public official
Hammett, Dashiell	2	Fiction writer
Hamsun, Knut	4	Fiction writer
Harding, Warren G.	1	Elected official
Hardy, Thomas	4	Fiction writer
Harkness, Rebecca West	1	Patron
Harlin, John Elvis, II	1	Explorer
Harris, Frank	2	Journalist
Harris, Jed	2	Producer
Hart, Lorenz Milton	3	Lyricist
Hastie, William Henry	2	Judge/Lawyer
Hawks, Howard Winchester	3	Director
Hays, Lee Elhardt	2	Performer
Haywood, Bill	1	Labor leader
Hayworth, Rita	3	Actor
Hearn, Lafcadio	2	Multimedia writer
Hearst, William Randolph	3	Publisher
Heggen, Orlo Thomas	3	Fiction writer
Held, John, Jr.	3	Caricaturist
Hellman, Lillian	3	Playwright
Hemingway, Ernest	4	Fiction writer
Hendrix, Jimi	3	Performer
Henri, Robert	3	Painter
Herbst, Josephine Frey	2	Fiction writer
Herzl, Theodor	4	Activist
Hesse, Hermann	4	Multimedia writer
Hickok, Lorena	1	Journalist
Higginson, Thomas W.	2	Reformer
Hill, Joe	1	Composer
Hindemith, Paul	4	Composer
Hitchcock, Alfred Joseph	4	Director
Hofmeyr, Jan	2	Elected official

Name	Quartile	Profession
Holland, John Philip	2	Inventor
Holliday, Judy	2	Actor
Holman, Libby	2	Singer
Holmes, Oliver Wendell	3	Judge
Holt, Hamilton	4	Educator
Homer, Winslow	3	Painter
Hoover, Herbert	3	Elected official
Hoover, J. Edgar	2	Public official
Hopkins, Harry	2	Public official
Hopper, Edward	4	Painter
Hopper, Hedda	2	Journalist
Horney, Karen	3	Mental Scientist
Houdini, Harry	4	Magician
Houselander, Caryll	1	Caricaturist
Housman, Alfred Edward	4	Poet
Houston, Charles Hamilton	3	Judge/Lawyer
Howe, Julia Ward	3	Multimedia writer
Howells, William Dean	2	Fiction writer
Hubbard, Elbert Green	3	Multimedia writer
Hudson, Rock	2	Actor
Hudson, W. H.	3	Scientist
Hughes, Howard	3	Businessman
Hughes, James Langston	3	Multimedia writer
Hulme, T. E.	3	Nonfiction writer
Humphrey, Hubert H., Jr.	1	Elected official
Humphrey, Doris	3	Choreographer
Hunt, H. L., Jr.	1	Businessman
Hunter, Alberta	2	Singer
Huntington, Collis Porter	1	Businessman
Hurston, Zora Neale	2	Fiction writer
Huston, John	4	Director
Hutchins, Robert Maynard	3	Educator
Huxley, Aldous	4	Fiction writer
Ibsen, Henrik	4	Playwright
Ickes, Harold Le Claire	1	Public official
Ingersoll, Ralph Mcallister	2	Journalist
Isaacs, Rufus Daniel	2	Public official
Jabotinsky, Vladimir	2	Activist
Jackson, Shirley	2	Fiction writer
James, Henry	4	Fiction writer
James, Robertson	1	Painter
James, William	4	Psychologist

Name	Quartile	Profession
Lowell, Robert	4	Poet
Lowenstein, Allard K.	1	Reformer
Lowry, Malcolm	2	Fiction writer
Luce, Henry Robinson	3	Publisher
Luhan, Mabel Dodge	1	Host
Lunt, Alfred, Jr.	3	Actor
Luxemburg, Rosa	2	Activist
MacArthur, Douglas	3	Soldier
Macdonald, Ross	2	Fiction writer
Macy, Anne Sullivan	1	Educator
Maeterlinck, Maurice	4	Playwright
Mahler, Alma Schindler	1	Companion
Mahler, Gustav	4	Composer
Malcolm X	2	Reformer
Mallory, George	1	Explorer
Malraux, Andre	4	Fiction writer
Mandelstam, Osip E.	3	Poet
Mankiewicz, Herman	2	Playwright
Mann, Heinrich Luiz	3	Fiction writer
Mann, Thomas	4	Fiction writer
Manning, William Thomas	1	Religious official
Mansfield, Katherine	4	Fiction writer
March, William	2	Fiction writer
Marciano, Rocky	1	Athlete
Marcus, David	1	Soldier
Marie, Queen Of Romania	1	Royalty
Markham, Beryl	3	Trainer (of horses)
Markievicz, Constance De	2	Activist
Marley, Bob	3	Singer
Marquand, John	3	Fiction writer
Marshall, George Catlett	3	Soldier
Marx, Groucho	3	Actor
Mary, Queen Of England	1	Royalty
Matisse, Henri	4	Painter
Maugham, Somerset	4	Fiction writer
Mayakovsky, Vladimir	3	Poet
Mayer, Louis B.	2	Producer
McCarthy, Joe	1	Elected official
McCay, Winsor	4	Caricaturist
McClure, Samuel S.	2	Publisher
McCormack, John	3	Singer
McCormick, Robert R.	2	Publisher
McCullers, Carson	2	Fiction writer
McDaniel, Hattie	2	Actor
McGill, Ralph	2	Journalist
McGraw, John	2	Coach

Name	Quartile	Profession
McPherson, Aimee Semple	1	Persuader
McQueen, Steve	2	Actor
Mead, Margaret	4	Anthropologist
Meinertzhagen, Richard	1	Soldier
Melba, Nellie	3	Singer
Melchior, Lauritz	3	Singer
Mencken, Henry Louis	3	Nonfiction writer
Menzies, Stewart	1	Public official
Mercer, Mabel	2	Singer
Merton, Thomas	3	Theologian
Metcalf, Willard L.	2	Painter
Mew, Charlotte	1	Poet
Meyer, Andre	2	Businessman
Meyer, Eugene	1	Businessman
Mies Van Der Rohe, Ludwig	4	Architect
Milk, Harvey	1	Reformer
Millay, Edna St. Vincent	3	Poet
Miller, Marilyn	2	Dancer
Mills, C. Wright	4	Sociologist
Mistral, Frederic	3	Poet
Mitchell, Lucy Sprague	3	Educator
Mitchell, Margaret	3	Fiction writer
Mitford, Nancy	2	Fiction writer
Mivart, St. George Jackson	1	Scientist
Modersohn-Becker, Paula	2	Painter
Monroe, Hector Hugh	3	Fiction writer
Monroe, Marilyn	3	Actor
Montesquiou, Count Robert De	1	Aesthete
Montgomery, Bernard	2	Soldier
Moore, George Edward	3	Philosopher
Moran, Thomas	2	Painter
More, Paul Elmer	2	Philosopher
Morgan, John Pierpont	1	Businessman
Morgan, Julia	3	Architect
Morley, Christopher	2	Fiction writer
Morrell, Ottoline	1	Host
Morrison, Jim	3	Singer
Mostel, Zero	2	Actor
Mountbatten, Lord	1	Royalty
Muir, John	3	Naturalist
Munby, Arthur J.	2	Poet
Munch, Edvard	4	Painter
Murphy, Gerald	2	Painter
Murrow, E. R.	3	Broadcaster
Murry, John Middleton	2	Nonfiction writer
Nabokov, Vladimir	4	Fiction writer

Name	Quartile	Profession
Nast, Condé	1	Publisher
Nation, Carry	1	Reformer
Nesbit, Edith	2	Fiction writer
Neutra, Richard	4	Architect
Newhouse, Samuel I.	1	Publisher
Niebuhr, Reinhold	4	Theologian
Niemoller, Martin	1	Theologian
Nietzsche, Elizabeth	1	Biographer
Nietzsche, Frederick	4	Philosopher
Nijinsky, Vaslav	4	Dancer
Nordica, Lillian	2	Singer
Normand, Mabel	2	Actor
Norris, George W.	3	Elected official
O'Casey, Sean	4	Playwright
O'Conner, Frank	3	Fiction writer
O'Flaherty, Hugh	1	Reformer
O'Hara, John	3	Fiction writer
O'Keeffe, Georgia	4	Painter
O'Neill, Eugene	4	Playwright
O'Shea, Kitty	1	Companion
Ochs, Phil	2	Singer
Odets, Clifford	3	Playwright
Oldfield, Barney	2	Sportsman
Olmstead, Frederick Law	4	Architect
Onassis, Aristotle	1	Businessman
Oppenheimer, J. Robert	4	Physicist
Orton, Joe	2	Playwright
Orwell, George	4	Fiction writer
Otero, Caroline	1	Dancer
Oughton, Diana	1	Activist
Owen, Wilfred	2	Poet
Owens, Jesse	2	Athlete
Paderewski, Ignacy Jan	4	Performer
Palmer, A. Mitchell	1	Public official
Palmer, Bertha Honore	1	Patron
Parker, Charlie	4	Composer
Parker, Dorothy	1	Fiction writer
Parrish, Maxwell	3	Painter
Parsons, Louella	2	Journalist
Pasolini, Pier Paolo	3	Multimedia writer
Pasternak, Boris	4	Poet
Patterson, Chippy	1	Judge/Lawyer
Patterson, Cissy	1	Editor
Patton, George, Jr.	1	Soldier
Pavlova, Anna	4	Dancer
Pearson, Drew	2	Journalist
Peary, Robert E.	2	Explorer
Perelman, S. J.	3	Nonfiction writer
Perez, Leander	1	Elected official
Perkins, Frances	1	Public official
Perkins, George W.	1	Businessman

Name	Quartile	Profession
Perkins, Maxwell	2	Editor
Pershing, John J.	2	Soldier
Piaf, Edith	2	Singer
Picabia, Francis	4	Painter
Picasso, Pablo	4	Painter
Pinchot, Gifford	2	Scientist
Pissarro, Jacob Camille	4	Painter
Pissarro, Lucien	2	Painter
Pittman, Key	1	Elected official
Plath, Sylvia	2	Poet
Plekhanov, G. V.	3	Political theorist
Pollock, Jackson	4	Painter
Porter, Cole	4	Composer
Porter, Katherine Anne	3	Fiction writer
Post, Marjorie Merriweather	2	Businesswoman
Potter, Beatrix	3	Fiction writer
Pound, Ezra	4	Poet
Powell, John Wesley	3	Scientist
Powell, Maud	2	Performer
Presley, Elvis	4	Singer
Primrose, Archibald	1	Public official
Prokofiev, Sergei	4	Composer
Proust, Marcel	4	Fiction writer
Przybyszewska, Stanislawa	1	Playwright
Puccini, Giacomo	4	Composer
Pulitzer, Joseph	2	Publisher
Quinn, John	1	Patron
Rachmaninoff, Sergei	4	Composer
Radnitsky, Emmanuel	4	Photographer
Rand, Ayn	3	Fiction writer
Rank, Otto	2	Psychoanalyst
Rankin, Jeannette	1	Elected official
Ransom, John Crowe	3	Poet
Rasputin, Grigorii	1	Persuader
Ravel, Maurice	4	Composer
Rawlings, Marjorie Kinnan	2	Fiction writer
Rayburn, Sam	1	Elected official
Rebay, Hilla	1	Aesthete
Reed, John	2	Nonfiction writer
Reich, Wilhelm	2	Psychoanalyst
Reitman, Ben	1	Reformer
Remington, Frederic	2	Painter
Renault, Louis	3	Businessman
Renoir, Pierre August	4	Painter
Reuther, Walter	1	Labor leader
Rhodes, Cecil	3	Elected official
Rhys, Jean	2	Fiction writer
Richardson, Dorothy	2	Fiction writer

Name	Quartile	Profession	Name	Quartile	Profession
Richthofen, Manfred Von	1	Soldier	Schamberg, Morton L.	2	Painter
			Schoenberg, Arnold	4	Composer
Rickenbacker, Edward	2	Soldier	Schreiner, Olive	2	Nonfiction writer
Rilke, Ranier Maria	4	Poet			
Rivera, Diego	4	Painter	Schreyvogel, Charles	1	Painter
Robertson, William	1	Soldier	Schulte, Edward	1	Reformer
Robeson, Paul	4	Actor	Schwab, Charles M.	1	Businessman
Robinson, Bill	3	Dancer	Schwartz, Delmore	4	Poet
Robinson, Edwin Arlington	3	Poet	Schweitzer, Albert	4	Philosopher
			Scott, Evelyn	1	Fiction writer
Robinson, Jackie	1	Athlete	Scott, Robert Falcon	2	Adventurer
Rockefeller, John D.	3	Businessman	Scriabin, Alexander	4	Composer
Rockefeller, John D., Jr.	2	Philanthropist	Seabury, Samuel	1	Judge/Lawyer
Rockefeller, Nelson	2	Elected official	Seberg, Jean	3	Actor
Rodin, Auguste	4	Sculptor	Sellers, Peter	3	Actor
Roethke, Theodore	3	Poet	Sereni, Enzo	1	Activist
Rogers, John	2	Sculptor	Sert, Misia	1	Patron
Rogers, Will	3	Actor	Seton, Ernest Thompson	2	Scientist
Rolfe, Frederick Williams	2	Fiction writer			
			Shackleton, Ernest	2	Explorer
Rommel, Erwin	2	Soldier	Shaw, Charlotte	1	Companion
Roosevelt, Anna	1	Host	Shaw, George Bernard	4	Playwright
Roosevelt, Eleanor	1	Companion	Shaw, Irwin	3	Fiction writer
Roosevelt, Franklin Delano	4	Elected official	Sheehy-Skeffington, Hanna	1	Reformer
Roosevelt, Theodore	4	Elected official	Sherwood, Robert E.	3	Playwright
Rose, Billy	2	Producer	Shostakovich, Dmitri	4	Composer
Rosenbach, Abe	1	Businessman	Shubert, Jacob	1	Businessman
Rosenberg, Isaac	2	Poet	Shubert, Lee	1	Businessman
Rothko, Mark	3	Painter	Shubert, Sam	1	Businessman
Royce, Josiah	4	Philosopher	Simenon, Georges	3	Fiction writer
Ruskin, John	3	Critic	Simpson, Wallis	1	Companion
Russell, Bertrand	4	Philosopher	Sinclair, Upton	3	Fiction writer
Ruth, Babe	2	Athlete	Sitwell, Edith	4	Poet
Ryan, John A.	1	Economist	Sloan, John	3	Painter
Sackville-West, Victoria	1	Hostess	Smedley, Agnes	1	Journalist
			Smith, Al	1	Elected official
Sackville-West, Vita	2	Poet	Smith, Bessie	3	Singer
Saint Gaudens, Augustus	3	Sculptor	Smith, Lillian	2	Fiction writer
			Smith, Red	2	Journalist
Saint-Exupery, Antoine De	3	Fiction writer	Smith, Stevie	3	Poet
			Smuts, Jan Christian	2	Elected official
Sandburg, Carl	4	Poet	Snow, Edgar	2	Journalist
Sanders, George	2	Actor	Sonnenberg, Benjamin	1	Publicist
Sanger, Margaret	2	Reformer	Spalding, A. G.	2	Athlete
Santayana, George	4	Philosopher	Spellman, Francis	1	Religious official
Santos-Dumont, Alberto	2	Sportsman			
			Spencer, Herbert	3	Sociologist
Sargent, John Singer	4	Painter	Spiegel, Sam	2	Producer
Sarnoff, David	3	Businessman	Springs, Elliott White	2	Businessman
Saroyan, William	3	Fiction writer	St. Denis, Ruth	4	Choreographer
Sartre, Jean-Paul	4	Philosopher	Stafford, Jean Wilson	2	Fiction writer
Savitch, Jessica	1	Broadcaster	Stanislavsky, Konstantin	4	Actor
Sayers, Dorothy	2	Fiction writer			

Name	Quartile	Profession
Stanton, Elizabeth Cady	1	Reformer
Steffens, Lincoln	3	Journalist
Stein, Edith	2	Theologian
Stein, Gertrude	3	Fiction writer
Steinbeck, John	4	Fiction writer
Stengel, Casey	1	Coach
Stephen, Leslie	3	Nonfiction writer
Stevens, Wallace	3	Poet
Stevenson, Adlai	3	Elected official
Stevenson, Fanny	1	Companion
Stieglitz, Alfred	4	Photographer
Stilwell, Joseph	1	Soldier
Stimson, Henry Lewis	1	Public official
Stokowski, Leopold	3	Conductor
Stout, Rex	3	Fiction writer
Strachey, John	2	Nonfiction writer
Strachey, Lytton	4	Biographer
Strauss, Richard	4	Composer
Stravinsky, Igor	4	Composer
Strindberg, Johan August	4	Playwright
Stuart, Jesse Hilton	2	Fiction writer
Sullivan, Arthur	4	Composer
Sullivan, Harry Stack	3	Psychiatrist
Sullivan, Louis	4	Architect
Susann, Jacqueline	2	Fiction writer
Sutcliffe, Frank	3	Photographer
Svero, Italo	3	Fiction writer
Swope, Herbert Bayard	2	Journalist
Szent-Gyorgyi, Albert	4	Biological scientist
Szold, Henrietta	1	Activist
Taft, Robert A.	1	Elected official
Tarbell, Ida	2	Nonfiction writer
Tausk, Victor	2	Psychiatrist
Tawney, Richard	2	Historian
Taylor, Frederick	2	Inventor
Taylor, Marshall W.	2	Athlete
Tchelitchew, Pavel	3	Painter
Teasdale, Sara	2	Poet
Teilhard De Chardin, Pierre	1	Anthropologist
Terry, Ellen	3	Actor
Tesla, Nikola	4	Inventor
Teyte, Maggie	2	Singer
Thalberg, Irving	2	Producer
Thomas, Dylan	4	Poet
Thomas, Norman	3	Reformer
Thompson, Dorothy	2	Journalist
Thurber, James	4	Fiction writer
Tiffany, Louis	4	Designer

Name	Quartile	Profession
Tilden, Bill	2	Athlete
Tillich, Paul	4	Theologian
Toklas, Alice B.	1	Companion
Tolkien, J. R. R.	4	Fiction writer
Tolstoy, Leo	4	Fiction writer
Tolstoy, Sonja	1	Companion
Toomer, Jean	1	Multimedia writer
Torres, Camillo	1	Activist
Toscanini, Arturo	3	Conductor
Toulouse-Lautrec, Henri	4	Painter
Toynbee, Arnold J.	4	Historian
Tracy, Spencer	3	Actor
Trefusis, Violet	1	Host
Tresca, Carlo	1	Activist
Trotsky, Leon	2	Activist
Troubridge, Una	1	Companion
Truman, Harry S.	2	Elected official
Trumbo, Dalton	3	Playwright
Tsvetayeva, Marina	2	Poet
Tucker, Preston	1	Businessman
Tucker, Richard	2	Singer
Tukhachevsky, Mikhail	2	Soldier
Turing, Alan	4	Physicist
Turner, Frederick Jackson	2	Historian
Turner, Reginald	1	Fiction writer
Twain, Mark	4	Fiction writer
Valentino, Rudolph	2	Actor
Van Vechten, Carl	2	Critic
Vanderbilt, Consuelo	1	Philanthropist
Vann, John Paul	1	Soldier
Varese, Edgard	4	Composer
Veeck, Bill	1	Businessman
Verdi, Giuseppe	4	Composer
Victoria, Queen	1	Royalty
Villard, Oswald Garrison	2	Journalist
Visconti, Luchino	3	Director
Von Moltke, Helmuth	1	Activist
Von Schrenk, Hermann	3	Scientist
Von Stroheim, Erich	3	Director
Vorse, Mary Heaton	2	Journalist
Wagner, Cosima	1	Companion
Wainwright, Jonathan M.	1	Soldier
Walker, Jimmy	1	Elected official
Wallace, Henry	3	Public official
Waller, Thomas Wright	3	Performer
Warburg, Siegmund	2	Businessman
Warhol, Andy	4	Painter
Waring, Julius Waites	1	Judge/Lawyer
Warren, Earl	3	Judge

Name	Quartile	Profession
Washington, Booker T.	2	Educator
Washington, Dinah	2	Singer
Watts, Alan	2	Philosopher
Waugh, Evelyn	3	Fiction writer
Weaver, Harriet Shaw	1	Patron
Webb, Beatrice Potter	2	Sociologist
Weber, Max	4	Sociologist
Webern, Anton Von	4	Composer
Weil, Simone	2	Nonfiction writer
Weill, Kurt	4	Composer
Weizmann, Chaim	4	Elected official
Welles, Orson	4	Director
Wells, H. G.	4	Fiction writer
West, Mae	3	Actor
West, Nathanael	3	Fiction writer
West, Rebecca	3	Journalist
Wharton, Edith	3	Fiction writer
Whistler, James Abbott McNeil	4	Painter
White, Katherine S.	1	Editor
White, T. H.	2	Fiction writer
White, William Allen	1	Editor
Whitehead, Alfred North	4	Philosopher
Whitney, Dorothy Payne	1	Patron
Whitney, Gertrude Vanderbilt	3	Patron
Whitney, William Collins	1	Businessman
Wilde, Oscar	4	Fiction writer
Wilder, Thornton	4	Playwright
Wiley, George A.	1	Reformer
Wilhelm II	1	Royalty
Wilkie, Wendell	2	Public official
Williams, Hank, Sr.	2	Singer

Name	Quartile	Profession
Williams, Charles	2	Editor
Williams, Tennessee	4	Playwright
Williams, Vaughan	3	Composer
Williams, William Carlos	4	Poet
Wilson, Edith	1	Companion
Wilson, Edmund	3	Critic
Wilson, Woodrow	4	Elected official
Wise, Isaac M.	2	Religious official
Wise, Jonah Bondi	1	Religious official
Wodehouse, P. G.	3	Multimedia writer
Wolf, Hugo	3	Composer
Wolfe, Thomas	4	Fiction writer
Wolfson, Harry Austryn	2	Educator
Woodhull, Victoria	3	Reformer
Woolf, Virginia	1	Fiction writer
Woollcott, Alexander	3	Nonfiction writer
Work, Monroe Nathan	1	Sociologist
Wright, Frank Lloyd	4	Architect
Wright, Orville	4	Inventor
Wright, Richard	2	Fiction writer
Wright, Wilbur	4	Inventor
Wurf, Jerome	1	Labor leader
Wylie, Elinor	2	Poet
Wyszynski, Stephen	1	Religious official
Yeats, John Butler	2	Painter
Yeats, William Butler	4	Poet
Young, Robert Ralph	1	Businessman
Zanuck, Darryl	2	Producer
Ziegfield, Florenz, Jr.	3	Producer
Zola, Emile	3	Fiction writer

APPENDIX B

Holland Classification*

Key: A = Artistic; E = Enterprising; C = Conventional; I = Investigative; R = Realistic; S = Social

Artistic Types

Actors (AES)
Architects (AIR)
Archivists (AES)
Art/Literary patrons (ASE)
Art collectors (ASE)
Art/Rare book dealers (ASE)
Biographers (ASE)
Cartoonists (AES)
Choreographers (AES)
Conductors (AES)
Comedians (AES)
Composers (ASE)
Critics (AES)
Cryptanalysts (AIE)
Dancers (AER)
Editors (AES)
Fashion designers (ASR)
Furniture designers (AES)
Illustrators (AES)
Interior designers (AES)
Lyricists (ASE)
Magicians (AES)
Motion picture set designers (AIR)
Musicians (ASI)
Painters (ASI)
Philosophers (ASI)
Photojournalists (AEC)
Photographers (AES)
Playwrights (ASE)

Poets (AES)
Reporters/Journalists (ASE)
Screenwriters (AEI)
Sculptors (AER)
Singers (AES)
Stage directors (AES)
Theatrical stage designers (AES)
Writers (fiction and nonfiction) (AES)

Enterprising Types

Advertising executives (ESA)
Airplane race/stunt pilots (ER)
Ambassadors (ESA)
Automobile racers (ER)
Cabinet members/Policy advisors (ESA)
Criminals (ERS)
Diplomats (ESA)
Entrepreneurs/Businessmen (ES)
Explorers (ER)
Financiers/Bankers (ESR)
Hunting/Fishing guides (ER)
Industrialists (ESR)
Judges (ESA)
Lawyers (ESA)
Literary agents (ESA)
Managers (ESC)
Military officers (ESR)
Motion picture producers (ESA)
Mountain climbers (ERI)
Museum directors (ESR)

*I am indebted to John L. Holland, Ph.D., and Gary D. Gottfredson, Ph.D. (personal correspondence, April, 1992), for taking the time to assign codes for certain occupations not listed in the *Dictionary of Holland Occupational Codes* (Odessa, FL: Psychological Assessment Resources, Inc., 1989). In addition, several minor coding adjustments were made to accommodate the special occupational activities of individuals. Labor leaders, such as Samuel Gompers and John L. Lewis, were grouped with social activists (SE) because they were politically active at the turn of the century. Historically, their roles were much like the civil rights and suffrage leaders in the study. Inventors, such as Alexander Graham Bell, Thomas Edison, Charles Kettering, and Bill Lear, instead of being coded RIE, were logically grouped with electrical engineers (IR). Barney Oldfield, as a race car driver, and Bror Blixen and Denys Finch Hatton, as hunting/fishing guides, who originally were coded RES, were grouped with adventurers/explorers (ER). And members of Royalty were grouped with ambassadors, diplomats, and ruling heads of state if they were politically involved, and with society/salon hosts if they were socially involved.

Political appointees/Administrators (ESA)
Politicians (ESA)
Publicists (ESA)
Publishers (ESR)
Royalty (ES)
Society/Salon hosts (ESA)
Theatrical producers (ESA)

Physicists (IRE)
Psychiatrists (ISA)
Physicians (ISE)
Sociologists (IES)
Surgeons (IRA)
Time-study engineers (IRE)
Zoologists (IRE)

Investigative Types

Aeronautical engineers (IRS)
Anthropologists (IRE)
Archaeologists (IRE)
Automotive engineers (IR)
Aviation pioneers (IRE)
Biochemists (IRS)
Biologists (ISR)
Botanists (IRS)
Chemists (IRE)
Civil engineers (IRE)
Economists (IAS)
Electrical engineers (IRE)
Ethnologists (IRE)
Geologists (IRE)
Inventors (IR)
Marine architect-engineers (IRE)
Mathematicians (IER)
Naturalists (IRS)
Paleontologists (ISR)

Social Types

Archbishops (SAI)
Athletes (professional) (SRC)
Coaches (SRE)
Conservationists (SEA)
Educators (SEI)
Evangelists (SEA)
Historians (SEI)
Homemakers (SE)
Labor leaders (SE)
Motion picture directors (SEC)
Philanthropists (SEA)
Political scientists (SEI)
Popes (SAI)
Psychologists (SIA)
Rabbis (reform leaders) (SAI)
Social activists (SE)
Teachers, elementary (SEC)
Teachers, deaf students (SEC)
Theologians (SIA)

APPENDIX C

Physical Handicaps of Individuals in the Sample

Speech

Clara Barton — lisp
André Bazin — stutter (age 23 failed oral exam)
Brendan Behan — stammer
Ruth Benedict* — stammer and "partially deaf"
Arnold Bennett — stammer
Aneurin Bevan — stammer
Truman Capote — high-pitched childish speech (and much anxiety)
George Washington Carver — "impaired vocal cords"; high-pitched voice all his life
Winston Churchill — stutter
Gary Cooper — stammer
Marion Davies — stammer
Edward VII — stammer
Anatole France — "slight" stammer
Cary Grant — lisp
D. W. Griffith — lisp until age 8
Helen Keller* — mute, deaf, blind
E. O. Lawrence — stammer
Joseph Lister — stammer
Henry Robinson Luce — stutter
Katherine Mansfield — stutter
Somerset Maugham — stammer
Phil Ochs — stutter
Jessica Savitch — lisp
Delmore Schwartz — lisp, stammer
Irwin Shaw — lisp
Konstantin Stanislavsky — speech impediment
Henri Toulouse-Lautrec* — crippled by accident, lisp, dwarfism
Thomas Wolfe — stuttered
Elinor Wylie — lisp

Hearing

Bernard Baruch — injury to left ear; partially deaf
Ruth Benedict* — partially deaf and stammer
Thomas Edison — partially deaf
Augustus John — partially deaf

Matthew Josephson — hearing problem
Alma Mahler — hearing loss (measles)
Steve McQueen — mastoid infection, partially deaf

Vision

Susan B. Anthony — crossed eyes
Cyril Burt — nearsighted (also delicate and underweight)
Henry Sloane Coffin — hereditary difficulty with one eyelid caused some vision problem
William O. Douglas — green–red color blindness
Bill Haywood — blind in one eye
Lafcadio Hearn — blind in one eye
Ernest Hemingway — left eye defective from birth
Aldous Huxley — age 17, staph infection in eye, near blindness for 18 months; vision problems all his life
Robinson Jeffers — right eye damaged at birth
Helen Keller* — blind, deaf, mute
Charles Kettering — serious eye condition since childhood
Le Corbusier — poor eyesight
William Lemke — blind in one eye
John Lennon* — astigmatism, myopic, dyslexia
Frederick Lindemann — long-sighted in one eye, short-sighted in the other; used a magnifying glass rather than eyeglasses
Malcolm Lowry — half blind from eye infection which caused some disfigurement for about four years
Anne Sullivan Macy — blind since age 5 (trachoma)
Sean O'Casey — poor eyesight, eyes often bandaged
Frederick Law Olmsted — sumac poisoning damaged eyesight and interrupted his education
Dorothy Richardson — very myopic; needed strong eyeglasses

*More than one disability.

232

Auguste Rodin — extremely nearsighted
Jean-Paul Sartre — could not use right eye
James Thurber — blind in one eye
Harry Truman — poor eyesight; wore
glasses at age 6
Dalton Trumbo — congenital drooping left
eyelid
Tennessee Williams* — illness damaged
kidneys and eyesight; could not walk,
pulled himself around for two years with
a handcar; because of long confinement
to bed, developed muscle weakness

Developmental

Albert Einstein — speculation suggests dys-
lexia; learned to speak late
J. Seward Johnson — dyslexia
Helen Keller* — deaf, mute, blind
John Lennon* — dyslexia, astigmatism,
myopia
George Smith Patton, Jr. — dyslexia
Norman Rockefeller — dyslexia
Woodrow Wilson — dyslexia

Deformities/Defects

Jane Addams — slight curvature of spine; pi-
geon-toed; head cocked to one side
Randolph Bourne — hunched back; stunted
growth; deformed face
Jane Bowles — crippled knee, from tubercu-
losis
Berthold Brecht — cardiac defect
Martin Buber — scarred mouth (forceps de-
livery); later wore mustache to hide scar
George Curzon — curvature of the spine

Claude Debussy — bony protuberances on
forehead
Charles Demuth — one bad hip; one leg
shorter than other
Allen Dulles — club foot
T. S. Eliot — congenital hernia (had to
wear truss all of his life)
Federico García Lorca — one leg shorter
than the other
E. H. R. Green — lame leg
Lord Halifax — born with one hand
W. H. Hudson — chronic heart condition
F. Tennyson Jesse — rickets; legs in braces
Frida Kahlo — limp (polio)
V. Khodasevich — born with six fingers on
each hand
Dorothea Lange — bad leg, limp (polio)
Ring Lardner — deformed foot, wore brace
till age 11; problem corrected with surgery
Rosa Luxemburg — deformed leg
Margaret Mitchell — slight limp
Boris Pasternak — leg injury; lifelong limp
Anna Roosevelt — spine injury
Eleanor Roosevelt — curvature of the spine
Henri Toulouse-Lautrec* — crippled by ac-
cident, lisp, dwarfism
Rudolph Valentino — cauliflower ear
Andy Warhol — albino
Wilhelm II — crippled left arm (wrenched
from socket during birth)
Tennessee Williams* — illness damaged
kidneys and eyesight; because of long con-
finement to bed, developed muscle weak-
ness (could not walk, pulled himself
around for two years with a handcar)
Jerome Wurf — leg pain and limp (polio);
often in a wheelchair

APPENDIX D

Incidental and Accidental Deaths

13 War Casualties (see also
Concentration Camp Victims below)

7 WWI

Hobey Baker
Julian Grenfell
T. E. Hulme
Hector Hugh Munro
Wilfred Owen
Manfred Von Richthofen
Isaac Rosenberg

2 WWII

Antoine De Saint-Exupéry
Frederick Faust

2 Vietnam

John Paul Vann
Robert Capa

2 South American Revolutionaries

Camilo Torres
Che Guevara

22 Political Executions/Murders

14 Assassinations

Rosa Luxemburg
Malcolm X
Harvey Milk
Lord Mountbatten
Rasputin
Carlo Tresca
Leon Trotsky
Franz Ferdinand
Jean Jaurès
John F. Kennedy
Robert F. Kennedy
Martin Luther King
Huey Long
Allard K. Lowenstein

2 Concentration Camp Victims

Edith Stein
Janusz Korczak ("probably")

3 Executions by Nazis

Helmuth Von Moltke

Marc Bloch
Dietrich Bonhoeffer

3 Political Executions

Federico García Lorca
Mikhail Tukhachevsky
Roger Casement

2 Accidental Shootings

David Marcus
Anton Von Webern

8 Murders

Robert Johnson
Marvin Gaye
Joe Orton
Pier Paolo Pasolini
Marc Blitzstein
Dian Fossey
Kit Lambert
John Lennon

1 Execution for Murder

Joe Hill

1 Train Accident

Sam Shubert

7 Airplane Crashes (does not include
wartime aircraft casualties)

Rocky Marciano
Walter Reuther
Will Rogers
Denys Finch Hatton
Dag Hammarskjöld
Carole Lombard
Kathleen Kennedy

14 Automobile/Motorcycle Accidents

Albert Barnes
Bror Blixen
Albert Camus

James Dean
Isadora Duncan
Jack Johnson
T. E. Lawrence
Grace Kelly
Margaret Mitchell
Jackson Pollock
Jessica Savitch
Bessie Smith
Italo Svevo
Nathanael West

8 Asphyxiation and Fire

1 Fire

Zelda Fitzgerald

3 Asphyxiation

John Cranko (under effect of sleeping pill)
Tennessee Williams (choked on a pill-bottle cap)
Émile Zola (suffocated while sleeping in a room with a blocked chimney)

1 Accidental Bomb Explosion

Diana Oughton

3 Drowning

E. G. Hubbard
George A. Wiley

Isabelle Eberhardt

2 Mountain Climbing

John Harlin
George Mallory

1 Electrocution

Thomas Merton

1 Food Poisoning

Jean Giraudoux (accidental or intentional)

6 Drug and Alcohol Related Deaths

Dinah Washington
John Belushi
Hank Williams
Rainer Werner Fassbinder (possibly cocaine induced)
Judy Garland

3 Deaths Resulting from Complications after a Fall

Eileen Gray (age 98)
Howard Hawks (age 81)
Alexander Kerensky (age 89)

APPENDIX E

CREATIVE ACHIEVEMENT SCALE
General Rating Instructions

All ratings pertain to assessment of recognized works, products, performances, accomplishments, creations (not personality, mental processes, or interpersonal relationships), *of a single individual* (not a group or organization) which contribute to or affect the lives of others within the context of Western civilization.

For persons who have not been dead for at least one generation, make best estimate on basis of available evidence and time frame. As much as possible, attempt to rate each item independent of others. If in doubt about level of rating for a particular item, rater should select the lower of the two levels.

MAJOR CRITERIA

ITEM #1

Are creations, products, performances, or works likely to be appreciated long after person's era even though person's actual name may not be remembered (probable or actual posthumous recognition or use, as defined 20 or more years after death)?

None (=0): By time of person's death, works or creations largely ignored or forgotten. Or, person shows no appreciable accomplishments during lifetime or has no references to him or her in general or specialty encyclopedias. Criminal or infamous activity (not socially sanctioned).

Minimal (=3): Works or products superseded by those of others. Athletic records broken by others. Products or policies supplanted or replaced by different or better ones. Works regarded as representative of a given trend rather than special or distinctive. Name recognition dimmed or absent among new professionals. Philanthropic organizations waning in influence. Person and/or works relatively unknown. Reputation based more on legend than accomplishments. Notoriety more than achievement.

Moderate (=6): Work regarded as representative of a time or era. Athletic records still stand but not regarded as unreachable. Representation in anthologies, collections. Individual viewed as important representative of a major movement or trend. Isolated works in major collections, galleries or museums. Work mentioned briefly in historical account. Product incorporated into rather than supplanted by newer one. Several articles or monographs on person's life and works. Credit for implementing rather than originating new policies. Artistic, social, political, or religious movement initiated by person still exists but waning. Works resurrected, displayed, or played on fewer and fewer occasions. Distinctive but not necessarily lasting contribution. Philanthropic organizations continue to exist but not necessarily grow.

236

Maximal (=9): Leader of still existing and thriving important movement. Athletic records regarded as out of reach. Sections in books devoted to accomplishments. Numerous articles, monographs, documentaries, and books about life and works. Writings, movies, performances regarded as "classics." Works collected and displayed in major museums. Products or processes still in use or likely to be. Followers still employ ideas, analyses, insights in work. Compositions still played in concerts or on record. Discovery or breakthrough regarded as representing an important building block rather than an evolving development in field. Philanthropic organizations have growing worldwide influence.

ITEM #2

Did personal product, ideas, or work have broad human application, apply to Western civilization in general, or embody universal values or ideals?

None (=0): No indication that product embodied universal values or had impact on others in any substantive or general way. Work largely has relevance to self or small numbers of individuals: e.g., banker, collector, spouse, etc. Work or ideas discredited during person's life.

Minimal (=3): Work regarded as regional, ethnic, or limited to special interest groups. Restricted technology. Work designed to address a specific but time-limited problem. Use of product highly specific or limited to certain times and places. Represents offshoot or by-product rather than an important development in field. Only minor or transient impact on accepted standards of beauty, truth, or usefulness. An interesting but not necessarily important way of interpreting reality. Validity of ideas or work may be controversial or not accepted by a segment of population or authorities. Work confined to a specific genre or subcategory of a general field.

Moderate (=6): Work limited to a given nation or countries with common language or social/political system. Achievement is culturally specific. Product designed for more immediate but not lasting needs. Development, discovery, or contribution affects only a portion of the field or discipline. Analysis or strategy applies only to a given society or subgrouping of humankind. Set new criteria for human accomplishment or performance in culturally relevant activity. Work affects one media or subcategory of expression in field rather than multimedia or entire field. Work may have detrimental impact on country even though accepted at time.

Maximal (=9): Work or standard applies to all Western society. An established standard of beauty, truth, or understanding of humankind or nature. An accepted classic. Product has potential universal use or aesthetic appeal. Writings translated into other languages. International tours. Collections in museums worldwide. Invention, discovery, new product utilized widely. Affects all media of expression within a particular field or discipline. Work appreciated worldwide by all societies. Commissions by other countries. Insights have value for all. Social, political, or aesthetic movement significantly has impact on all Western countries. Development or discovery influences entire field.

ITEM #3

Did person rise above limitations of his or her society or era by setting new directions, anticipating social needs or foreseeing future?

None (=0): Work or products completely traditional and molded by all the limitations of the individual's society and era.

Minimal (=3): Only a small part of work, technology or ideas at forefront of field. Most of work or productions are traditional. Works readily incorporated within body of field. Works, products, services, or productions generally regarded as respectable and acceptable by colleagues or general public. Works or ideas represent somewhat better variations on the same theme. Body of work of uneven or mixed quality. Works largely of a popular rather than a substantive nature.

Moderate (=6): Work, technologies, or ideas at forefront of field. Change is more evolutionary than revolutionary, quantitative rather than qualitative in nature. Antagonism or resistance to change minimal. Negligible lag time between introduction of product or performance and professional or public acceptance. Ideas or product ahead of its time but not discontinuous from prior trends or views. Work or ideas extend frontiers.

Maximal (=9): Work, technologies, or ideas significantly in advance of field with respect to noticeably changing its direction or nature. Design or introduction to new service or product significantly ahead of its time. Arousal of resistance, controversy, rejection, antipathy, or apathy prior to eventual acceptance of ideas. A lag time of variable duration between introduction of new ideas or works and eventual acceptance. Ideas are revolutionary and radical in nature. Accurate prediction of future, either through science fiction, economic forecast, musical trends, architecture, experimental theater, etc. Work represents entirely different way of interpreting reality.

ITEM #4

How influential was person on contemporary and subsequent professionals (protégés, disciples, adherents)?

None (=0): No indication that person's special point of view or contribution had a significant impact on work of others.

Minimal (=3): Highly respected among a small circle of professionals or within a fairly narrow specialty. Regarded as competent and proficient with special expertise in a particular area. Influence on broader field minimal. Attracts graduate students but leaves no distinctive marks. Awards from local, regional, professional societies or organizations. Citations and references in literature for solid but not innovative work. A respected journeyman or practitioner of trade. Ideas or works attract both adherents and detractors.

Moderate (=6): Highly respected in field as an accomplished professional. Among the elite but not at the top. National leadership and honors. Professional supporters but not necessarily followers. Recognized for honorary offices in professional organizations. Editorships. Honorary degrees. Legislative leadership. Sponsor important bills. National or professional society awards, such as Pulitzer Prize, Booker Prize, Academy Award. Command performance for royalty or head of government. Limited mention of subject in lectures or classes. Leader of a sectarian religious or political movement.

Maximal (=9): Many imitators, elaborators, followers, disciples, or adherents. International leadership, statesmanship, expertise, innovation in field. Accomplished individuals study under, emulate, quote widely. Highest honors and awards by fellow professionals or social superiors, such as knighthood, Nobel Prize, retrospective exhibition at MOMA or at Louvre, Lasker award. Impact of work profoundly affects the professional activities of others. Numerous biographies and articles written about person and his or her work. Classes or significant lecture time devoted to person and his or her work or ideas.

ITEM #5

How original was the person's main work, product, or accomplishment?

None (=0): Negligible indication of originality or innovation in person's main work or production. Implements basic ideas of others or of time. Finished works or products not particularly distinctive.

Minimal (=3): Achievement within the context of tradition but with occasional new twist or perspective. Work characterized by distinctive style but without representing significant innovation or advance in field. Work may be clever but not necessarily original. Accomplishment represents progress, extension, or achievement beyond what existed before (e.g., setting new record). New but not necessarily novel. Work may be original and imaginative but of dubious validity or quality.

Moderate (=6): Work exemplifies a new emphasis or dimension. Modification in (but no fundamental change of) basic principles, concepts, theories. Invention, breakthrough, or innovation pertains to a component of a whole system rather than the entire system itself. Innovation also may pertain to new uses, rearrangements, or combinations of old parts or to exploiting unusual relationships. The development of novel strategies.

Maximal (=9): Work represents a major discovery. New basic conceptualization or theory. Formulation of new principles. Monumental work representing extraordinary accomplishment. Scientific or conceptual breakthrough. Product qualitatively different rrom what existed before. Change in fundamental laws or perspectives. Invention or breakthrough revolutionizes entire field. Represents a radical change in interpreting reality. Ingenious strategy for solving a previously insoluble problem. Open new frontiers. Establish new discipline.

ITEM #6

Extent of innovative accomplishments by person over his or her adult lifetime in his or her field? (A "field" represents a general category which may include a variety of related professions or media of expression. For example, the general category [field] of "artist" includes painting, sculpting, photography, and so on. The field of "writing" includes editing, poetry, biography, fiction, and so on. A person who is an editor and poet, therefore, potentially may qualify as making distinctive contributions in only one field, whereas, an artist and writer, as making distinctive contributions in two.)

None (=0): Not noted for any trend-setting works, masterpieces, discoveries, breakthroughs, or innovative accomplishments or original achievements within a particular field. (To qualify as "innovative," the [body of] work or product should be regarded as having novel or original features. Success, recognition, distinctiveness, popularity or competence per se does not automatically qualify as innovative.)

Minimal (=3): Noted for at least one or more original, innovative or novel achievements within *one* particular field.

Moderate (=6): Noted for at least one or more original, innovative or novel achievements within *two* particular fields.

Maximal (=9): Noted for at least one or more original, innovative or novel achievements within *three* particular fields.

INTERMEDIATE CRITERIA

ITEM #7

How versatile and many-sided (i.e., active in many fields and different media) was person?

None (=0): Competency/proficiency, if any, within a field confined mostly to only one medium of expression (e.g., painting but not sculpting). Here competency/ proficiency pertains to general ability and *need not* be related to original, distinctive, or innovative accomplishments in the field. For example, if a writer becomes a businessman, he should receive a "Moderate" rating for two fields even if he has not made major contributions in either. If an artist becomes an architect, competency pertains to two related media rather than two separate fields.

Minimal (=2): Competency/proficiency in two or more *related* media of expression within a particular field (e.g., poetry and playwrighting; painting and sculpture; dancing and choreography; composing and performing).

Moderate (=4): Competency/proficiency displayed in at least two *separate* fields (e.g., art and writing, politics and business).

Maximal (=6): Competency/proficiency displayed in three or more separate fields (e.g., science, business, and art; composing, performing, and writing) or two or more different media within at least one of two fields (e.g., publisher, editor, journalist, and businessman).

ITEM #8

How prolific and/or sustained was productivity (finished *personal* products or works) over adult lifetime? Assume "Moderate" productivity for individual in a creative profession unless otherwise indicated (e.g., shortened or lengthened longevity for field or meager or prodigious output for field). Assume "Minimal" productivity for individual in professions yielding no visible or tangible personal products (e.g., business, finance, politics, etc.) even if person highly successful. Assume "None" rating if products of individual have no broader social application or are of a more idiosyncratic nature (e.g., homemaker, mystic, spouse/lover, member of royal family).

None (=0): No evidence of personal works, products or performances in a given field.

Minimal (=2): Works, products, or performances of individual are relatively small in number for average person in particular field over normal life span. Limitations in number of works may be due to prolonged illnesses, premature death, career changes, low motivation, writing blocks, hospitalizations, overcompulsivity, imprisonment, or other circumstances.

This category also pertains to individuals with reasonable "productivity" in professions in which personal products are not so evident (e.g., business, politics, administration, etc.), regardless of success.

Moderate (=4): Productivity within average range for a given field. Neither meager nor prodigious output. Person produces a "normal" body of work over normal life span. It is assumed that if person has significant outside, nonvocational interests or activities, he or she will not qualify for "Maximal" productivity rating. This category also pertains to persons whose enormous outputs during certain periods are counterbalanced by fallow periods. Normal longevity for athletes or dancers should be regarded as less than that for a writer or composer.

Maximal (=6): Person has been very productive and turned out an enormous amount of work in field over entire adult life span. Reputation of individual may be based on multiple contributions, entire body of work or prodigious output, even if has not accomplished breakthroughs, discoveries, innovations, or classical works. Person prolific within context or constraints of field. Quantity rather than quality of output per se represents primary basis for judgment. Person appears driven over lifetime.

ITEM # 9

Was work admired, accepted, or appreciated beyond person's own country (popularity, fame, recognition, acceptance)? If person rejected or denounced by country of origin but praised by an adopted country (e.g., spy, traitor, etc.), rate work as though it came from the adopted country.

None (=0): Work, products, or performances, if any, have only limited acceptance or limited audience within country or are not known or appreciated outside person's country. Works regarded as having only narrow, regional, ethnic, racial, religious relevance or indicative of a culture-bound genre. Works pertain only to special groups or cliques within own country (e.g., American Indians, etc.). Works may be highly controversial with negative reception in own country.

Minimal (=2): Works, products, or performances mostly admired or accepted essentially in own country by appropriate audience with only limited acceptance elsewhere. When works do appear elsewhere, they are regarded as representative of a broader national rather than regional outlook without possessing multinational relevance. Works regarded as distinctly "American," "Russian," etc. in nature.

Moderate (=4): Works, products, or performances admired and appreciated in several countries but usually limited to those with same language or similar cultures. Works distributed, for example, only in English-speaking countries or only within Soviet Union cultures. Limited translations available. Little attempt to bridge language or culture gaps.

Maximal (=6): Works, products, or performances accepted and appreciated throughout Western world as evidenced by translations of writings; international collections of art; use of inventions, product, or ideas; performance tours; subtitles to movies; application of methods; spread of beliefs; and so on. Individual regarded as international celebrity, star, or genius.

MINOR CRITERIA

ITEM #10

How great was the person's technical competence or skill with respect to his or her work or activity (facility, proficiency, talent, special ability, etc.)? ("Skill" pertains to special ability with music, memory, mimicry, mathematics, physical agility, color, drawing, spatial sense, mechanical ingenuity, writing, etc., usually manifested by the late teens. Skill, however, need not be associated with innovation or creativity or originality.) Assume "competency" (Minimal rating) unless evidence to the contrary. Interpersonal ability or shrewdness which relies on force of character, personal conviction, opportunism, status, or the prevalent social climate, should be included under this category if no case can be made that individual utilizes "exceptional" or special personal skill. An attempt should be made to distinguish among "competency," "exceptional" skill, and "virtuoso" ability.

None (=0): No special skills or talent in medium or field evident over lifetime. Position or achievement mostly because of luck, circumstance, birthright, etc.

Minimal (=1): Person regarded as "competent" but not necessarily exceptional in talent, facility, or skill in field or medium of expression. Craftsmanship. Motivation, leadership, or other factors may compensate for ordinary skill.

Moderate (=2): Person regarded as possessing "exceptional" skill or talent in field or medium of expression. An expert in a particular technique. Accomplished. Talent usually evident by late teens or early twenties.

Maximal (=3): Person regarded as a "master" or "genius" with respect to a particular talent. Virtuoso. A rare talent. Unexcelled in a given ability. Extraordinary memory, musical ability, verbal fluency, artistic ability, physical agility, interpersonal skills, or other rare talents often evident before age 17 (i.e., prodigy) which appear to contribute to person's success.

ITEM #11

Did person show creative involvement in nonvocational pursuits (hobbies, interests, secondary activities) outside chosen field or career over the course of lifetime? Individuals associated with any of the aesthetic professions, involving creative expression, automatically receive a "Maximal" rating.

None (=0): No or minimal interest or involvement in aesthetic activities.

Minimal (=1): Person displays *avid interest* in at least one of the following: literature, art, music, photography, dance, theater, or other aesthetic pursuit. Interest is more than passive appreciation; it involves being actively knowledgeable in a particular area.

Moderate (=2): Person displays *amateur involvement* in at least *one* of the following: writing, painting, performing, dancing, photography, or other aesthetic pursuit. Amateur involvement indicates actual participation in the given activity but without remuneration or professional status.

Maximal (=3): Person displays *amateur involvement* in at least *two* or *professional involvement* in at least *one* of the following: writing, composing, painting, performing, dancing, photography, or other aesthetic pursuits.

METHOD AND STATISTICS: CHAPTER 2

S1: General Overview of Data Collection and Statistical Methods

Comprehensive information forms were used to record all relevant biographical data about subjects and, when available, their immediate relatives as well. Project personnel received extensive training and supervision on the recording of appropriate biographical materials. Appropriate materials were mainly "hard data," behavioral observations and judgments based on scientific evidence or expert sources. Opinions and interpretations by the biographers or others for which there was no documented evidence were ignored.

Based on the extensive material contained in the information forms, a data form, consisting of 240 items, was filled out for each subject. An Instruction Manual provided detailed guidelines for the interpretation and recording of information.

Reliability checks were conducted for each stage of the information processing and coding procedures prior to data entry in the computer. In order to determine the adequacy of information transferred from a standard biographical source to the information form, four raters independently read the same biographies on six different individuals and filled out separate information forms, each consisting of 116 general categories of information. Each form was then independently coded on a categorical basis as to whether or not it contained the requisite information. Cross-tabulations were then performed to determine the extent of agreement among raters. Cohen's kappa statistic, which ranged from .69 to .75 (mean = .71), indicated high levels of agreement (see D. G. Altman, *Practical Statistics for Medical Research*, London: Chapman and Hall, 1991). The percentage of agreement between pairs of raters ranged from 81.9 to 88.4% (mean = 86.3%).

To determine the extent to which bias or error potentially affected the coding of material from the information form to the data form, four raters independently filled out data forms on eight different subjects using the same information forms on each. Because the 228 designated items represented a mixture of nominal, ordinal, and fixed interval data, interrater reliability was determined on the basis of the percentage the agreement between pairs of raters. These values ranged from 84.2 to 87.4% (mean = 85.9%).

An automatic verification program was used during double data entry in the computer to detect and eliminate errors. The SPSS-PC, SPSS for Windows and Absurv Plus for personal computers were the main statistical software packages employed for data analysis.

Statistical Procedures

Aside from the specific analyses described above for evaluating interrater reliability, other statistical procedures were used to test the general hypotheses under investigation.

Differences among the groups for dichotomous variables were analyzed by using chi-square statistics on *the raw data or actual frequencies*. Posthoc tests for significant chi square between individual pairs of groups were undertaken only if the overall chi square proved statistically significant. Between-group comparisons were interpreted as "meaningful" only if one group differed significantly from at least two others. For instances in which the proportion of responders was too small for chi-square analysis, Fisher's exact test was used. Multivariate analyses were based on logistic regression models that estimated the probability that an event occurred in relation to various categorical variables. These analyses were used when appropriate to control for the effects of gender and race if chi-square results were significant.

One-way analyses of variance were used to compare mean responses among professions for interval level variables. Posthoc tests for significant F ratios were based on Scheffé's multiple comparison procedure, which was undertaken only if the omnibus ANOVA proved statistically significant. Multivariate analyses were based on two-way or three-way analyses of variance (i.e., gender, race, and profession as independent variables) or multiple regression models. In certain instances, factor analyses and other special procedures, such as analyses of correspondence or calculations of survival probabilities, were performed. More detailed explanation of these procedures will be given when appropriate.

Unless otherwise specified, all comparative results reported in the text were statistically significant (i.e., $p < .05$, two-tailed test of probability). The actual values for these statistical comparisons are included in the corresponding Method and Statistics section for each chapter. In order to simplify most data tables, I included only summary percentages or mean scores (plus standard deviations). In many instances, the numbers of subjects in groups varied because of missing information. This naturally was taken into account in all statistical analyses.

METHOD AND STATISTICS: CHAPTER 3

S1. Correlations between Father's Success (FS), Social Status (SS), and Family Income Level (FI)

	SS	FI
FS	.46*	.33*
SS		.46*

*p < .000; n = 925/926

S2. Social Status (by Percentage) (n = 966)

Level I	Upper class	Cert. prof.	Noncert. prof.	Skilled	Un-skilled	Unem-ployed	Total
Architecture	9	14	68	0	9	0	2
Art	9	16	57	6	12	1	7
Business	17	10	39	3	29	1	7
Exploration	10	40	20	10	20	0	1
Sports	0	6	44	6	39	6	2
Composing	6	17	56	2	19	0	5
Entertainment	2	17	41	2	38	0	4
Military	5	32	47	5	11	0	2
Public office	20	27	35	0	11	7	11
Natural sciences	3	38	41	0	8	11	4
Social activism	9	20	41	3	17	10	6
Social figure	52	7	38	0	3	0	3
Companion	29	29	35	0	6	0	2
Social sciences	9	52	29	0	7	3	7
Theater	3	17	48	5	23	3	7
Nonfiction	5	26	48	3	12	7	6
Fiction	11	26	45	5	12	1	18
Poetry	11	36	38	2	11	2	6

Chi square = 230.3   df = 85   p = .000

Level II							
Artistic	9	23	48	4	15	2	57
Enterprising	19	20	38	2	16	5	22
Investigative	3	50	30	0	11	6	7
Social	13	26	38	2	17	5	14

Chi square = 56.6   df = 15   p = .000

Level III							
Creative arts	8	23	48	4	16	2	55
Other	16	27	37	2	15	5	45

Chi square = 31.2   df = 5   p = .001

Key: Cert. prof. = Certified professional; Noncert. prof. = Noncertified professional

S3. Vocational Activities of Mothers (by Percentage) (n = 957)

Level I	Home-maker	Un-skilled	Skilled	Business	Applied prof.	Creative prof.	Other	Total
Architecture	87	4	0	0	0	9	0	2
Art	88	2	3	5	2	0	2	7
Business	86	3	2	5	3	0	2	7
Exploration	91	0	0	0	9	0	0	1
Sports	82	12	0	6	0	0	0	2
Composing	72	6	4	4	4	6	2	5
Entertainment	50	18	5	11	0	11	5	5
Military	85	10	0	0	0	0	5	2
Public office	81	2	2	1	13	0	1	11
Natural sciences	84	0	0	5	5	3	3	4
Social activism	80	5	0	13	2	0	0	6
Social figure	93	0	0	0	0	7	0	3
Companion	83	6	6	0	0	6	0	2
Social sciences	83	3	0	4	10	0	0	7
Theater	63	9	0	9	6	11	2	7
Nonfiction	88	0	2	2	3	5	0	1
Fiction	82	6	2	3	4	2	1	6
Poetry	85	2	2	0	8	4	0	18

Chi square = 174.9 df = 102 p = .000

Level II

	Home-maker	Un-skilled	Skilled	Business	Applied prof.	Creative prof.	Other	Total
Artistic	79	5	2	4	4	5	1	58
Enterprising	84	3	1	1	9	1	1	22
Investigative	81	2	0	6	9	2	2	7
Social	84	5	1	7	2	1	0	13

Chi square = 40.6 df = 18 p = .002

Level III

	Home-maker	Un-skilled	Skilled	Business	Applied prof.	Creative prof.	Other	Total
Creative arts	78	6	2	4	4	5	1	56
Other	84	3	1	4	6	1	1	44

Chi square = 21.3 df = 6 p = .002

Key: Prof. = Profession

S4. Occupational Success of Fathers (by Percentage) (n = 949)

Level I	Unsuc-cessful	Steady work	Successful	Limited fame	Eminence	Total
Architecture	5	10	65	10	10	2
Art	5	19	65	9	3	7
Business	21	16	41	16	6	7
Exploration	10	30	50	0	10	1
Sports	0	68	26	5	0	2
Composing	13	23	55	6	2	5
Entertainment	27	29	37	7	0	4
Military	17	6	61	17	0	2
Public office	7	20	43	14	16	11
Natural sciences	5	22	51	19	3	4
Social activism	16	18	54	12	0	6
Social figure	3	3	70	17	7	3
Companion	13	0	69	13	6	2
Social sciences	12	10	59	15	4	7
Theater	24	22	41	6	6	7
Nonfiction	15	15	53	15	3	7
Fiction	22	14	48	14	2	18
Poetry	6	14	62	16	2	5

Chi square = 155.9 df = 68 p = .000

Level II						
Artistic	16	17	53	11	3	57
Enterprising	11	17	46	15	11	22
Investigative	12	15	53	16	4	7
Social	10	22	50	14	3	13

Chi square = 33.2 df = 12 p = .001

Level III						
Creative arts	17	18	52	11	3	55
Other	11	17	51	14	7	45

Chi square = 13.7 df = 4 p = .008

S5. Family Income Level (by Percentage) (n = 975)

Level I	Lower	Middle	Upper	Total
Architecture	5	86	9	2
Art	12	71	17	7
Business	10	70	20	7
Exploration	20	70	10	1
Sports	5	84	11	2
Composing	13	79	8	5
Entertainment	29	71	0	4
Military	11	84	5	2
Public office	10	66	24	11
Natural sciences	3	86	11	4
Social activism	8	75	17	6
Social figure	0	31	69	3
Companion	6	59	35	2
Social sciences	4	76	20	7
Theater	13	81	6	7
Nonfiction	8	82	10	7
Fiction	13	72	15	18
Poetry	11	66	23	5

Chi square = 113.4 $df = 34$ $p = .000$

Level II	Lower	Middle	Upper	Total
Artistic	13	73	14	58
Enterprising	9	67	23	22
Investigative	6	85	9	7
Social	6	74	20	13

Chi square = 19.1 $df = 6$ $p = .004$

Level III	Lower	Middle	Upper	Total
Creative arts	13	75	12	55
Other	8	70	22	45

Chi square = 21.4 $df = 2$ $p = .000$

S6. Nonconformity of Fathers (by Percentage) (n = 947)

Level I	Conformity	Some nonconformity	Nonconformity	Total
Architecture	95	0	5	2
Art	93	4	3	7
Business	81	17	1	7
Exploration	90	10	0	1
Sports	94	6	0	2
Composing	83	15	2	5
Entertainment	69	26	5	4
Military	80	20	0	2
Public office	94	5	1	11
Natural sciences	89	11	0	4
Social activism	91	9	0	6
Social figure	93	7	0	3
Companion	81	19	0	2
Social sciences	93	7	0	7
Theater	71	24	5	7
Nonfiction	88	8	3	6
Fiction	81	16	3	18
Poetry	84	14	2	5

Chi square = 51.50   *df* = 34   *p* = .028

Level II

	Conformity	Some nonconformity	Nonconformity	Total
Artistic	84	13	3	57
Enterprising	88	11	1	23
Investigative	88	12	0	7
Social	88	11	1	13

Chi square = 7.5   *df* = 6   *p* = N.S.

Level III

	Conformity	Some nonconformity	Nonconformity	Total
Creative arts	83	14	3	55
Other	90	10	1	45

Chi square = 14.4   *df* = 2   *p* = .001

S7. Same General Profession as Father (by Percentage) (n = 1,004)

Level I
___

Architecture (13); Art (10); Business (44); Exploration (0); Sports (5); Musical composition (19); Musical entertainment (11); Military (30); Public office (31); Natural sciences (15); Social activism (10); Social figure (7); Companion (0); Social sciences (18); Theater (13); Nonfiction (13); Fiction (6); Poetry (4).

Chi square = 101.9 $df = 17$ $p = .000$

Level II
___

Artistic (9); Enterprising (31); Investigative (17); Social (13).

Chi square = 62.1 $df = 3$ $p = .000$

Level III
___

Creative arts (10); Other (22).

Chi square = 29.3 $df = 1$ $p = .000$

S8. Marked Aesthetic Interests in Family Members (by Percentage)

Level I	Mothers	Fathers	Any siblings
Architecture	60	50	44
Art	44	67	61
Business	19	20	22
Exploration	29	17	20
Sports	20	0	0
Composing	61	72	66
Entertainment	63	57	58
Military	0	22	17
Public office	21	13	11
Natural sciences	26	18	19
Social activism	15	26	26
Social figure	33	20	21
Companion	50	63	9
Social sciences	39	24	30
Theater	46	49	48
Nonfiction	41	39	44
Fiction	38	37	47
Poetry	53	42	34
n	511	561	606
Chi square	74.6	93.3	78.9
df	34	34	17
p	.000	.000	.000

Level II			
Artistic	46	47	48
Enterprising	21	13	19
Investigative	27	15	23
Social	35	40	21
Chi square	37.1	55.2	50.7
df	6	6	3
p	.000	.000	.000

Level III			
Creative arts	47	49	50
Other	25	20	19
Chi square	23.3	45.3	60.9
df	2	2	1
p	.000	.000	.000

S9. Because the Level I results were not statistically significant, only results for the Level II classification are provided.

Age at Father's Death (by Percentage)

	Artistic	Enterprising	Investigative	Social
1 to 6 years	8	7	9	6
7 to 13 years	8	9	0	11
14 to 20 years	11	11	7	16
> 21 years	72	72	84	67
n	368	152	44	81

Chi square = 8.6   df = 9   p = .48

Age at Mother's Death (by Percentage)

	Artistic	Enterprising	Investigative	Social
1 to 6 years	6	4	2	7
7 to 13 years	9	12	6	6
14 to 20 years	8	6	9	9
> 21 years	77	78	83	78
n	353	137	46	82

Chi square = 6.7   df = 9   p = .66

S10. Pearson product–moment correlations between age at mother's death and lifetime adjustment problems, alcoholism, drug abuse, anxiety, depression, mania, psychoses, somatization, suicide attempts, and other problems range from −.07 to .08 ($n = 618$, p = N.S.). Pearson product–moment correlations between age at father's death and lifetime adjustment problems, alcoholism, drug abuse, anxiety, depression, mania, psychoses, somatization, suicide attempts, and other problems range from −.06 to .06 ($n = 645$, p = N.S.).

S11. Percentage of Intact Parental Marriages ($n = 967$)

Level I

Architecture (91); Art (97); Business (91); Exploration (90); Sports (77); Musical composition (89); Musical entertainment (71); Military (90); Public office (97); Natural sciences (95); Social activism (93); Social figure (83); Companion (83); Social sciences (92); Theater (74); Nonfiction (90); Fiction (86); Poetry (77).

Chi square = 52.3   df = 17   p = .000

Level II

Artistic (85); Enterprising (93); Investigative (90); Social (89).

Chi square = 9.5   df = 3   p = .023

Level III

Creative arts (85); Other (92).

Chi square = 11.4   df = 1   p = .001

S12. Results of one-way analyses of variance with the status of parental marriage as the independent variable and total Creative Achievement Scale score as the dependent variable were not statistically significant.

$F = .71$ $df = 1, 965$ $p = .40$

S13. Percentages of Subjects from Broken or Intact Homes Who Displayed Various Forms of Psychopathology ($n = 967$)

Problem in subject	Broken home (%)	Intact home (%)	Chi square	$p =$
Alcohol	35	25	5.0	.03
Drugs	23	11	14.7	.00
Depression	41	38	0.5	.47
Mania	8	7	0.2	.64
Psychosis	11	5	8.2	.00
Adjustment	40	36	1.1	.30
Anxiety	11	8	1.3	.26
Somatization	8	11	1.4	.24
Suicide attempt	16	10	3.8	.05
Other	5	5	0.0	.99
Any problem	80	68	7.2	.01

S14. One-way analysis of variance between the marital status of parents and the combined total psychopathology scores of the mother and father.

	Mean	SD
Divorced/Separated	.65	1.03
Intact marriage	.37	.73
Total	.41	.78

$F = 13.0$ $df = 1, 965$ $p = .000$

One-way analysis of variance between the marital status of parents and the total psychopathology score of the mother.

	Mean	SD
Divorced/Separated	.32	.71
Intact marriage	.16	.50

$F = 9.2$ $df = 1, 965$ $p = .000$

One-way analysis of variance between the marital status of the parents and the total psychopathology score of the father.

	Mean	SD
Divorced/Separated	.33	.65
Intact marriage	.21	.51

$F = 5.2$ $df = 1, 965$ $p = .023$

S15. Family Size: Means (Standard Deviations) (n = 981)

Level I

Architecture = 3.3 (1.5); Art = 4.0 (2.3); Business = 4.1 (2.5); Exploration = 4.4 (3.0); Sports = 4.5 (2.5); Composing = 3.9 (2.5); Entertainment = 3.7 (2.8); Military = 4.9 (2.5); Public office = 5.1 (2.7); Natural sciences = 4.3 (2.3); Social activism = 5.1 (2.9); Social figure = 4.3 (2.7); Companion = 3.8 (2.9); Social sciences = 4.1 (2.7); Theater = 3.3 (2.3); Nonfiction = 3.4 (1.8); Fiction = 3.8 (2.3); Poetry = 3.4 (1.9).

$SD = 2.5$ Total mean = 4.0 $df = 17, 963$ $F = 3.2$ $p = .000$

Level II

Artistic = 3.7 (2.3); Enterprising = 4.5 (2.6); Investigative = 4.2 (2.7); Social = 4.7 (2.8)

$df = 3, 977$ $F = 10.6$ $p = .000$

Level III

Creative Arts = 3.6 (2.2); Others = 4.5 (2.7)

$df = 1, 979$ $F = 33.2$ $p = .000$

S16. The following analysis was provided by Richard J. Kryscio, Ph.D., Department of Biostatistics, University of Kentucky.

To determine if the first born is more likely to be famous, we used a method similar to that used by N. Mantel and M. Halperin ("Analyses of Birth Rank Data," *Biometrics*, 19[1963]: 324–340), when analyzing birth rank data. In this method, a table is formed with rows indexed by R, the total number of children in a family. Other entries in the Rth row include: N, the total number of families having R children; O, the number of famous first borns among these families; and the mean and variance of the expected number of famous first borns under the null hypothesis of randomness. Randomness states that O is a binomial variate with mean N/R and variance $NR (1 - 1/R)$. Hence, given R children in a family the first born has a probability of $1/R$ to be famous; that is, the first born is no more likely to be famous than any of the other $R - 1$ children. A test of this hypothesis is obtained by squaring the difference between the total observed famous first borns and total expected divided by the total variance. This yields a chi-square statistic having one degree of freedom. Statistical significance is determined at the .05 level.

Notice in the table, which was formed by using the procedure outlined above, that except for single children families and for the few very large families, in every row the observed number of families with famous first borns is larger than the hypothesized mean. Since this excess is highly significant ($p < 0.0001$), there is evidence that the first born is more likely to be famous even after adjusting for the number of children in a family.

Table: R, the number of children in a family; N, the number of families with R children; O, the observed number of famous first borns among the N families; M, the mean; and V, the variance of the number of famous first borns under randomness.

R	N	O	M	V
1	138	138	138.000	0.0000
2	176	102	88.000	44.0000
3	177	63	59.000	39.3333
4	137	42	34.250	25.6875
5	117	33	23.400	18.7200
6	82	23	13.667	11.3889
7	49	9	7.000	6.0000
8	49	11	6.125	5.3594
9	23	6	2.556	2.2716
10	18	1	1.800	1.6200
11	7	1	0.636	0.5785
12	5	1	0.417	0.3819
13	3	0	0.231	0.2130
16	1	0	0.063	0.0586
Total	982	430	375.14	155.61

Chi square = $(430 - 375.14)^2/155.61 = 19.34 \ (p < .0001)$

S17. Percentage of Subjects with Psychopathology

	Only born	First born	Later born	Chi square	$p =$
Alcohol	37	23	25	9.9	.007
Drugs	22	12	10	14.9	.001
Depression	41	39	37	0.9	.627
Mania	15	6	6	12.6	.002
Psychosis	9	5	5	5.8	.055
Anxiety	15	7	8	9.6	.008
Adjustment	33	33	39	4.1	.127
Somatization	13	9	11	1.7	.418
Suicide attempt	15	10	10	2.9	.233
Other problem	7	4	5	2.5	.286
Any problem	76	68	68	4.0	.137
Forced treatment	9	4	3	7.7	.021
Psychotherapy	15	7	10	6.8	.033

Analyses of covariance for birth order were run for each form of psychopathology with social status, time period of parental death, and gender as covariates. For these analyses, the extent of psychopathology represented the dependent measure, with scores ranging from 0 to 2 based on whether the particular problem existed before age 40 and after age 40. Except for alcoholism, all other significant findings remained.

S18. Average Psychopathology Score for Mothers of Subjects (SD in Parentheses)

Only children = .34 (.72); First born = .17 (.50); Later born = .14 (.47).

$df = 2, 978$ $F = 7.9$ $p = .000$

Percentage of Subjects Whose Parents Remained Married

Only children (67%); First born (92%); Later born (91%).

Chi square = 71.4 $df = 6$ $p = .000$

S19. Representation in Different Professions by Birth Order in Males (by Percentage) (n = 739)

Level I	Only children	First born	Later born
Architecture	13	31	56
Art	16	38	46
Business	14	32	54
Exploration	33	11	56
Sports	0	41	59
Composing	12	28	60
Entertainment	22	26	52
Military	5	15	80
Public office	5	27	68
Natural sciences	9	31	60
Social activism	0	29	71
Social figure	0	38	62
Companion	100	0	0
Social sciences	16	36	47
Theater	26	21	53
Nonfiction	18	34	48
Fiction	17	29	54
Poetry	15	46	39
Total %	14	30	56

Chi square = 53.8 $df = 34$ $p = .017$

Level II			
Artistic	18	31	51
Enterprising	9	28	63
Investigative	11	32	57
Social	6	31	63

Chi square = 15.7 $df = 6$ $p = .015$

Level III			
Creative arts	18	31	51
Other	9	30	61

Chi square = 12.7 $df = 2$ $p = .002$

S20. Physical Problems in Subjects during Childhood (by Percentage)

Level I	Handicaps	Sickliness	Major illness
Architecture	9	4	9
Art	10	4	11
Business	6	10	4
Exploration	0	0	9
Sports	0	5	5
Composing	4	8	2
Entertainment	2	4	4
Military	5	5	0
Public office	11	8	3
Natural sciences	21	10	10
Social activism	12	7	8
Social figure	3	7	0
Companion	11	11	6
Social sciences	8	14	7
Theater	11	6	11
Nonfiction	6	14	8
Fiction	12	13	13
Poetry	15	17	13
Chi square	21.7	17.7	25.8
df	17	17	17
p	N.S.	N.S.	N.S.

S21. Either Handicaps, Sickliness, or Major Illness during Childhood (by Percentage)

Level I

Architecture (17); Art (19); Business (16); Exploration (9): Sports (11); Composing (13); Entertainment (11); Military (10); Public office (20); Natural sciences (31); Social activism (20); Social figure (10); Companion (22); Social sciences (23); Theater (24); Nonfiction (20); Fiction (31); Poetry (38).

Mean = 22%   Chi square = 33.2 *df* = 17   *p* = .01

S22. Behavioral Attributes of Subjects during Childhood (by Percentage)*

Level I	Solitary/Sociable	Moody/Stable	Odd/Normal
Architecture	25/58	36/64	6/82
Art	40/31	29/43	7/78
Business	25/50	20/63	0/90
Exploration	38/50	40/60	0/100
Sports	25/42	18/46	7/79
Composing	39/42	19/76	3/87
Entertainment	29/55	27/47	5/82
Military	8/67	20/60	6/88
Public office	27/57	15/72	1/96
Natural sciences	43/19	18/65	3/84
Social activism	24/55	25/44	6/85
Social figure	37/47	25/69	0/88
Companion	15/69	20/60	0/69
Social sciences	60/22	40/57	6/84
Theater	26/54	24/42	12/75
Nonfiction	34/51	30/46	8/80
Fiction	41/36	39/38	9/71
Poetry	42/40	37/30	2/77
n	686	567	821
Chi square	54.0	60.5	49.8
df	34	34	34
p	.016	.003	.039

Level II			
Artistic	38/41	33/44	7/77
Enterprising	26/56	19/68	1/93
Investigative	54/26	26/60	4/83
Social	26/54	24/51	6/83
Chi square	21.4	21.6	24.6
df	6	6	6
p	.002	.001	.000

Level III			
Creative arts	36/43	32/44	7/77
Other	33/47	23/61	3/88
Chi square	1.1	17.0	19.1
df	2	2	2
p	N.S.	.000	.000

*Percentages for "Equivocal" ratings not included

S23. Evidence of Precocity (by Percentage) (n = 1,004)

Level I

Architecture (17); Art (23); Business (14); Exploration (9); Sports (26); Musical composition (48); Musical entertainment (40); Military (0); Public office (14); Natural sciences (31); Social activism (8); Social figure (7); Companion (6); Social sciences (18); Theater (21); Nonfiction (12); Fiction (21); Poetry (28).

Chi square = 91.8 df = 34 p = .000

Level II

Artistic (25); Enterprising (12); Investigative (22); Social (12).

Chi square = 25.2 df = 6 p= .000

Level III

Creative arts (25); Other (14).

Chi square = 18.3 df = 2 p = .000

S24. Love of Reading as a Child (by Percentage) (n = 1,004)

Level I

Architecture (22); Art (24); Business (19); Exploration (27); Sports (16); Musical composition (15); Musical entertainment (4); Military (30); Public office (32); Natural sciences (41); Social activism (34); Social figure (33); Companion (39); Social sciences (40); Theater (27); Nonfiction (55); Fiction (57); Poetry (68).

Chi square = 121.1 df = 17 p = .000

Level II

Artistic (41); Enterprising (26); Investigative (41); Social (32).

Chi square = 17.4 df = 3 p= .000

Level III

Creative arts (40); Other (32).

Chi square = 7.8 df = 1 p = .005

S25. Conflicts with Teachers (n = 1,004)

Artistic (12%); Enterprising (6%); Investigative (3%); Social (7%).

Chi square = 10.4 df = 3 p = .016

S26. The analysis of correspondence (ANACOR) procedure analyzes any two-way table whose cells contain some measurement of correspondence between the rows and columns. The advantage of this procedure is that it graphically examines the relationship between the nominal variables in multidimensional space. It computes row and column scores and produces plots based on those scores. Categories that are dissimilar appear far away and categories that are similar are closer to each other in the plots. This allows a visual determination of which categories of the two variables are related.

S27. Highest Level of Education Completed (by Percentage) ("Other" Educational Experiences Not Included) (n = 960)

Level I	None	Grade school	High school	Special/ Technical	College	Graduate school	Total
Architecture	5	18	36	23	9	9	2
Art	0	9	19	63	6	3	7
Business	1	36	41	1	12	9	7
Exploration	0	27	27	9	36	0	1
Sports	0	50	31	0	19	0	2
Composing	0	9	22	61	4	4	5
Entertainment	7	47	14	30	2	0	5
Military	0	5	10	20	40	25	2
Public office	2	6	11	1	34	46	11
Natural sciences	0	10	18	8	13	51	4
Social activism	5	21	18	7	11	38	6
Social figure	4	32	39	11	4	11	3
Companion	12	47	24	12	6	0	2
Social sciences	3	4	7	3	23	61	7
Theater	5	43	32	13	6	2	7
Nonfiction	0	5	33	6	44	11	7
Fiction	1	20	36	3	30	10	18
Poetry	0	14	35	6	25	21	5

Chi square = 698.0   df = 85   p = .000

Level II							
Artistic	2	20	29	20	20	10	58
Enterprising	1	17	24	5	26	27	22
Investigative	3	12	17	1	10	57	7
Social	4	26	18	9	16	27	13

Chi square = 143.7   df = 15   p = .000

Level III							
Creative arts	2	20	30	21	20	8	55
Other	3	18	20	5	20	34	45

Chi square = 135.1   df = 5   p = .000

S28. General Academic Performance in High School/College (by Percentage) (n = 413)

Level I	Failing	Below average	Average	Above average	Some superior	Superior	Total
Architecture	0	33	0	50	0	17	2
Art	6	12	24	47	12	0	4
Business	0	8	27	50	8	8	6
Exploration	0	20	20	20	20	20	1
Sports	0	20	40	40	0	0	1
Composing	6	18	24	29	18	6	4
Entertainment	0	0	29	57	14	0	1
Military	0	0	30	50	0	20	2
Public office	0	7	21	40	1	30	17
Natural sciences	0	0	19	19	6	56	4
Social activism	0	5	19	48	5	24	5
Social figure	0	17	17	50	0	17	2
Companion	0	0	0	100	0	0	1
Social sciences	0	8	11	33	8	39	9
Theater	17	11	39	22	0	11	4
Nonfiction	0	5	28	49	5	13	9
Fiction	1	13	30	30	12	14	21
Poetry	0	4	33	30	15	19	7

Chi square = 122.1 $df = 85$ $p = .005$

Level II							
Artistic	2	11	29	35	10	14	55
Enterprising	0	7	23	44	4	23	28
Investigative	0	4	15	22	11	48	6
Social	2	9	16	43	5	25	11

Chi square = 34.8 $df = 15$ $p = .003$

Level III							
Creative arts	3	11	29	36	10	12	53
Other	0	7	20	40	5	28	47

Chi square = 28.2 $df = 5$ $p = .000$

S29. Academic Honors and Awards (by Percentage) (n = 1,004)

Level I

Architecture (9); Art (16); Business (9); Exploration (9); Sports (5); Musical composition (25); Musical entertainment (6); Military (20); Public office (34); Natural sciences (36); Social activism (16); Social figure (10); Companion (0); Social sciences (37); Theater (9); Nonfiction (20); Fiction (18); Poetry (32).

Chi square = 69.4 df = 17 p = .000

Level II

Artistic (18); Enterprising (22); Investigative (27); Social (19).

Chi square = 3.9 df = 3 p = N.S.

Level III

Creative arts (17); Other (23).

Chi square = 5.0 df = 1 p = .026

S30. With such differences existing among these professionals in the extent of their educational levels and their academic performance, we may wonder what the relationship of these variables is to the lifetime creative achievement. Fortunately, we are in a position to determine this by correlating these variables with the Creative Achievement Scale (CAS) scores (described in Chapter 6), which represents a reliable indicator of relative eminence. When these correlations were run for the entire sample, there was a statistically significant but very weak relationship for both education level and academic performance with Creative Achievement Scale scores.

	Academics	CAS scores
Education	.39 (n = 408)**	.11 (n = 960)**
Academics		.10 (n = 413)*

$*p < .05; **p < .00$

However, when this relationship was examined separately for members of the creative arts and those in the other professions, certain intriguing results were found. Members of the creative arts showed absolutely no relationship between the amount of education they received or their academic performance and their lifetime creative achievement scores (r = .06 and –.03, respectively). Nor was any curvilinear or unusual relationship noted on inspection of scatterplots. But with the members of the noncreative arts professions, the relationship was highly significant (r = .32, p = .00; r = .33, p = .00; respectively). The higher the level of education, the greater the creative achievement.

S31. Mentors (by Percentage) (n = 1,004)

Level I

Architecture (26); Art (27); Business (20); Exploration (9); Sports (32); Musical composition (31); Musical entertainment (36); Military (30); Public office (15);

Natural sciences (26); Social activism (31); Social figure (10); Companion (0); Social sciences (40); Theater (21); Nonfiction (25); Fiction (16); Poetry (15).

Chi square = 43.6   *df* = 17   *p* = .000

Level II

Artistic (22); Enterprising (18); Investigative (37); Social (28).

Chi square = 12.9   *df* = 3   *p* = .005

Level III:

Creative arts (23); Other (23).

Chi square = .1   *df* = 1   *p* = N.S.

S32. First Notable Accomplishment before Age 21 (by Percentage) (*n* = 958)

Level I

Architecture (9); Art (8); Business (5); Exploration (0); Sports (32); Musical composition (35); Musical entertainment (51); Military (0); Public office (4); Natural sciences (5); Social activism (3); Social figure (4); Companion (0); Social sciences (1); Theater (31); Nonfiction (8); Fiction (14); Poetry (25).

Chi square = 152.9   *df* = 34   *p* = .000

Level II

Artistic (19); Enterprising (4); Investigative (4); Social (9).

Chi square = 41.2   *df* = 6   *p* = .000

Level III

Creative arts (20); Other (5).

Chi square = 50.0   *df* = 2   *p* = .000

S33. Age of Initial Professional Success (by Means) (*n* = 924)

Level I

Architecture (26.9); Art (25.0); Business (27.8); Exploration (29.3); Sports (23.6); Musical composition (22.3); Musical entertainment (18.5); Military (41.2); Public office (32.9); Natural sciences (29.4); Social activism (29.8); Social figure (29.8); Companion (27.5); Social sciences (30.2); Theater (21.2); Nonfiction (25.1); Fiction (25.7); Poetry (24.4).

F = 23.1   *df* = 17, 906   *p* = .000

Level II

Artistic (24.2); Enterprising (31.3); Investigative (30.4); Social (29.4).

F = 62.8   *df* = 3, 920   *p* = .000

Level III

Creative arts (24.0); Other (30.6).

F = 198.3   *df* = 1, 922   *p* = .000

S1. Adult Attributes (by Percentage)

Level I	Moody	Nonaff.	Sol.	Diff.	Athletic	Aes-thetic	Confid.
Architecture	35	35	23	22	0	57	35
Art	49	57	29	48	11	44	31
Business	40	36	11	19	13	12	43
Exploration	30	46	36	18	9	36	46
Sports	47	50	11	26	26	26	58
Composing	48	38	24	17	2	15	48
Entertainment	48	59	15	35	4	17	43
Military	23	10	25	10	10	25	35
Public office	22	9	7	9	7	21	44
Natural sciences	31	40	27	18	15	51	36
Social activism	37	10	9	38	3	23	39
Social figure	36	43	17	31	3	33	17
Companion	47	41	0	22	0	51	22
Social sciences	24	16	22	24	0	26	38
Theater	47	60	0	29	10	39	34
Nonfiction	31	19	10	30	2	25	33
Fiction	55	43	20	34	5	31	35
Poetry	59	35	25	49	2	31	40
n	904	976	945	996	1,001	999	1,004
Total %	42	35	17	28	6	29	36
Chi square	79.6	177.4	72.1	64.0	96.4	90.1	30.6
df	34	34	34	17	34	34	17
p	.000	.000	.000	.000	.000	.000	.022
Level II							
Artistic	49	44	20	35	5	32	34
Enterprising	30	21	12	12	10	18	40
Investigative	27	31	26	23	7	35	32
Social	37	22	9	27	7	32	40
Chi square	35.8	69.3	24.6	42.2	32.7	19.1	4.9
df	6	6	6	3	6	6	3
p	.000	.000	.000	.000	.000	.004	N.S.
Level III							
Creative arts	50	45	19	34	5	31	33
Other	31	23	14	21	8	26	39
Chi square	38.9	67.0	10.0	22.4	15.3	2.8	3.7
df	2	2	2	1	2	2	1
p	.000	.000	.007	.000	.000	N.S.	N.S.

Key: Nonaff. = Nonaffiliative; Sol. = Solitary; Diff. = Different; Confid. = Expressed confidence

S2. Religious Beliefs (by Percentage) (n = 869)

Level I	Atheist	Agnostic	Unorth.	Nonprac.	Irreg. church	Regular church
Architecture	5	24	14	33	5	19
Art	15	32	9	22	0	22
Business	7	12	5	33	15	28
Exploration	11	11	0	56	11	11
Sports	0	0	8	31	31	31
Composing	15	18	10	33	5	18
Entertainment	3	8	11	41	5	32
Military	6	11	6	22	6	50
Public office	2	13	2	16	7	60
Natural sciences	11	25	19	19	11	14
Social activism	12	14	8	18	6	42
Social figure	9	17	4	17	9	44
Companion	0	24	6	24	6	41
Social sciences	15	19	12	23	6	26
Theater	2	22	13	33	13	18
Nonfiction	5	38	10	20	7	20
Fiction	9	28	17	27	6	14
Poetry	9	20	22	22	7	22
Total %	8	21	11	25	7	28

Chi square = 191.1 $\quad$ *df* = 85 $\quad$ *p* = .000

Level II

	Atheist	Agnostic	Unorth.	Nonprac.	Irreg. church	Regular church
Artistic	9	25	14	28	6	19
Enterprising	4	14	5	23	9	45
Investigative	12	20	17	25	9	17
Social	8	15	5	19	10	43

Chi square = 88.4 $\quad$ *df* = 15 $\quad$ *p* = .000

Level III

	Atheist	Agnostic	Unorth.	Nonprac.	Irreg. church	Regular church
Creative arts	8	26	14	27	6	19
Other	8	15	7	23	9	39

Chi square = 56.5 $\quad$ *df* = 5 $\quad$ *p* = .000

Key: Unorth. = Unorthodox; Nonprac. = Nonpracticing believer; Irreg. = Irregular

S3. Relations to Authority and Legal System (by Percentage)

Level I	Anger at father	Anger at mother	Antag. toward emplr.	Defend-ant	Plaintiff	Nonpol. jail	Pol. jail
Architecture	13	8	15	9	9	4	0
Art	25	20	38	10	6	6	4
Business	33	16	20	39	19	6	4
Exploration	14	11	11	9	9	9	0
Sports	13	20	39	32	5	37	11
Composing	11	6	16	10	10	4	6
Entertainment	33	24	33	26	13	26	9
Military	14	13	12	5	0	5	5
Public office	12	6	10	6	2	2	3
Natural sciences	15	0	32	8	5	5	8
Social activism	13	8	44	31	5	21	46
Social figure	14	14	0	10	7	3	0
Companion	0	29	17	6	0	0	6
Social sciences	9	20	20	4	0	4	14
Theater	33	41	36	24	19	16	4
Nonfiction	21	17	29	19	3	8	9
Fiction	41	31	34	12	6	12	13
Poetry	38	19	30	4	6	11	21
n	632	667	590	1,004	1,004	1,004	1,004
Total %	25	19	27	15	7	10	11
Chi square	60.2	77.7	58.9	87.2	47.9	63.6	115.7
df	34	34	34	17	17	17	17
p	.004	.000	.005	.000	.000	.000	.000

Level II							
Artistic	30	24	31	13	8	11	10
Enterprising	17	12	15	16	7	5	3
Investigative	25	14	20	6	1	6	9
Social	12	14	36	24	4	15	26
Chi square	22.6	17.3	21.8	16.3	7.3	12.9	46.9
df	6	6	6	3	3	3	3
p	.001	.008	.001	.001	N.S.	.005	.000

Level III							
Creative arts	31	25	32	14	8	11	10
Other	17	12	22	16	5	8	11
Chi square	20.8	24.9	11.4	.5	3.3	3.7	.7
df	2	2	2	1	1	1	1
p	.000	.000	.003	N.S.	N.S.	N.S.	N.S.

Key: Antag. = Antagonism; Emplr. = Employer/Superior; Nonpol. = Civil/Criminal; Pol. = Political

S4. Sexual Orientation (by Percentage)

	Homosexual	Bisexual	Hyposexual	Heterosexual	n
Females	5	12	10	73	37
Males	5	3	5	87	749

Chi square = 36.0   *df* = 3   *p* = .000

S5. Sexual Orientation (by Percentage) (n = 985)

Level I	Homosexual	Bisexual	Hyposexual	Heterosexual
Architecture	0	9	9	83
Art	6	9	6	79
Business	4	0	0	96
Exploration	0	0	0	100
Sports	6	0	6	89
Composing	6	6	4	83
Entertainment	2	13	4	81
Military	0	0	6	94
Public office	0	2	8	90
Natural sciences	3	0	14	84
Social activism	3	2	13	82
Social figure	10	3	3	83
Companion	11	0	0	89
Social sciences	1	3	17	79
Theater	3	9	2	87
Nonfiction	3	3	8	86
Fiction	11	10	3	76
Poetry	14	10	8	69
Total %	5	6	6	83

Chi square = 106.0   *df* = 51   *p* = .000

Level II				
Artistic	7	8	5	80
Enterprising	2	1	3	95
Investigative	2	3	18	78
Social	5	2	11	82

Chi square = 59.1   *df* = 9   *p* = .000

Level III				
Creative arts	7	9	5	80
Other	3	1	8	87

Chi square = 39.7   *df* = 3   *p* = .000

S6. Personal Family Variables (by Percentage)*

Level I	Married	Divorced	Affairs	Children	Death of child	Death of spouse	Spouse same prof.	Spouse creat.
Architecture	78	25	13	65	21	33	11	50
Art	76	28	39	54	35	23	24	76
Business	91	37	37	81	18	23	8	48
Exploration	91	10	50	73	25	0	0	50
Sports	79	27	47	53	20	33	0	50
Composing	83	35	46	65	39	28	28	86
Entertainment	87	56	36	51	13	24	17	67
Military	90	18	18	70	29	44	0	60
Public office	90	15	27	77	29	35	11	21
Natural sciences	80	26	19	62	33	16	10	14
Social activism	79	34	32	67	37	46	19	37
Social figure	80	33	38	60	33	54	4	25
Companion	94	47	35	72	69	65	20	63
Social sciences	74	33	26	52	35	32	19	52
Theater	94	59	56	59	15	15	56	88
Nonfiction	89	38	41	66	17	46	21	63
Fiction	83	44	45	56	26	24	15	72
Poetry	74	35	49	49	19	15	21	67
n	1,004	807	807	1,001	620	841	844	366
Total %	84	36	38	62	27	29	18	58
Chi square	31.4	55.7	37.1	39.4	31.2	56.2	91.7	97.4
df	17	17	17	17	17	17	17	34
p	.018	.000	.003	.002	.019	.000	.000	.000

Level II								
Artistic	83	42	43	57	25	26	23	73
Enterprising	93	22	31	79	26	33	10	31
Investigative	76	38	25	52	35	19	13	26
Social	79	35	33	62	35	42	18	55
Chi square	19.5	24.5	14.7	37.4	4.4	15.2	17.1	55.2
df	3	3	3	3	3	3	3	6
p	.000	.000	.002	.000	N.S.	.002	.001	.000

Level III								
Creative arts	84	42	44	57	24	25	24	74
Other	84	28	31	68	31	34	11	36
Chi square	.1	19.0	15.2	12.8	3.5	8.3	23.4	51.9
df	1	1	1	1	1	1	1	2
p	N.S.	.000	.000	.000	N.S.	.004	.000	.000

*Key: Prof. = Profession; Creat. = Creative

S7. Average Number of Marriages

Level I

Architecture (1.2); Art (1.0); Business (1.6); Exploration (1.0); Sports (1.4); Musical composition (1.4); Musical entertainment (1.7); Military (1.3); Public office (1.2); Natural sciences (1.2); Social activism (1.1); Social figure (1.3); Companion (1.7); Social sciences (1.1); Theater (2.1); Nonfiction (1.5); Fiction (1.4); Poetry (1.1).

$F = 4.6$ $df = 17, 983$ $p = .000$

Level II

Artistic (1.4); Enterprising (1.3); Investigative (1.2); Social (1.2).

$F = 1.8$ $df = 3, 997$ $p = $ N.S.

Level III

Creative arts (1.4); Other (1.3).

$F = 6.9$ $df = 1, 999$ $p = .009$

S8. Average Number of Divorces

Level I

Architecture (0.5); Art (0.4); Business (0.6); Exploration (0.1); Sports (0.7); Musical composition (0.6); Musical entertainment (1.0); Military (0.2); Public office (0.2); Natural sciences (0.4); Social activism (0.4); Social figure (0.5); Companion (0.7); Social sciences (0.5); Theater (1.4); Nonfiction (0.5); Fiction (0.7); Poetry (0.5).

$F = 5.6$ $df = 17, 789$ $p = .000$

Level II

Artistic (0.7); Enterprising (0.3); Investigative (0.6); Social (0.5).

$F = 7.5$ $df = 3, 803$ $p = .000$

Level III

Creative arts (0.7); Other (0.4).

$F = 20.4$ $df = 1, 805$ $p = .000$

S9. Divorce Rate (by Percentage)

	Women	Men
%	49	32
n	183	624

$df = 1$; Chi square $= 19.1$; $p = .000$

Extramarital Affairs (by Percentage)

	Women	Men
%	45	36
n	183	624

$df = 1$; Chi square $= 5.0$; $p = .03$

S10. Spouse Employment in Relation to Marriage (by Percentage) (n = 362)

Level I	None	Before	Before/ During	After	Other
Architecture	0	40	40	20	0
Art	22	22	56	0	0
Business	41	36	23	0	0
Exploration	50	0	25	25	0
Sports	50	25	25	0	0
Composing	25	8	67	0	0
Entertainment	12	12	77	0	0
Military	67	0	33	0	0
Public office	65	15	15	4	0
Natural sciences	46	9	46	0	0
Social activism	29	8	63	0	0
Social figure	7	7	86	0	0
Companion	0	7	93	0	0
Social sciences	28	22	50	0	0
Theater	5	15	78	3	0
Nonfiction	21	10	69	0	0
Fiction	21	8	68	2	2
Poetry	28	6	67	0	0
Total %	27	14	58	2	0

Chi square = 134.1   *df* = 68   *p* = .000

Level II	None	Before	Before/ During	After	Other
Artistic	17	12	69	1	1
Enterprising	51	21	26	2	0
Investigative	33	4	58	4	0
Social	24	13	61	2	0

Chi square = 52.5   *df* = 12   *p* = .000

Level III	None	Before	Before/ During	After	Other
Creative arts	17	12	69	2	1
Other	39	16	44	2	0

Chi square = 27.2   *df* = 4   *p* = .000

S11. Occupations of Spouses (by Percentage) (*n* = 690)

Level I	Home-maker	Unskilled	Skilled	Business	Applied prof.	Creat. prof.
Architecture	59	0	0	12	6	18
Art	57	2	0	2	6	32
Business	76	6	0	6	2	11
Exploration	56	11	0	11	0	22
Sports	92	0	0	8	0	0
Composing	54	0	0	0	6	40
Entertainment	32	11	0	18	7	32
Military	94	0	0	0	6	0
Public office	80	0	3	0	14	2
Natural sciences	70	0	4	0	19	7
Social activism	44	0	8	6	31	6
Social figure	11	0	0	26	42	11
Companion	0	0	0	20	47	33
Social sciences	51	0	2	2	33	9
Theater	11	2	4	6	9	64
Nonfiction	42	2	7	9	20	18
Fiction	42	2	5	10	9	32
Poetry	47	3	3	6	9	31
Total %	52	2	3	6	14	22

Chi square = 334.0   *df* = 102   *p* = .000

Level II						
Artistic	42	2	3	8	11	33
Enterprising	75	2	2	3	12	5
Investigative	51	0	4	7	29	9
Social	41	0	5	6	25	19

Chi square = 113.7   *df* = 18   *p* = .000

Level III						
Creative arts	41	3	3	8	10	35
Other	64	1	3	5	19	8

Chi square = 87.9   *df* = 6   *p* = .000

S12. Mental Illness in Spouse (by Percentage) (n = 841)

Level I

Architecture (11); Art (6); Business (2); Exploration (0); Sports (13); Musical composition (13); Musical entertainment (10); Military (6); Public office (7); Natural sciences (10); Social activism (13); Social figure (4); Companion (13); Social sciences (9); Theater (11); Nonfiction (16); Fiction (19); Poetry (15).

Chi square = 25.0 $df = 17$ $p = .100$

Level II

Artistic (13); Enterprising (5); Investigative (9); Social (13).

Chi square = 11.4 $df = 3$ $p = .010$

Level III

Creative arts (14); Other (7.4).

Chi square = 9.2 $df = 1$ $p = .002$

S13. Average Number of Children

Level I

Architecture (2.4); Art (1.9); Business (2.7); Exploration (2.1); Sports (1.2); Musical composition (1.7); Musical entertainment (1.2); Military (1.9); Public office (2.6); Natural sciences (1.8); Social activism (2.0); Social figure (1.4); Companion (2.8); Social sciences (1.6); Theater (1.4); Nonfiction (1.4); Fiction (1.5); Poetry (1.1).

$F = 3.3$ $df = 17, 983$ $p = .000$

Level II

Artistic (1.5); Enterprising (2.5); Investigative (1.6); Social (1.9).

$F = 13.2$ $df = 3, 997$ $p = .000$

Level III

Creative arts (1.5); Other (2.1).

$F = 21.6$ $df = 1, 999$ $p = .000$

S14. Children in Same General Profession as Subjects (by Percentage) (n = 363)

Architecture (50); Art (50); Business (45); Exploration (0); Sports (0); Musical composition (29); Musical entertainment (27); Military (33); Public office (56); Natural sciences (50); Social activism (46); Social figure (17); Companion (10); Social sciences (19); Theater (67); Nonfiction (50); Fiction (36); Poetry (46).

Chi square = 33.6 $df = 17$ $p = .009$

S15. Health Status and Cause of Death (by Percentage)

Level I	Chronic illness		Cause of death*		
	Before 50	After 50	Natural	Accidental	Suicide
Architecture	17	24	96	4	0
Art	29	38	91	3	6
Business	11	24	91	3	6
Exploration	27	0	56	44	0
Sports	42	30	79	16	5
Composition	44	57	90	10	0
Entertainment	28	35	77	15	8
Military	20	21	70	25	5
Public office	25	34	94	6	0
Natural sciences	26	36	95	0	5
Social activism	41	39	69	29	2
Social figure	7	32	93	7	0
Companion	22	21	100	0	0
Social sciences	23	32	89	7	4
Theater	27	39	80	13	7
Nonfiction	30	33	97	1	2
Fiction	43	49	88	8	4
Poetry	34	28	72	8	20
n	1,004	674	990		
Total %	30	36	87	9	4
Chi square	51.1	24.3	117.0		
df	17	17	34		
p	.000	N.S.	.000		
Level II					
Artistic	34	40	87	8	5
Enterprising	20	28	89	9	2
Investigative	28	25	90	1	9
Social	31	40	81	18	1
Chi square	16.0	11.0	28.8		
df	3	3	6		
p	.001	.012	.000		
Level III					
Creative arts	35	40	86	8	6
Other	24	31	87	10	3
Chi square	13.2	6.5	6.2		
df	1	1	2		
p	.000	.011	.050		

*Percentages calculated after exclusion of those who died from unknown causes.

S16. Longevity (Average Age)

Level I

Architecture (75.9); Art (69.8); Business (73.4); Exploration (51.4); Sports (60.2); Musical composition (65.1); Musical entertainment (57.2); Military (67.9); Public office (72.3); Natural sciences (71.5); Social activism (66.0); Social figure (74.4); Companion (77.4); Social sciences (73.5); Theater (63.4); Nonfiction (70.6); Fiction (66.1); Poetry (59.6).

$F = 6.8$ $df = 17, 986$ $p = .000$

Level II

Artistic (66.0); Enterprising (71.3); Investigative (71.2); Social (69.2).

$F = 7.2$ $df = 3, 1000$ $p = .000$

Level III

Creative arts (65.7); Other (70.9).

$F = 25.6$ $df = 1, 1002$ $p = .000$

S17. Factor Analysis

Bartlett's Test of Sphericity (= 1,605.145, significance = .0000) and the Kaiser–Meyer–Olkin Measuring of Sampling Adequacy (= .68607) revealed that the data were adequate for factor analysis. A Principal Components factor analysis with a varimax rotation was then run on all 48 variables with automatic replacement of missing values with the mean. In order to incorporate certain important categorical variables in the analysis, they were recoded beforehand and transformed into dichotomous or interval level variables. A scree test was used to identify four factors with eigenvalues above 2.00, which accounted for 21.8% of the total variance. The four regression factor scores were then saved and later used as dependent variables for one-way analyses of variance, employing posthoc modified LSD (Bonferroni) tests to determine the relative status of Level I and Level II professions on this measure.

The factor loadings for each variable and other pertinent information are given below.

	Factor I	Factor II	Factor III	Factor IV
Eigenvalue	3.84	2.28	2.10	2.01
% total variance	8.2	4.8	4.5	4.3

S18. The correlations below are illustrative of the magnitude of the relationships among selected childhood and adult behavior variables.

Correlations between Adult and Youthful Attributes

Adult attributes	Child attributes		
	Oddness	Moody	Sociable
Different	.36*	.24	.12
	(818)	(547)	(683)
Moody	.23	.54	.27
	(754)	(533)	(640)
Affiliative	.15	.14	.13
	(801)	(553)	(667)
Sociable	.17	.24	.50
	(786)	(549)	(666)

*Pearson r values are underlined (total numbers in parentheses)

All probability values < .001

S1. Distribution of Groups in Different Professions (by Percentage)

Level I	Females	Blacks	Jews	Bisexuals/ Homosexuals
Architecture	30	0	13	9
Art	20	0	14	15
Business	6	0	36	4
Exploration	18	0	0	0
Sports	11	26	0	6
Composing	6	4	15	13
Entertainment	40	30	12	15
Military	0	0	7	0
Public office	7	2	11	2
Natural sciences	8	5	9	3
Social activism	41	10	29	5
Social figure	73	0	8	13
Companion	94	0	6	11
Social sciences	22	3	19	4
Theater	37	3	16	12
Nonfiction	28	0	14	6
Fiction	25	3	11	21
Poetry	25	0	8	24
n	1,004	1,002	863	985
Total %	24	4	15	11
Chi square	166.6	129.3	117.8	55.5
df	17	17	68	17
p	.000	.000	.000	.000
Level II				
Artistic	27	4	14	15
Enterprising	10	1	16	3
Investigative	21	4	16	5
Social	35	9	17	7
Chi square	37.2	13.8	20.5	30.8
df	3	3	12	1
p	.000	.003	.058	.000
Level III				
Creative arts	26	4	13	16
Other	22	4	17	4
Chi square	2.5	0.1	15.4	33.8
df	1	1	4	1
p	.114	.774	.004	.008

S2. Effects of Gender (by Percentage)

	Female	Male	Chi square	df	p =
Avid reader (as child)	35	37	0.2	1	N.S.
School honors	9	23	25.2	1	.000
Conflicts with teachers	5	10	5.4	1	.021
Conflicts with students	3	5	0.6	1	N.S.
Superior grades	11	21	9.4	5	N.S.
College/Graduate school	20	45	69.8	6	.000
Extracurricular (marked)	18	35	4.3	2	N.S.
Parent marriage (intact)	82	90	14.2	3	.003
Handicap (as child)	8	10	0.6	1	N.S.
Sickly (as child)	7	10	2.3	1	N.S.
Major illness (as child)	10	7	2.4	1	N.S.
Death of mother (<13)	16	14	1.1	3	N.S.
Death of father (<13)	15	17	0.3	3	N.S.
Precocity	17	21	4.6	2	N.S.
Solitary (as youth)	35	35	0.0	2	N.S.
Moodiness (as youth)	33	27	2.8	2	N.S.
Oddness (as youth)	8	4	4.3	2	N.S.
Success before 21	17	13	5.0	2	N.S.
Nonaffiliative	41	33	7.2	2	.028
Creative hobby	33	28	3.1	2	N.S.
Athletic	8	20	18.0	2	.000
Sociable	55	48	2.9	2	N.S.
Moody (as adult)	41	42	0.0	2	N.S.
Expressed confidence	30	38	4.7	1	.030
Different	38	25	16.8	1	.000
Urban background	60	56	3.3	4	N.S.
Defendant	12	16	2.4	2	N.S.
Plaintiff	8	7	0.4	1	N.S.
Jail/Fine—nonpolitical	6	11	4.3	1	.039
Jail/Fine—political	10	11	0.0	1	N.S.
Antagonism father	22	26	2.0	2	N.S.
Antagonism mother	30	15	18.9	2	.000
Antagonism employer	27	27	0.6	2	N.S.
Mentor	23	23	0.0	1	N.S.
Homosexual/Bisexual	18	8	16.6	1	.000
Married	81	85	2.2	1	N.S.
Divorced (of married)	49	32	19.1	1	.000
Affair (of married)	46	37	5.3	1	.022
Mother homemaker	78	81	7.7	6	N.S.
Mother creative interest	38	39	0.7	2	N.S.
Mother nonconform (some)	17	10	11.9	2	.003
Mother mental problem	17	11	7.2	1	.007
Father college	63	68	3.1	5	N.S.
Father creative profession	10	6	16.0	6	.014

		Female	Male	Chi square	df	p =
Father creative interest		42	37	1.2	2	N.S.
Father nonconform (some)		19	13	11.0	2	.004
Father mental problem		18	17	0.2	1	N.S.
Sibling mental problem		21	13	8.0	1	.005
Parents upper income		27	14	22.0	2	.000
Parents upper class		20	9	33.1	5	.000
Father successful		76	66	17.0	4	.002
Cause of death				2.2	2	N.S.
Accident/Incident		7	10			
Suicide		5	4			
Religious beliefs				9.8	5	N.S.
Atheist		5	9			
Agnostic		20	21			
Idiosyncratic		14	10			
Medical problems < 50		31	30	0.1	1	N.S.
Medical problems > 50		31	38	1.9	1	N.S.
Adjustment problem		46	33	14.6	1	.000
Alcohol		23	28	2.2	1	N.S.
Drugs		17	10	7.7	1	.005
Depression		40	38	0.4	1	N.S.
Mania		7	7	0.0	1	N.S.
Psychosis		7	5	2.9	1	N.S.
Somatization		14	10	3.1	1	N.S.
Suicide attempt		17	8	16.0	1	.000
Anxiety		12	7	5.7	1	.017
Other		9	4	10.5	1	.001
Any problem		74	67	3.8	1	.051
Any psych. treatment		35	23	14.5	1	.000
# children	Mean	SD	df		F	p =
Females	1.2	1.8	.999		24.8	.000
Males	2.0	2.2				
Age of death	Mean	SD	df		F	p =
Females	70.5	17.1	1, 1,002		7.8	.005
Males	67.2	16.0				
Education level	Mean	SD	df		F	p =
Females	3.2	1.4	1, 984		59.0	.000
Males	4.1	1.4				
CAS total score	Mean	SD	df		F	p =
Females	31.8	14.1	1, 1,002		66.0	.000
Males	40.1	14.7				

S3. Effects of Race (by Percentage)

	Black	White	Chi square	df	p =
Avid reader (as child)	18	37	6.5	1	.011
School honors	20	20	0.0	1	N.S.
Conflicts with teachers	10	9	0.0	1	N.S.
Conflicts with students	3	4	0.3	1	N.S.
Superior grades	31	19	5.9	5	N.S.
College/Graduate school	29	39	21.4	6	.002
Extracurricular (marked)	50	32	1.5	2	N.S.
Parent marriage (intact)	61	89	32.4	3	.000
Handicap (as child)	3	10	2.4	1	N.S.
Sickly (as child)	8	10	0.2	1	N.S.
Major illness (as child)	3	8	1.7	1	N.S.
Death of mother (< 13)	20	14	10.3	3	.017
Death of father (< 13)	35	16	6.7	3	N.S.
Precocity	23	20	1.2	2	N.S.
Solitary (as youth)	29	35	0.6	2	N.S.
Moodiness (as youth)	17	29	2.7	2	N.S.
Oddness (as youth)	3	6	0.3	2	N.S.
Success before 21	28	13	7.9	2	.019
Nonaffiliative	32	35	0.2	2	N.S.
Creative hobby	10	30	8.1	2	.018
Athletic	5	18	4.6	2	N.S.
Sociable	49	50	3.3	2	N.S.
Moody (as adult)	36	42	2.0	2	N.S.
Expressed confidence	65	64	0.0	1	N.S.
Different	39	28	2.2	1	N.S.
Urban background	65	56	3.4	4	N.S.
Defendant	35	14	13.6	2	.001
Plaintiff	8	7	0.0	1	N.S.
Jail/Fine—nonpolitical	40	8	44.5	1	.000
Jail/Fine—political	20	10	4.0	1	.045
Antagonism father	42	24	3.6	2	N.S.
Antagonism mother	19	19	2.6	2	N.S.
Antagonism employer	27	27	6.2	2	.044
Mentor	35	22	3.5	1	N.S.
Homosexual/Bisexual	13	11	0.2	1	N.S.
Married	90	84	1.1	1	N.S.
Divorced (of married)	55	35	5.2	1	.022
Affair (of married)	47	38	1.1	1	N.S.
Mother homemaker	38	82	119.0	6	.000
Mother creative interest	40	38	0.3	2	N.S.
Mother nonconform (some)	16	11	0.7	2	N.S.
Mother mental problem	3	13	3.7	1	N.S.
Father college	44	68	11.3	5	.047
Father creative profession	10	7	37.3	6	.000
Father creative interest	44	38	1.1	2	N.S.

	Black	White	Chi square	df	p =
Father nonconform (some)	26	14	3.1	2	N.S.
Father mental problem	10	18	1.6	1	N.S.
Sibling mental problem	0	16	7.3	1	.007
Parents upper income	0	17	8.1	2	.017
Parents upper class	0	12	60.1	5	.000
Father successful	30	70	35.0	4	.000
Cause of death			6.3	2	.042
Accident/Incident	20	9			
Suicide	3	4			
Religious beliefs			5.7	5	N.S.
Atheist	0	8			
Agnostic	13	21			
Idiosyncratic	16	11			
Medical problems < 50	23	30	1.1	1	N.S.
Medical problems > 50	52	35	2.7	1	N.S.
Adjustment problem	38	36	0.0	1	N.S.
Alcohol	33	26	0.8	1	N.S.
Drugs	25	11	6.9	1	.009
Depression	25	39	3.0	1	N.S.
Mania	5	7	0.3	1	N.S.
Psychosis	8	5	0.4	1	N.S.
Somatization	5	11	1.4	1	N.S.
Suicide attempt	20	10	4.0	1	.045
Anxiety	0	9	3.7	1	N.S.
Other	0	5	2.2	1	N.S.
Any problem	73	69	0.2	1	N.S.
Any psych. treatment	15	26	2.5	1	N.S.

# children	Mean	SD	df	F	p =
Black	1.6	2.0	1, 997	0.3	N.S.
White	1.8	2.1			

Age of death	Mean	SD	df	F	p =
Black	56.6	16.8	1, 1,000	20.7	.000
White	68.4	16.1			

Education level	Mean	SD	df	F	p =
Black	3.4	1.7	1, 982	4.0	.045
White	3.9	1.4			

CAS total score	Mean	SD	df	F	p =
Black	38.5	10.6	1, 1000	0.0	N.S.
White	38.4	15.1			

S4. Effects of Religious Background (by Percentage)

	Cath.	Jewish	Prot.	Chi square	df	p =
Avid reader (as child)	30	40	38	4.6	2	N.S.
School honors	17	17	22	3.4	2	N.S.
Conflicts with teachers	11	12	8	2.2	2	N.S.
Conflicts with students	3	6	4	0.8	2	N.S.
Superior grades	10	26	23	15.9	10	N.S.
College/Graduate school	31	44	44	26.6	12	.003
Extracurricular (marked)	20	33	35	15.4	4	.004
Parent marriage (intact)	87	92	91	9.7	6	N.S.
Handicap (as child)	9	9	10	0.3	2	N.S.
Sickly (as child)	8	7	10	1.4	2	N.S.
Major illness (as child)	8	6	7	0.7	2	N.S.
Death of mother (< 13)	13	10	14	1.9	6	N.S.
Death of father (< 13)	19	10	15	15.5	6	.017
Precocity	21	24	17	17.1	4	.002
Solitary (as youth)	34	32	36	2.0	4	N.S.
Moodiness (as youth)	31	37	27	4.8	4	N.S.
Oddness (as youth)	4	1	6	5.0	4	N.S.
Success before 21	20	8	12	11.3	4	.023
Nonaffiliative	47	26	31	20.3	4	.000
Creative hobby	23	23	31	5.4	4	N.S.
Athletic	15	11	18	3.6	4	N.S.
Sociable	53	55	48	8.8	4	N.S.
Moody (as adult)	48	49	37	16.1	4	.003
Expressed confidence	43	44	31	12.0	2	.003
Different	27	24	27	0.6	2	N.S.
Urban background	60	80	51	41.2	8	.000
Defendant	15	17	13	2.1	4	N.S.
Plaintiff	6	6	7	0.4	2	N.S.
Jail/Fine—nonpolitical	9	13	9	2.9	2	N.S.
Jail/Fine—political	14	20	6	25.2	2	.000
Antagonism father	25	24	24	7.5	4	N.S.
Antagonism mother	17	15	17	12.9	4	.012
Antagonism employer	30	33	20	8.2	4	N.S.
Mentor	76	76	77	0.2	2	N.S.
Homosexual/Bisexual	10	11	10	0.1	2	N.S.
Married	81	83	86	2.2	2	N.S.
Divorced (of married)	34	41	34	2.2	2	N.S.
Affair (of married)	48	42	33	11.2	2	.004
Mother homemaker	79	85	81	17.5	12	N.S.
Mother creative interest	42	25	40	5.2	4	N.S.
Mother nonconform (some)	10	8	10	0.6	4	N.S.
Mother mental problem	10	12	12	0.9	2	N.S.
Father college	68	55	69	8.1	10	N.S.

		Cath.	Jewish	Prot.	Chi square	df	p =
Father creative profession		11	6	3	64.7	12	.000
Father creative interest		51	28	33	13.7	4	.008
Father nonconform (some)		15	11	14	3.2	4	N.S.
Father mental problem		18	11	20	5.3	2	N.S.
Sibling mental problem		11	17	17	4.0	2	N.S.
Parents upper income		16	6	20	25.7	4	.000
Parents upper class		14	3	13	53.8	10	.000
Father successful		56	63	74	27.4	8	.001
Cause of death					8.5	4	N.S.
Accident/Incident		10	12	6			
Suicide		3	6	4			
Religious beliefs					36.7	10	.000
Atheist		10	10	4			
Agnostic		11	21	21			
Idiosyncratic		12	8	9			
Medical problems < 50		36	32	26	6.6	2	.037
Medical problems > 50		44	31	35	3.7	2	N.S.
Adjustment problem		36	38	35	0.6	2	N.S.
Alcohol		28	19	25	3.2	2	N.S.
Drugs		13	10	10	0.9	2	N.S.
Depression		41	40	37	1.0	2	N.S.
Mania		6	9	6	1.1	2	N.S.
Psychosis		6	2	6	2.7	2	N.S.
Somatization		12	14	9	2.8	2	N.S.
Suicide attempt		11	11	10	0.2	2	N.S.
Anxiety		9	7	9	0.3	2	N.S.
Other		6	6	5	0.7	2	N.S.
Any problem		73	72	66	4.4	2	N.S.
Any psych. treatment		22	35	25	6.7	2	.035

# children	Mean	SD	df	F	p =
Catholic	1.7	2.2	2, 787	0.5	N.S.
Jewish	1.7	2.1			
Protestant	1.9	2.2			

Age of death	Mean	SD	df	F	p =
Catholic	66.9	15.9	2, 790	2.1	N.S.
Jewish	66.8	16.5			
Protestant	69.3	15.9			

Education level	Mean	SD	df	F	p =
Catholic	3.8	1.4	2, 778	0.9	N.S.
Jewish	4.0	1.5			
Protestant	4.0	1.5			

CAS total score	Mean	SD	df	F	p =
Catholic	40.7	16.7	2, 790	3.4	.035
Jewish	36.8	14.1			
Protestant	37.6	14.7			

S5. Effects of Sexual Orientation (by Percentage)

	Bisex./ Homosex.	Hypo./ Hetero.	Chi square	df	p =
Avid reader (as child)	42	36	1.4	1	N.S.
School honors	15	21	1.6	1	N.S.
Conflicts with teachers	13	9	2.4	1	N.S.
Conflicts with students	10	4	8.0	1	.005
Superior grades	10	21	14.5	5	.013
College/Graduate school	33	40	6.7	6	N.S.
Extracurricular (marked)	24	35	2.7	2	N.S.
Parent marriage (intact)	76	89	15.9	3	.001
Handicap (as child)	10	9	0.0	1	N.S.
Sickly (as child)	12	9	1.1	1	N.S.
Major illness (as child)	17	7	14.2	1	.000
Death of mother (<13)	18	14	1.1	3	N.S.
Death of father (<13)	15	17	5.1	3	N.S.
Precocity	27	20	3.0	2	N.S.
Solitary (as youth)	33	35	7.2	2	.028
Moodiness (as youth)	41	27	12.7	2	.002
Oddness (as youth)	17	4	40.9	2	.000
Success before 21	22	13	7.3	2	.026
Nonaffiliative	48	33	20.1	2	.000
Creative hobby	40	28	7.0	2	.030
Athletic	13	18	3.6	2	N.S.
Sociable	48	51	0.4	2	N.S.
Moody (as adult)	21	40	17.6	2	.000
Expressed confidence	29	37	2.8	1	N.S.
Different	56	25	44.4	1	.000
Urban background	67	56	7.2	4	N.S.
Defendant	17	15	0.6	2	N.S.
Plaintiff	9	7	0.5	1	N.S.
Jail/Fine—nonpolitical	16	9	5.8	1	.016
Jail/Fine—political	10	11	0.1	1	N.S.
Antagonism father	40	23	10.7	2	.005
Antagonism mother	35	17	25.4	2	.000
Antagonism employer	36	26	2.3	2	N.S.
Mentor	23	23	0.0	1	N.S.
Married	46	89	135.8	1	.000
Divorced (of married)	50	34	4.2	1	.040
Affair (of married)	83	36	43.1	1	.000
Mother homemaker	76	81	8.8	6	N.S.
Mother creative interest	44	38	4.1	2	N.S.
Mother nonconform (some)	17	10	5.5	2	N.S.

		Bisex./ Homosex.	Hypo./ Hetero.	Chi square	df	p =
Mother mental problem		15	12	1.0	1	N.S.
Father college		55	69	14.5	5	.013
Father creative profession		9	7	6.0	6	N.S.
Father creative interest		41	38	1.2	2	N.S.
Father nonconform (some)		26	13	14.5	2	.001
Father mental problem		27	16	7.1	1	.008
Sibling mental problem		21	14	3.4	1	N.S.
Parents upper income		19	16	1.9	2	N.S.
Parents upper class		12	11	3.6	5	N.S.
Father successful		76	68	8.8	4	N.S.
Cause of death				21.9	2	.000
Accident/Incident		15	8			
Suicide		12	4			
Religious beliefs				8.3	5	N.S.
Atheist		9	8			
Agnostic		17	21			
Idiosyncratic		15	10			
Medical problems < 50		31	30	0.2	1	N.S.
Medical problems > 50		44	35	1.9	1	N.S.
Adjustment problem		48	35	6.8	1	.009
Alcohol		42	25	14.3	1	.000
Drugs		31	10	38.1	1	.000
Depression		50	37	6.8	1	.009
Mania		11	7	3.3	1	N.S.
Psychosis		6	5	0.0	1	N.S.
Somatization		8	11	1.0	1	N.S.
Suicide attempt		20	9	11.4	1	.001
Anxiety		13	8	4.3	1	.039
Other		3	5	1.1	1	N.S.
Any problem		84	67	12.1	1	.000
Any psych. treatment		41	24	14.4	1	.000

# children	Mean	SD	df	F	p =
Bisex./Homosex.	0.3	0.8	1, 980	57.7	N.S.
Hypo./Hetero.	2.0	2.2			

Age of death	Mean	SD	df	F	p =
Bisex./Homosex.	62.1	17.3	1, 983	16.4	.000
Hypo./Hetero.	68.8	16.0			

Education level	Mean	SD	df	F	p =
Bisex./Homosex.	3.8	1.3	1, 966	0.7	N.S.
Hypo./Hetero.	3.9	1.5			

CAS total score	Mean	SD	df	F	p =
Bisex./Homosex.	38.4	15.0	1, 983	0.0	N.S.
Hypo./Hetero.	38.4	15.1			

S1. Creative Achievement Scale Mean Scores ($n = 1,004$)

Level I	CAS items*										
	1	2	3	4	5	6	7	8	9	10	11
Architecture	6.0	5.2	4.8	6.5	4.7	4.0	3.9	5.0	3.8	1.6	3.0
Art	6.2	6.2	5.3	5.7	4.6	3.2	2.8	4.5	3.6	1.5	3.0
Business	4.3	3.1	2.7	5.0	1.8	1.1	2.4	2.6	2.2	1.2	1.0
Exploration	3.8	1.9	2.5	5.7	1.4	0.0	2.4	2.0	3.1	1.0	1.5
Sports	4.1	2.7	1.9	6.0	1.4	0.8	1.8	3.5	3.5	1.8	0.6
Composing	7.3	7.2	5.4	7.0	5.1	3.2	2.8	4.8	5.2	2.2	3.0
Entertainment	5.6	5.0	3.7	6.5	3.8	2.2	2.2	4.0	4.4	1.9	3.0
Military	4.1	3.6	2.0	5.6	1.8	1.1	2.7	2.8	2.2	1.2	0.8
Public office	4.3	4.5	2.5	5.4	1.5	1.2	2.4	3.1	1.9	1.3	0.8
Natural sciences	6.9	7.1	6.3	7.1	5.3	3.5	3.2	4.8	4.6	1.6	1.6
Social activism	4.5	4.1	4.1	4.8	2.0	1.2	2.7	3.1	1.9	1.1	1.1
Social figure	3.0	2.8	0.9	2.1	0.9	0.5	1.7	1.9	0.5	0.8	1.7
Companion	1.2	1.5	0.2	0.3	0.0	0.0	0.6	1.0	0.2	0.7	1.7
Social sciences	5.6	6.0	4.9	6.1	4.4	3.3	2.6	4.8	3.6	1.3	1.4
Theater	5.7	5.4	3.2	6.1	3.3	2.5	2.5	4.0	3.8	1.6	3.0
Nonfiction	4.3	4.4	3.5	4.9	2.9	2.2	2.9	4.6	2.3	1.3	2.6
Fiction	6.2	5.5	4.5	6.0	4.0	3.2	2.7	4.5	3.5	1.5	3.0
Poetry	5.6	5.6	5.0	5.7	4.6	3.2	2.3	3.9	3.0	1.5	3.0
Total mean	5.3	5.0	3.9	5.6	3.3	2.3	2.6	3.9	3.1	1.4	2.1
F ratio	15.9	24.9	28.0	16.8	39.0	31.5	3.9	23.3	22.6	14.4	98.7
df = 17, 986											
p	.000	.000	.000	.000	.000	.000	.000	.000	.000	.000	.000

Level II											
Artistic	5.8	5.5	4.3	5.9	4.0	2.9	2.7	4.3	3.5	1.6	2.9
Enterprising	4.2	3.8	2.5	5.2	1.7	1.1	2.4	2.8	2.0	1.2	0.9
Investigative	6.4	6.5	5.8	6.7	5.0	3.2	2.8	4.7	4.3	1.5	1.3
Social	4.2	3.9	3.2	4.7	2.0	1.5	2.3	3.3	2.2	1.2	1.4
Total mean	5.3	5.0	3.9	5.6	3.3	2.3	2.6	3.9	3.1	1.4	2.1
F ratio	39.8	54.1	62.8	17.7	123.6	84.1	2.7	63.4	49.4	23.5	412.5
df = 3, 1,000											
p	.000	.000	.000	.000	.000	.000	.045	.000	.000	.000	.000

*1 = Posthumous fame; 2 = Universality; 3 = New directions; 4 = Influence; 5 = Originality; 6 = Extent of innovation; 7 = Versatility; 8 = Productivity; 9 = Contemporary fame; 10 = Skill; 11 = Aesthetics

S2. Creative Achievement Scale Scores (n = 1,004)

Level I	No.	Mean	SD
Architecture	23	48.7	10.8
Art	70	46.7	13.6
Business	70	27.3	12.9
Exploration	11	25.2	10.7
Sports	19	28.0	7.2
Composing	48	53.1	9.8
Musical entertainment	47	43.5	11.4
Military	20	27.7	9.5
Public office	108	28.8	12.5
Natural sciences	39	51.9	14.1
Social activism	61	30.7	12.4
Social figure	30	16.9	10.5
Companion	18	7.3	6.4
Social sciences	73	44.0	14.5
Theater	70	41.1	9.2
Nonfiction	64	35.8	7.8
Fiction	180	44.5	10.7
Poetry	53	43.5	11.4

$df = 17, 986$ $F = 43.3$ $p = .000$

Level II	No.	Mean	SD
Artistic	576	43.2	12.3
Enterprising	221	27.8	12.6
Investigative	71	48.1	14.1
Social	136	29.9	16.0

$df = 3, 1,000$ $F = 106.8$ $p = .000$

METHOD AND STATISTICS: CHAPTER 7

S1. Prevalence of Any Psychopathology (n = 1,004)

			Time periods		
Level I	< 13	13–20	21–40	41–60	60
Architecture	4	4	26	44	47
Art	6	16	59	70	52
Business	0	9	29	45	41
Exploration	0	9	36	44	33
Sports	0	5	68	63	25
Composing	8	21	63	59	55
Entertainment	4	30	70	63	32
Military	0	5	25	26	15
Public office	2	7	23	34	23
Natural sciences	3	15	18	34	24
Social activism	8	15	43	43	37
Social figure	3	7	37	28	29
Companion	0	22	33	31	38
Social sciences	3	14	41	47	35
Theater	6	26	66	70	62
Nonfiction	5	16	61	59	51
Fiction	5	29	70	74	65
Poetry	9	34	77	81	58
Total %	4	18	51	55	44
Chi square	17.1	55.9	148.7	101.6	66.3
$df = 17$					
p	.449	.000	.000	.000	.000
Level II					
Artistic	5	24	64	67	55
Enterprising	1	8	27	37	29
Investigative	4	13	32	41	26
Social	4	14	43	46	40
Chi square	6.3	29.5	102.2	66.9	41.7
$df = 3$					
p	.097	.000	.000	.000	.000
Level III					
Creative arts	6	24	65	68	56
Other	2	11	33	39	31
Chi square	6.7	30.3	104.8	76.3	47.3
$df = 1$					
p	.010	.000	.000	.000	.000

S2. Lifetime Prevalence of Psychiatric Syndromes (n = 1,004)

Level I	Permissive criteria*									
	1	2	3	4	5	6	7	8	9	10
Architecture	22	4	17	13	4	13	13	9	9	52
Art	29	10	50	9	4	10	34	14	9	73
Business	17	7	26	6	3	11	27	3	6	49
Exploration	27	0	0	0	0	0	27	0	0	27
Sports	32	0	16	0	11	5	58	0	11	53
Composing	23	13	46	6	10	13	44	4	10	60
Entertainment	40	36	32	9	4	15	23	4	17	68
Military	10	0	5	5	0	5	25	5	5	30
Public office	14	2	21	4	0	4	28	2	1	35
Natural sciences	3	0	15	3	0	3	36	5	8	28
Social activism	10	10	34	5	5	15	41	7	10	49
Social figure	10	13	20	3	7	10	27	7	10	37
Companion	17	0	28	0	0	11	39	6	11	44
Social sciences	10	7	32	1	4	8	38	8	1	51
Theater	60	24	34	17	6	7	34	14	23	74
Nonfiction	27	9	47	11	8	13	39	16	8	72
Fiction	41	19	59	9	7	14	46	11	14	77
Poetry	34	17	77	13	17	17	38	13	26	87
Total %	26	12	38	7	5	11	36	8	11	59
Chi square $df = 17$	118.6	77.0	133.2	28.8	32.0	19.8	30.4	29.5	52.8	128.5
p	.000	.000	.000	.036	.015	.286	.024	.030	.000	.000

Level II	1	2	3	4	5	6	7	8	9	10
Artistic	35	18	50	10	8	13	38	11	14	72
Enterprising	15	4	20	5	1	6	26	3	4	39
Investigative	6	1	24	0	4	6	39	7	7	41
Social	19	6	27	3	3	12	40	6	6	49
Chi square $df = 3$	58.1	42.7	77.4	19.4	16.5	9.9	11.7	14.2	23.2	92.3
p	.000	.000	.000	.000	.001	.020	.009	.003	.000	.000

Level III	1	2	3	4	5	6	7	8	9	10
Creative arts	37	18	50	11	7	13	38	11	15	73
Other	13	5	24	3	3	8	33	5	5	42
Chi square $df = 1$	75.0	37.6	72.8	18.6	11.0	6.6	2.1	15.6	24.7	101.8
p	.000	.000	.000	.000	.001	.010	.146	.000	.000	.000

*1 = Alcohol; 2 = Drugs; 3 = Depression; 4 = Mania; 5 = Psychosis; 6 = Somatic; 7 = Adjustment; 8 = Anxiety; 9 = Suicide attempt; 10 = Any problem (includes #'s 1–6, 8, 9, and "other" mental problems)

S3. Comparisons of Survival Probability Using the Wilcoxon (Gehan) Statistic

a. Survival variable: Alcohol   Statistic = 65.5; *df* = 3; *p* = .000

Overall comparison

Group	n	Uncen.	Cen.	% cen.	Mean score
Artistic	504	130	374	74.2	−77.2
Enterprising	200	12	188	94.0	98.2
Investigative	69	2	67	97.1	128.6
Social	119	9	110	92.4	87.4

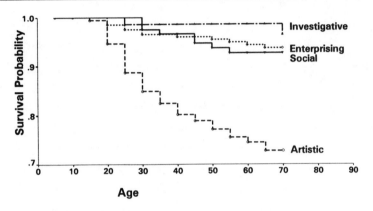

b. Survival variable: Drug abuse   Statistic = 26.8; *df* = 3; *p* = .000

Overall comparison

Group	n	Uncen.	Cen.	% cen.	Mean score
Artistic	540	65	475	88.0	−35.5
Enterprising	220	8	212	96.4	44.3
Investigative	71	1	70	98.6	57.7
Social	133	5	128	96.2	40.0

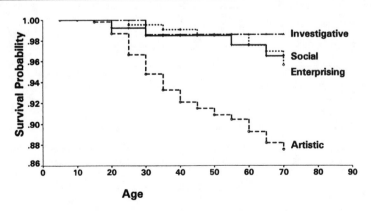

c. Survival variable: Depression   Statistic = 59.0; *df* = 3; *p* = .000

Overall comparison

Group	*n*	Uncen.	Cen.	% cen.	Mean score
Artistic	484	197	287	59.3	–94.1
Enterprising	208	33	175	84.1	130.3
Investigative	69	15	54	78.3	85.7
Social	125	25	100	80.0	100.2

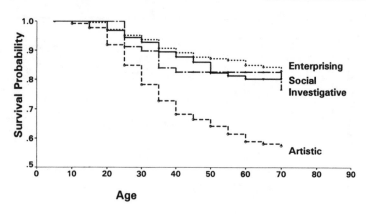

d. Survival variable: Mania   Statistic = 13.4; *df* = 3; *p* = .004

Overall comparison

Group	*n*	Uncen.	Cen.	% cen.	Mean score
Artistic	543	26	517	95.2	–15.9
Enterprising	215	4	211	98.1	13.7
Investigative	71	0	71	100.0	28.5
Social	133	1	132	99.3	27.4

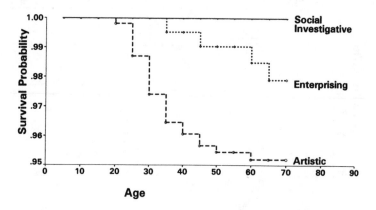

e. Survival variable: Psychosis   Statistic = 20.1; *df* = 3; *p* = .000

Overall comparison

Group	n	Uncen.	Cen.	% cen.	Mean score
Artistic	566	35	531	93.8	−20.3
Enterprising	220	1	219	99.6	30.4
Investigative	70	2	68	97.1	6.6
Social	133	1	132	99.3	32.6

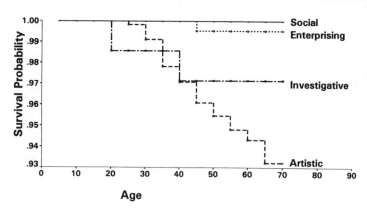

f. Survival variable: Anxiety   Statistic = 9.9; *df* = 3; *p* = .020

Overall comparison

Group	n	Uncen.	Cen.	% cen.	Mean score
Artistic	557	46	511	91.7	−19.0
Enterprising	220	6	214	97.3	31.9
Investigative	70	4	66	94.3	11.3
Social	134	6	128	95.5	20.7

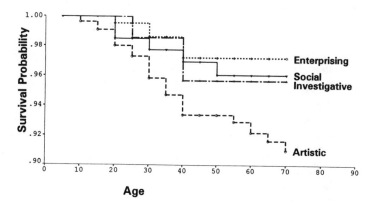

g. Survival variable: Suicide   Statistic = 10.7; df = 3; p = .013

Overall comparison

Group	n	Uncen.	Cen.	% cen.	Mean score
Artistic	569	31	538	94.6	−12.0
Enterprising	219	5	214	97.7	20.2
Investigative	69	6	63	91.3	−23.3
Social	133	1	132	99.3	30.1

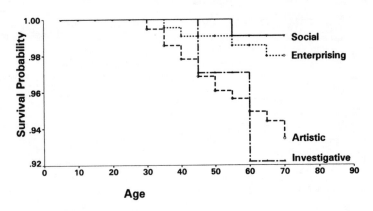

S4. See S15 (Chapter 4)

S5. Comorbidity (≥ 2 Syndromes) by Percentage (n = 1,004)

Level I

Architecture = 30; Art = 49; Business = 29; Exploration = 18; Sports = 32; Composing = 48; Musical performance = 45; Military = 15; Public office = 19; Natural sciences = 13; Social activism = 33; Social figure = 27; Companion = 33; Social sciences = 30; Theater = 51; Nonfiction = 47; Fiction = 59; Poetry = 68.

Mean = 40   Chi square = 106.3 df = 17 p = .000

Level II

Artistic = 52; Enterprising = 22; Investigative = 23; Social = 28

Chi square = 82.3 df = 3 p = .000

Level III

Creative arts = 53; Other = 25

Chi square = 81.0 df = 1 p = .000

S6. Lifetime Prevalence of Mental Health Care (n = 1,004)

Level I	Forced hosp.	Voluntary hosp.	Out-patient	Psycho-therapy	Unorth-odox	Other	Any care
Architecture	9	9	4	9	0	0	26
Art	3	10	10	7	7	4	26
Business	0	11	9	4	1	1	19
Exploration	0	0	0	0	0	0	0
Sports	5	5	5	0	0	0	16
Composing	6	17	8	13	4	0	31
Entertainment	6	19	9	4	6	4	30
Military	0	0	0	0	0	0	0
Public office	0	3	0	2	1	1	6
Natural sciences	0	5	5	5	0	5	15
Social activism	2	5	7	2	3	7	20
Social figure	3	13	7	17	3	0	30
Companion	0	6	11	6	0	0	17
Social sciences	3	14	4	16	1	0	27
Theater	11	19	20	17	3	1	34
Nonfiction	2	8	9	16	3	3	27
Fiction	8	21	15	15	3	4	39
Poetry	11	25	15	11	6	6	42
Total %	5	13	9	10	3	3	26
Chi square $df = 17$	37.6	46.5	38.8	42.6	15.3	18.3	68.3
p	.003	.000	.002	.001	.572	.372	.000

Level II							
Artistic	7	17	13	13	4	3	33
Enterprising	0	6	3	3	1	1	10
Investigative	1	13	3	14	1	3	25
Social	2	5	7	4	2	3	18
Chi square $df = 3$	25.4	26.0	22.8	22.8	7.3	3.5	48.5
p	.000	.000	.000	.000	.062	.315	.000

Level III							
Creative arts	7	17	13	13	4	3	34
Other	1	7	5	6	1	2	16
Chi square $df = 1$	21.5	22.4	20.9	13.4	6.3	2.6	39.7
p	.000	.000	.000	.000	.012	.110	.000

Key: Hosp. = Hospitalization

S7. Percentages of Family Members with Any Form of Psychopathology

Level I	Mother	Father	Any sibling
Architecture	4	4	31
Art	14	12	26
Business	9	16	21
Exploration	18	27	0
Sports	0	11	13
Composing	4	13	13
Entertainment	11	17	26
Military	5	5	0
Public office	8	11	13
Natural sciences	8	16	4
Social activism	7	7	13
Social figure	10	10	33
Companion	6	28	20
Social sciences	19	18	33
Theater	27	30	31
Nonfiction	5	24	29
Fiction	22	28	40
Poetry	14	19	33
n	965	983	598
Total %	13	18	25
Chi square	45.6	39.9	40.8
df	17	17	17
p	.000	.001	.001

Level II			
Artistic	15	21	32
Enterprising	9	14	14
Investigative	15	17	16
Social	9	13	20
Chi square	7.9	8.1	19.3
df	3	3	3
p	.048	.044	.000

Level III			
Creative arts	16	21	31
Other	10	14	17
Chi square	7.3	10.2	15.6
df	1	1	1
p	.007	.001	.000

S8. Since the lifetime prevalence of certain forms of psychopathology in biological relatives was so low, a logistic regression model was not suitable, largely because it produced artificially inflated significance levels simply by predicting that all subjects would not display the event of interest. For this reason, I chose to employ a multiple regression model, substituting continuous outcome measures for categorical ones. The results of the forward stepwise multiple regression analyses with pairwise deletions (PIN = .05 and POUT = .10) are given below. The outcome variables for these particular analyses represented additive scores for the presence or absence of specific psychopathology for both before and after age 40, with potential scores being 0, 1, 2. These scores represented the extent to which individuals suffered from that particular form of psychopathology over the course of their lives. The Total Symptom Score represented a sum of the different categories of psychopathology experienced by subjects (i.e., alcohol, drugs, depression, mania, somatization, suicide attempts, unspecified problems, psychosis, anxiety). And the Total Time Score represented the number of time periods (i.e., 0–13 years, 14–20 years, 21–40 years, 41–60 years, 61 years to death) during which individuals suffered from any major form of psychopathology.

Here is a summary of stepwise multiple regression results, for the subjects' different psychopathology scores as dependent variable, and the mother's and father's psychopathology scores as independent variables.

Dependent Variable = Lifetime Alcohol Abuse

Independent variables	ß	SE	Beta	R^2	T	$p =$
Father alcoholism	.61	.10	.25	.08	6.1	.000
Mother alcoholism	.80	.28	.12	.09	2.9	.000

Dependent Variable = Lifetime Drug Abuse

Independent variables	ß	SE	Beta	R^2	T	$p =$
Mother alcoholism	.77	.12	.20	.05	6.3	.000
Mother psychosis	.43	.13	.10	.06	3.3	.001
Father unspecified	.18	.09	.07	.07	2.1	.033
Father alcoholism	.11	.05	.07	.07	2.1	.033

Dependent Variable = Lifetime Depression

Independent variables	ß	SE	Beta	R^2	T	$p =$
Father alcoholism	.26	.09	.10	.01	3.0	.003
Mother psychosis	.44	.22	.06	.01	2.0	.049

Dependent Variable = Lifetime Mania

Independent variables	ß	SE	Beta	R^2	T	$p =$
Mother unspecified	.23	.10	.09	.01	2.2	.029
Father depression	.13	.08	.08	.02	2.0	.043

Dependent Variable = Lifetime Psychosis

Independent variables	ß	SE	Beta	R^2	T	$p =$
Mother highs	.68	.13	.22	.04	5.2	.000
Father highs	.34	.14	.10	.05	2.5	.015
Mother unspecified	.18	.07	.10	.05	2.5	.015
Mother depression	−.12	.05	−.09	.06	−2.2	.025

Dependent Variable = Lifetime Somatization

Independent variables	ß	SE	Beta	R^2	T	$p =$
Mother somatization	.45	.15	.13	.01	3.9	.002
Mother psychosis	.60	.23	.11	.03	2.6	.009

Dependent Variable = Lifetime Anxiety

Independent variables	ß	SE	Beta	R^2	T	$p =$
Mother alcoholism	.48	.15	.13	.02	3.3	.001
Father unspecified	.24	.09	.11	.03	2.6	.009

Dependent Variable = Suicide Attempts

Independent variables	ß	SE	Beta	R^2	T	$p =$
Mother drug abuse	.56	.19	.12	.01	2.9	.004
Father suicide	.33	.13	.10	.02	2.6	.011

Dependent Variable = Total Psychopathology

Independent variables	ß	SE	Beta	R^2	T	$p =$
Father alcoholism	.39	.12	.13	.03	3.2	.001
Mother alcoholism	1.04	.34	.13	.05	3.1	.002
Mother unspecified	.56	.21	.11	.06	2.7	.007
Father depression	.31	.15	.08	.06	2.1	.040

Dependent Variable = Total Time with Mental Problems

Independent variables	ß	SE	Beta	R^2	T	$p =$
Father alcoholism	.60	.18	.14	.03	3.3	.001
Mother alcoholism	1.12	.52	.09	.04	2.2	.031
Mother psychosis	1.46	.67	.09	.05	2.2	.030
Father depression	.47	.23	.08	.06	2.0	.044

METHOD AND STATISTICS: CHAPTER 8

S1. Significant differences existed among the professions with regard to when psychopathology occurred (chi square = 29.8; df = 6; p < .000). A one-way analysis of variance also was run to determine if these different temporal patterns of psychopathology were associated with significantly different lifetime creative achievement scores. The result indicated that they were not.

$F = 1.9$ $\qquad\qquad$ $df = 2, 629$ p = N.S.

S2. In order to determine the relationship of psychopathology to creative achievement across all professions, a stepwise multiple regression analysis was run (PIN = .05; POUT = .10) with pairwise deletion of missing data, utilizing CAS total scores as the dependent variable and the indicated psychopathology scores as independent variables. Beta coefficients, R^2 values, and significance levels are given below.

Variable	ß	SE	Beta	R^2	T	$p =$
Total time disturbed	1.89	.42	.17	.044	4.48	.000
Depression	2.45	1.15	.08	.049	2.13	.034
(Constant)	34.48	.72			48.16	.000

(Comparable analyses run separately for the artistic types and investigative types failed to reveal any significant predictors of creative achievement.)

METHOD AND STATISTICS: CHAPTER 9

S1. Percentage in Upper Quartile

Level I

Architecture (93); Art (81); Business (10); Exploration (0); Sports (0); Musical Composition (94); Musical Performance (92); Military (0); Public Office (12); Natural Sciences (89); Social Activism (17); Social Figure (0); Companion (0); Social Sciences (72); Theater (77); Nonfiction (27); Fiction (82); Poetry (86).

Chi square = 285.1 $\quad\quad\quad$ $df = 17$ $\quad\quad$ $p = .000$

Level II

Artistic (78); Enterprising (10); Investigative (81); Social (23).

Chi square = 202.6 $\quad\quad\quad$ $df = 3$ $\quad\quad$ $p = .000$

S2. Percentages and Significance Levels for Selected Measures

	CAS quartile				
	Low	High	Chi square	df	$p =$
Gender (male)	41	59	50.5	1	.000
Only child	11	13	0.7	2	.713
Creative parents	33	65	30.8	1	.000
Nonconforming parents	5	3	2.0	1	.159
Religious background			4.2	2	.124
Catholic	23	32			
Jewish	15	12			
Protestant	61	56			
Urban background	57	58	1.8	4	.771
Conflicts with teachers	5	9	3.7	1	.055
Conflicts with students	2	7	6.8	1	.009
Special schooling (academy, conservatory, etc.)	8	22	29.0		
Superior grades	13	26	13.5	5	.019
Academic awards	14	26	11.3	1	.001
Extracurricular activities	39	32	6.1	2	.048
Avid reader	25	42	14.9	1	.000
Parents' marriage intact	87	90	4.1	3	.246
Succesful father	72	69	4.5	4	.340
Mother's death <13	18	16	1.0	3	.840
Father's death <13	18	18	0.5	3	.914
Mother homemaker	81	82	4.9	6	.556
Father college	57	67	7.3	5	.200
Father creative profession	5	8	11.9	5	.036
Handicap as child	8	16	6.1	1	.014

| | CAS quartile | | Chi square | df | p = |
	Low	High			
Sickly as child	5	15	13.5	1	.000
Major illness as child	5	10	4.3	1	.039
Precocious	8	32	46.6	1	.000
Solitary as child	20	44	31.1	2	.000
Moody as child	21	34	7.3	2	.026
Odd as child	3	8	9.5	2	.009
Creative arts profession	16	73	165.1	1	.000
First success < 21	5	19	25.5	2	.000
Nonaffiliative	27	46	21.1	2	.000
Aesthetic interests	22	37	14.3	2	.001
Athletic	22	14	5.6	2	.061
Solitary	9	22	25.7	2	.000
Moody	35	47	13.1	2	.001
Expressed confidence	35	41	2.1	1	.149
Different	28	32	0.9	1	.339
Defendant	17	8	9.0	1	.011
Plaintiff	6	9	1.4	1	.236
Jail (nonpolitical)	6	8	1.1	1	.305
Jail/Harassment (political)	10	9	0.4	1	.534
Antagonism toward father	20	26	6.8	2	.033
Antagonism toward mother	17	16	0.9	2	.652
Antagonism toward employer	22	22	2.3	2	.324
Mentor	18	26	4.1	1	.042
Homosexual/Bisexual	12	11	0.4	3	.946
Homosexual/Bisexual	40	14	17.0	3	.001
(creative arts)					
Atheist/Agnostic/	25	53	56.5	5	.000
Idiosyncratic					
Married	82	84	0.4	1	.511
Divorced	30	34	0.7	1	.401
Affairs	32	41	3.1	1	.080
Mental problems < 13	2	8	7.9	1	.005
Mental problems 13–20	10	23	14.5	1	.001
Mental problems 21–40	37	54	15.3	1	.000
Mental problems 41–60	39	64	28.4	1	.000
Mental problems > 60	33	56	20.1	1	.000
Adjustment disorder	29	42	8.8	1	.003
Alcoholism	17	25	4.7	1	.030
Anxiety	5	10	3.5	1	.062
Depression	25	46	24.3	1	.000
Drugs	8	14	3.4	1	.065
Mania	5	9	2.5	1	.118
Psychosis	4	7	2.4	1	.112
Somatization	8	13	4.1	1	.042

	CAS quartile		Chi square	df	p =
	Low	High			
Suicide attempt	9	8	0.1	1	.742
Other	5	5	0.0	1	.992
Any mental problem	55	78	29.4	1	.000
Any mental health treatment	15	30	15.5	1	.000
Chronic illness < 50	21	36	13.9	1	.000
Chronic illness ≥ 50	27	40	6.6	1	.010
Cause of death			15.8	2	.000
Natural	83	94			
Accidental/Incidental	13	4			
Suicide	4	2			

S3. Mean Scores (SD) for Selected Measures

	CAS quartile		F	df	p =
	Low	High			
Father mental problems	0.2(0.4)	0.2(0.5)	3.4	1, 497	.067
Mother mental problems	0.1(0.4)	0.2(0.6)	4.4	1, 497	.036
Sibling mental problems	0.3(0.7)	0.3(0.7)	0.4	1, 425	.518
Total time with mental problems	1.1(1.2)	1.9(1.4)	46.4	1, 497	.000
Total psychopathology	0.7(0.8)	1.1(0.9)	27.7	1, 497	.000
Level of education	3.8(1.6)	4.1(1.4)	5.0	1, 481	.026
Parents' social status	2.7(1.4)	2.9(1.1)	1.5	1, 480	.214
Parents' income level	2.3(0.5)	2.0(0.5)	29.9	1, 482	.000

S4. Classification Table for Prediction of Creative Achievement

	Predicted by model		
Actually observed	1st quartile	4th quartile	% correct
1st quartile	172	12	93
4th quartile	19	77	90
Overall			92

INDEX

Munch, Edvard, 1, 46, 70, 103
Murders, 79
Murry, John Middleton, 50
Musical performers and entertainers; *see also*
  Composers, 3, 5, 6, 9, 27, 33, 34, 38,
  41, 44, 46, 47, 49, 51, 57, 61, 63, 69,
  70, 73, 74, 76, 79, 81, 82, 84, 86, 88,
  89, 91, 97, 106, 108, 112, 113, 116,
  120, 121, 124, 132, 133–137, 148, 150,
  151, 152, 162, 167, 171, 178, 182, 189
Musicians; *see* Musical performers and entertainers

Nabokov, Vladimir, 117, 183
Names of subjects, 219–230
Nation, Carry, 72, 120, 132,
National Comorbidity Survey, 148–150
Natural scientists and sciences, 3, 27, 40, 45,
  47, 51, 52, 65, 68, 73, 76, 79, 81, 82,
  86, 89, 91, 105, 106, 108, 110, 112,
  116, 120, 121, 123, 124, 132, 133, 134,
  138, 142, 148, 149, 153, 162; *see also*
  Sciences
Nervous breakdown, 77, 129, 145, 155; *see*
  also Mental Illness
"Networks of enterprise," 211n
Nietzsche, Frederick, 1, 188
Nijinsky, Vaslav, 58, 189
Nobel laureates, 18, 53, 61, 90, 113, 114,
  134, 182, 198n
Nonconformity, 5, 6, 7, 15, 29, 34, 42, 44,
  47, 48, 60–61, 64–70, 75, 81–82, 84–
  87, 94, 111
Noncreative arts professions, 29–30; *see also*
  Creative arts professions
Nonfiction writers, 5, 7, 27, 44, 48, 51, 68,
  76, 79, 91, 112, 116, 124, 132, 138,
  139, 143, 148, 151, 162, 178; *see also*
  Fiction writers, Poets, and Writers

O'Hara, John, 169, 174
O'Keeffe, Georgia, 103, 111
O'Neill, Eugene, 1, 9, 52, 78, 134, 168, 171,
  174
Ochs, Phil, 171
"Oddness"; *see* Nonconformity
Oldfield, Barney, 71
Oppenheimer, J. Robert, 50
Organizers of behavior, 32
Organizing principle, 58
Originality, 8, 65, 101, 102, 108–112, 124;
  see also Innovativeness
Ortega hypothesis, 20
Ortega y Gasset, Jose, 20
Orwell, George, 46, 52, 187

Parental loss during childhood, 35–40, 202–
  203n
  relationship to mental illness and creativ-
    ity, 37, 40
Parents
  characteristics of, 12, 32–34, 41–45, 77–
    78, 178, 182–187
  death of, 35–40
  divorce of, and effects on children, 41, 86
  mental illness of, 41, 153–157
  relationship to, 182–184; *see also* Author-
    ity figures and Mentors
  social status of, 33
Pareto's law of universal inequality, 19
Park, Robert E., 84
Parker, Charlie, 71
Parker, Dorothy, 62, 66, 165
Parker, Charlie, 71, 135
Pasternak, Boris, 132
Pathological anxiety, 143–144
Pavlov, Ivan, 186
Personal seal, 189–190
Phaëthon complex, 35–36, 40
Philoctetes, 126
Piaf, Edith, 58
Picabia, Francis, 117, 170, 173, 185
Picasso, Pablo, 50, 52, 58, 59, 103, 118, 173,
  189
Pissarro, Lucien, 3, 50, 53, 62, 117
Pittman, Key, 37
Plath, Sylvia, 3, 164
Plato, 1, 19
Poets, 1, 3, 5–7, 9, 20–21, 27, 34, 36, 41, 45,
  47, 49, 50–53, 61–65, 68–69, 72–76,
  79, 81–83, 89, 91, 99, 106, 109–114,
  116–117, 120, 123–124, 132–134, 138–
  139, 142–143, 146, 148–154, 162, 164,
  167, 178, 184, 191
Politicians, 6, 7, 19, 27, 32, 40, 50, 58, 62–
  64, 73, 79, 82, 88, 96, 102, 105, 110,
  112, 115, 119, 120, 124, 132, 142, 143,
  148, 150, 170, 177; *see also* Public office
Porter, Cole, 103, 110
Posthumous recognition, 102–103
Pound, Ezra, 62, 72, 120, 141, 191
Precocity, 48–51, 206n; *see also* Giftedness
Prediction model, 179, 180
Predictive equation, 11
Presley, Elvis, 135
Productivity, 115–119
Professions
  classification of, 26–30; *see also* Holland
    classification
  types of, 68, 75, 80, 83, 131, 153, 162,
    176, 200n
Prokofiev, Sergei, 58, 116